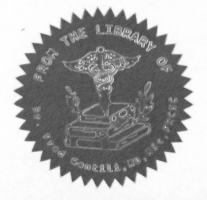

PRINCIPLES
OF
CHEST X-RAY DIAGNOSIS

PRINCIPLES
OF
CHEST X-RAY DIAGNOSIS

THIRD EDITION

GEORGE SIMON, M.D., F.R.C.P., F.F.R.

Lately Director, X-ray Department, Brompton Hospital, London;
Radiologist, St. Bartholomew's Hospital, London;
Demonstrator, Radiological Anatomy, St. Bartholomew's Hospital, London;
Curator of the Radiological Museum and Teacher of Radiology,
The Institute of Diseases of the Chest, University of London;
Kodak Research Scholar, National Heart Hospital, London

LONDON
BUTTERWORTHS

ENGLAND: BUTTERWORTH & CO. (PUBLISHERS) LTD.
                LONDON: 88 Kingsway, WC2B 6AB

AUSTRALIA: BUTTERWORTH & CO. (AUSTRALIA) LTD.
                SYDNEY: 20 Loftus Street
                MELBOURNE: 343 Little Collins Street
                BRISBANE: 240 Queen Street

CANADA: BUTTERWORTH & CO. (CANADA) LTD.
                TORONTO: 14 Curity Avenue, 374

NEW ZEALAND: BUTTERWORTH & CO. (NEW ZEALAND) LTD.
                WELLINGTON: 49/51 Ballance Street
                AUCKLAND: 35 High Street

SOUTH AFRICA: BUTTERWORTH & CO. (SOUTH AFRICA) (PTY.) LTD.
                DURBAN: 33/35 Beach Grove

First Edition   *1956*
Second Edition   *1962*
Reprinted   *1966*
Reprinted   *1969*
Third Edition   *1971*

Suggested UDC Number: 616–073·75:616·1/·2

ISBN 0 407 36322 X

PRINTED AND BOUND IN GREAT BRITAIN BY R. J. ACFORD LTD., INDUSTRIAL ESTATE, CHICHESTER, SUSSEX.

TABLE OF CONTENTS

LIST OF TABLES

PREFACE TO THE THIRD EDITION

In this third edition some of the original text has been retained, some changes of order have been made, and much of the text has been re-written. Either new knowledge has necessitated these changes, or there has been a need to present the information more clearly, partly to enable the student to learn more easily and partly to make it easier for the student to understand the x-ray appearances, their possible clinical importance or the pathological states which they might represent.

There are 141 new illustrations of radiographs, 6 new blocks to improve the quality of the old illustrations, and 24 charts, tables and diagrams have been added to supplement the text.

LONDON, 1971   GEORGE SIMON

ACKNOWLEDGEMENTS

I wish to acknowledge the help and encouragement I have received from all the clinicians whose cases have enabled me to learn something about the causes of the various shadows seen in radiographs.

I am also particularly indebted to the pathologists who have spent much time and trouble on correlating the abnormal shadows seen with the morbid anatomy and the histological features of the lesion; namely to R. J. R. Cureton and W. J. Hanbury for the histology of the various tuberculous lesions and the lung changes associated with bronchial carcinoma; to G. J. Cunningham for tuberculosis and bronchiectasis; and to Lynne M. Reid for bronchiectasis, chronic bronchitis, emphysema, bullae, idiopathic pulmonary fibrosis, unilateral transradiancy, certain basal line shadows, and certain cases of mitral stenosis in which line shadows are seen above the costophrenic recess.

I am indebted to St. Thomas's Hospital for Fig. 314, and to the authors and publishers for their permission to use the following illustrations: Figs. 14–16 from *Clinical Radiology*, **20,** 231 (Simon and colleagues); Fig. 22 from *Britisn Journal of Radiology*, **41,** 863 (Simon); Fig. 25 from *Surface and Radiological Anatomy* (Hamilton, Hamilton and Simon; Cambridge, Heffer); Figs. 183, 210, 224 and 225 from *The Pathology of Emphysema* (Reid; London, Lloyd-Luke); Fig. 232 from *Thorax,* **20,** 214 (Waddell, Simon and Reid); Fig. 330 from Foster-Carter in *Chest Diseases* (Perry and Holmes Sellors; London, Butterworths).

The old illustrations are from photographs prepared from the original radiographs by D. F. Kemp and A. C. Curd in the photographic department of the Institute of Diseases of the Chest, the Brompton Hospital. The new illustrations are from photographs prepared from the original radiographs by the department of medical illustration, St. Bartholomew's Hospital, the Royal Marsden Hospital and the Institute of Cardiology at the National Heart Hospital.

The bibliography and references given are only a faint indication of my debt to written works. Most of the references are key ones which themselves refer to the work of others on that particular subject.

LONDON, 1971   GEORGE SIMON

INTRODUCTION

THIS BOOK is written for the student radiologist and for the clinician who is particularly concerned with chest diseases, whether he interprets the radiographs himself or has the co-operation of a radiologist.

The material has been arranged under headings descriptive of the x-ray shadows rather than under the clinical disease labels. The author has found this grouping more useful not only in teaching clinical students or radiologists in training but also in the actual day-to-day work. Frequently no firm clinical disease label is available when the first radiographs are inspected, while in many cases the x-ray appearances themselves have led to reconsideration of the initial clinical diagnosis. Nor is the initial clinical diagnosis always relevant to the sphere in which the radiograph may be of use in a particular case. For instance, in mitral stenosis the radiograph is not needed for diagnosis, but is often of help in indicating the haemodynamic effects of the stenosis.

Confronted with an abnormal shadow, the observer's first obligation is to give a factual report on what he sees or thinks he sees in regard to its size, shape, position, and other characteristics, and also its effect on surrounding or nearby normal shadows. A statement of this kind, or an equivalent diagrammatic drawing, is necessary in the patient's interest, since it is a record of what was seen at the time, should the radiographs be mislaid, and an indication of the basis from which diagnostic conclusions were drawn. A certain amount of " observer error " is inevitable at this stage.

In the second stage—that of interpretation—the pitfalls are legion. There is usually an obligation to define the anatomical site or the nature of the underlying pathological process, and finally to correlate any tentative conclusions thus drawn with the clinical picture. This done, the final diagnosis may be at once apparent, or may be arrived at gradually after further clinical and radiological investigations.

The sections in this book take this same course, each type of shadow being in turn described factually and then discussed from the point of view of interpretation and misinterpretation. It is the author's hope that this particular approach to the subject of chest radiology may help the reader to extract the maximum value from what is, after all, an important ancillary aid to diagnosis.

DEFINITION OF TERMS

" Then you should say what you mean," the March Hare went on.
" I do," Alice hastily replied; " at least—at least I mean what I say—that's the same thing, you know."
" Not the same thing a bit ! " said the Hatter.

Lewis Carroll

That the writer of an x-ray report does not always say what he means is often due to confusion over the precise meaning of the terms which he uses. Certain words are expected to convey a quantity of subsidiary ideas, which is not justified, and many words are used to describe x-ray shadows which properly pertain to morbid histology. " There is atelectasis of the left upper lobe " will be frequently found in an x-ray report. Does this mean that there is a shadow giving evidence of lobar shrinkage ? Does it imply only that the lobe is airless with the alveolar walls more or less in apposition, or does it also suggest that the airlessness is due to bronchial occlusion ? Does it exclude or allow for some alveolar exudate or transudate, that is, consolidation, or even dilated mucus-filled bronchi ?

It is not unknown for expressions to be deliberately vague or even misleading. " There is infiltration (or infiltrate—U.S.A.) in the right upper zone ", for example, is a favourite way of shelving the problem only too prominent in the writer's mind, of whether shadows are tuberculous before there is any clinical proof of this, or whether there is any radiological proof that they are in the lung at all.

There are of course sources of confusion other than verbal ones to account for the high observer-error figures found in so many carefully controlled experiments (Garland, 1950; Newell and his colleagues,

1954). False conclusions are drawn from correct observations. Observers may be asked to determine from an initial radiograph whether there is an abnormal shadow present or not, and may interpret a shadow as a pathological lesion, when in fact it is a normal shadow accentuated by slight rotation of the patient. Or again, observers may be asked to discover from a pair of radiographs taken at an interval of 3 months, whether the patient's condition is better, worse, or unchanged. In the last of the two radiographs, the shadow may be smaller, and may be thus recorded by two observers; but whereas one observer may conclude that this indicates improvement, the other may conclude that it indicates bronchostenosis and atelectasis, and therefore deterioration.

Finally, some errors may occur through failure to notice the shadow at all, because it is indistinct or partly obscured by superimposed normal shadows, because inspection of the radiograph was too hurried, or because the observer's attention was distracted by other shadows or blunted by being focused too long on normal radiographs during a rushed session of work. Errors due to this cause can be greatly reduced if all radiographs are seen by two observers, and less reliance is placed on a single observer and a single anterior-view radiograph to exclude a significant lesion.

Humility is certainly required regarding the supposed accuracy of all observers in detecting and describing common abnormal shadows in radiographs. To deal with only one side of the problem, it would be an advantage if certain words commonly used in x-ray reports could be given a more definite meaning by general agreement. In the meantime, pending this happier state of affairs, a definition of terms is given below for use when reading this book.

Atelectasis

Synonyms—collapse, incomplete expansion

In this book the word will be used only in the sense of absorption atelectasis, meaning that the air is absorbed from the alveoli, which may occur if a bronchus is occluded (Kerley, 1951). It will not be used in relation to passive collapse or relaxation, as under a pneumothorax.

The pathological state of a lobe distal to occlusion of the lobar bronchus is variable. In acute atelectasis, as may occur if a lobar bronchus is blocked by an endotracheal tube during anaesthesia, the lobe shrinks and becomes opaque within seconds, and there may then be just airlessness. In atelectasis lasting more than a few hours there will be additional changes. One is varying degrees of bronchial dilatation beyond the stenosis due to the altered forces acting on the bronchial wall, and the bronchi will soon become full of mucus which may still be secreted, but which cannot escape because of the bronchial occlusion. Also, there will be some intra-alveolar oedema, and perhaps some alveolar wall oedema because of the hypoxia. Finally, in some cases there may be infection and inflammatory exudate. In fact, unless these latter conditions are present, or unless the degree of shrinkage is very great, no shadow will be seen (Dornhorst and Pierce, 1954).

Atelectasis is, broadly speaking, airlessness with shrinkage. In either case there may or may not be main or lobar bronchial occlusion, and the most that the radiologist can do when confronted with such a shadow is to see whether there is an associated shadow which might indicate the possibility of bronchial occlusion, or to try to demonstrate or exclude this by tomography or bronchography, unless it is about to be, or already has been, demonstrated by bronchoscopy.

Lobar shrinkage without occlusion of the lobar bronchus is illustrated in Fig. 88, and bronchial occlusion with little lobar shrinkage in Fig. 97.

If bronchial obstruction has already been demonstrated, the term " obstructive atelectasis " may be used in reference to the radiographic appearance of a homogeneous shadow with evidence of lung shrinkage.

Prefixes to the word " atelectasis " which will not be used in this book

The following prefixes are often attached to the word " atelectasis " in x-ray reports, but are considered an unsatisfactory way of describing an x-ray shadow because the underlying pathology is variable and cannot be deduced with any certainty from the radiograph. They will not be used in this book.

Compression atelectasis.—Synonyms—passive collapse, collapse. Used in relation to the state of the lung under a pneumothorax. The increase in external pressure is only relative and, since there is still a negative intrapleural pressure, the word " compression " is really unsuitable. The condition will be referred to as " relaxation of the lung ". The term could be used in a tension pneumothorax.

Mantle atelectasis.—Zones of airless alveoli, some with evidence of lung shrinkage, and some with oedema and consolidation without shrinkage, are seen by the morbid histologist round nearly every lesion, be it a pneumonic focus, a cavity (" mantle atelectasis ") or a neoplasm. These airless zones are often microscopic in size, and too small to be demonstrable in a radiograph. Whenever a shadow is described in this book, only the main pathology will be indicated, and very small airless areas will be ignored.

Focal atelectasis.—Small areas of airless lung are found histologically in chronic bronchitis, emphysema, some pneumoconioses, and many other conditions. They may be small areas of absorption atelectasis, or of relaxed lung compressed by surrounding bullae or areas of consolidation. They are usually either invisible in the radiograph or are masked by the more spectacular surrounding lesions, so that there would be no occasion to use the expression to describe multiple small shadows in an x-ray report. Nor is it possible from the radiograph, when numerous small ill-defined shadows are seen, to decide whether these represent small areas of consolidation or areas of focal atelectasis.

Plate or linear atelectasis.—This description has been given to a long linear or band-like shadow which is often seen running horizontally in a lower zone (Fleischner, 1941). The pathology of these lesions, however, is mixed and the range of change is evenly balanced between airlessness, alveolar exudates with or without lung shrinkage, fibrotic organization and indrawn or thickened pleura. No useful purpose is served by labelling the shadow after one set of changes rather than another. In fact, the majority of these puzzling long line shadows are due to a local vascular occlusion of an artery by an embolus or to thrombosis in a vein either intrinsic or secondary to an arterial embolus. Associated with the vascular occlusion or with a scar from a healed infarct there may be some indrawing of the pleura towards the lesion which may be responsible for a part of the line shadow (*see* p. 112).

Congenital atelectasis.—This condition differs from " absorption atelectasis " in that there never has been air in the affected alveoli. The area of opacity is caused by the failure of a lobe or the whole of one lung to aerate and expand when breathing was first initiated. The term " failure to aerate " is more descriptive in such a case.

Bronchial occlusion

Synonym—complete obstruction of the bronchus

This may be the result of an intraluminal foreign body; or of an organic disease of the bronchial wall, particularly tuberculous endobronchitis and neoplasm; or of extrinsic pressure, most often from an enlarged or healing gland. The result of the occlusion of a main, lobar or sometimes segmental bronchus is airlessness with atelectasis (collapse) of the lung distal to it. The occlusion may be permanent or temporary; should it be relieved the lung recover, unless there is irreversible damage from infection.

Bronchiectasis

The term " bronchiectasis " originally referred to bronchial dilatation only, but is now used to include the many associated pathological changes seen either in the plain radiographs, such as the opacities of a thickened bronchial wall which may actually have a narrowed lumen, or in the bronchograms, such as the narrowing and occlusion of the smaller bronchi as well as the dilatation of the more proximal bronchi. Since occlusion is commonly present both of the side branches and the end of a dilated bronchus (Fig. 336), the term " bronchitis obliterans " can be used synonymously with bronchiectasis, and describes better the functional consequences of the lesion.

Bronchostenosis

Synonym—partial obstruction of the bronchus

This condition may have the same causes as bronchial occlusion. It may be present without any distal lung changes, or it may be associated with a variety of changes in the radiograph, such as evidence of lobar shrinkage without an opacity, hypertransradiancy due to a check-valve over-inflation, or evidence of distal inflammation or bronchiectasis. It also often causes airlessness, the x-ray picture being then the same as that beyond a total occlusion. Since it is not often possible to distinguish between partial or complete obstruction of the bronchus from the radiographs, and since a bronchus may be intermittently occluded, the term " bronchostenosis " is used to cover all degrees of obstruction unless complete bronchial occlusion is known to exist.

Bulla

The term bulla is derived from the Latin meaning a blister (or the amulet worn around the neck by Roman girls).

Pathologically it refers to a local elevation of the pleura above the general contour of the lung (best seen when the lung is removed from the body) filled with air. This subpleural collection of air may have replaced destroyed alveoli or may contain distended but architecturally intact alveoli, but in either case its wall consists of pleura and to a varying degree connective tissue septa and compressed lung.

Radiologically a bulla appears as a relatively transradiant zone with either narrow, too few, or no vessels within it which is partly demarcated by a fine hair-line shadow representing its wall.

Bullous area

A bullous area describes an x-ray appearance in which a transradiant and avascular area is seen but there is no hair-line shadow representing its wall. The wall may in fact be present but not shown in the particular projection used, or it may be too thin to be shown, or it may consist of candy floss lung which is invisible.

A similar x-ray appearance may be seen, and the same term used, if the transradiant zone is the result of an emphysematous area of lung. In this case some of the larger vessel shadows may be seen running across the transradiant zone, but the loss of smaller vessel shadows will still be apparent.

Circular or oval shadows

These are purely descriptive terms and will cover all shadows of this shape whether the pathological lesion is believed to be an infiltration, an infiltrate, an exudate, a productive lesion, a nodule, or so forth. If the shadow is visible in two planes, it may be styled a " spherical shadow ".

Very small circular shadows.—Shadow 1·5 mm or less. Synonyms—if multiple: fine mottling, pin-point or micro-nodular shadows.

Small circular shadow.—Shadow up to 2 cm. Synonyms—if multiple and individual shadows 1·5–3 mm: mottling, nodular shadows; if 3–8 mm: coarse mottling, coarse nodular shadows.

Large circular shadow.—A shadow measuring 2 cm or more in diameter.

Consolidation

This is a pathological term indicating the state of the lung where the alveolar air has been replaced by fluid, cells or a cellular exudate, and there is airlessness without shrinkage as in all types of pneumonia. It includes replacement of the air by a transudate as in pulmonary oedema and by blood whether due to trauma, inhalation, or infarction. It also includes replacement of the alveolar air by neoplastic cells, the alveoli remaining intact, a condition which occurs in some kinds of carcinoma.

Difficulties arise in the use of the term because the x-ray appearances are the same whatever the cause and often whatever the stage of consolidation. In the earliest stages the radiograph may show patchy clouding, but the shadow soon becomes homogeneous with little or no lobar shrinkage. If lobar shrinkage occurs at a later date, the appearances will be those of atelectasis or collapse, and can be so designated.

When a homogeneous shadow is seen with only slight or moderate lung shrinkage, the compromise term " collapse-consolidation " or " consolidation-collapse " can be used, though it is scarcely worth while since it does not indicate the most important feature, namely whether or not bronchostenosis is present.

Density

Unless it is qualified as " number per unit area " the word " density " will refer to the radio-opacity of the lesion. Judged from the radiograph this radio-opacity will be relative. The shadow of the heart will be as white as that of some calcified pericardium in a lightly exposed film, but in a film taken with more exposure, the heart will be grey, and the denser more radio-opaque calcified pericardium will remain white. A shadow will therefore be considered dense if it remains more or less white on the radiograph, while a nearby shadow of somewhat similar or larger size is grey.

Low density.—Small shadows caused by cells or body fluids.

Fairly high density.—Larger shadows—particularly those due to fluids.

Dense or very high density.—Shadows produced by lesions containing a lot of relatively radio-opaque atoms, such as iron, or calcium derived from the body fluids, or atoms of high atomic weight introduced from without, such as iron, calcium, barium, tin or iodine.

Disseminated or diffused circular shadows

Shadows which are widely disseminated more or less uniformly over a considerable area, or throughout both lung fields.

Effusion

This usually refers to a pleural effusion, whether serous, purulent, haemorrhagic, fibrinous or transudate and includes semi-solid states of any of these. In the case of a pleural effusion, especially if encysted, the x-ray appearances may be the same whether the exudate is still fluid or whether it has in the course of time been invaded by fibroblasts and thus converted into a solid mass of fibrous tissue. The actual pleural cells rarely proliferate and the term " pleural thickening " usually refers to the shadow caused by an organizing exudate. Fluid in other sites will be denoted with a prefix, for example, mediastinal, extrapleural, pericardial.

Honeycomb shadow, or small ring shadows

Synonym—cystic lung

These are fine white ring shadows enclosing a transradiant zone, and measuring up to, say, 5 mm in diameter. If the ring shadows are larger, the condition is described as " coarse honeycomb shadow " (Figs. 1 and 138).

Ill-defined opacity

Synonym—area of patchy clouding

This is a poorly demarcated or diffuse shadow, often amorphous, but may be roughly circular or oval. If multiple, they can be described as blotchy shadows.

Linear or band-like shadow (includes tooth paste and gloved-finger shadow)

This is a descriptive term. Linear shadows vary from " hair-line " to 2 mm in thickness; there are also band-like shadows varying from 2 mm to 2 cm in thickness. Relatively wide band-like shadows, some 5–8 mm in width, are described as " tooth paste " shadows being in appearance like a column of tooth paste after extrusion on a flat surface (Figs. 1 and 195).

A band-like shadow with an expanded and rounded end as in Figs. 1 and 196 is described as a "gloved-finger " shadow.

Patchy clouding

Amorphous shadows, 1–2 cm in size, so not oval or circular in shape, and with poorly defined margins.

Potter–Bucky diaphragm

Synonyms—Potter–Bucky, Bucky, moving grid

These two names have come into common use to describe a piece of apparatus, the essential component of which is a grid interposed between the patient and the film with the object of absorbing some of the unwelcome scatter radiation. (It is said that Bucky invented the grid, and Potter made it move.) It will be used as a generic term to cover any type of such grid, whether moving or stationary, and whatever mechanism is used for moving it during the exposure.

Reticulation

This term is used to describe a fine linear shadowing with an interlacing pattern, usually spaced 5–8 mm apart, although a coarser pattern is possible. No pathological basis directly corresponds with this network, which is the result of more or less linear shadows, circular shadows, and small ring shadows being superimposed on each other. In the author's experience such a pattern is very rare and often the shadow thus described is not truly reticular but on close inspection is seen to be due to a mixture of nodular, linear and small ring (honeycomb) shadows; and when this is so the term reticular is probably best avoided.

Ring shadow

Synonym—cavity

A transradiant space surrounded by a zone of opacity representing its wall. Ring shadows can be classified by the diameter of the ring and by the thickness of the shadow representing the wall around the air space. The ring shadow or wall may enclose nothing but a relatively transradiant air space or there may be a shadow of some contents additional to the transradiant zone.

Septal lines

Synonym—Kerley " B " lines

Septal lines are used to suggest the cause of several horizontal line shadows usually about 1–3 mm wide and 1 cm apart in the region just above a costophrenic recess (Figs. 1 and 188).

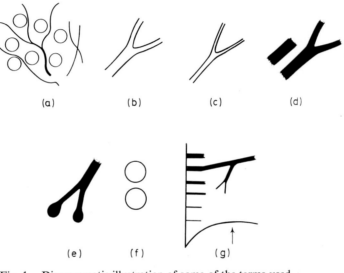

Fig. 1.—Diagrammatic illustration of some of the terms used.
(*a*) Honeycomb shadows (*see* Fig. 136). (*b*) Tubular shadow; parallel line shadow (*see* Fig. 200). (*c*) Tram line shadow (*see* Fig. 199). (*d*) Tooth paste shadow (*see* Fig. 195). (*e*) Gloved-finger shadow (*see* Fig. 196). (*f*) Ring shadow (*see* Fig. 355). (*g*) Septal line shadow (arrow points to diaphragm) (*see* Fig. 188).

Thickened pleura

The term is used to denote a widening of a normal pleural hair-line shadow such as the horizontal fissure or, in a lateral view, the main fissure, or in either view the visibility of a part of the pleura not ordinarily seen such as that over an apex or just above the costophrenic recess in the lower axillary region. Histological examination may show an exudate between the layers of the pleura, which may be fluid, semi-fluid or even solid and cellular in the course of time, without any increase in the width of the layer of pleural cells over it. Therefore there may be no actual pleural cell thickening corresponding to this x-ray description.

Tubular shadow

A shadow with two fine white linear walls which are more or less parallel and which enclose a central transradiancy about 3–8 mm wide (Figs. 1 and 200). If the parallel line shadow is in the position of a bronchus and the transradiant zone between the lines is of the appropriate diameter for a bronchus at that level, the term "tram line" shadow may be used (Figs. 1 and 199).

CHAPTER 1

ANATOMICAL LANDMARKS AND VARIATIONS

THE BASIC ANATOMICAL LANDMARKS

When inspecting a chest radiograph it is very useful to identify some basic anatomical landmarks and record the findings systematically. A suggested routine is as follows.

(1) Read the request form to note the name, age and sex of the patient, and then inspect the radiograph for consistency with this data.

(2) Inspect diaphragm for rib levels and relative levels of the two domes, their shape and clarity of outline (*see* below).

(3) Check orientation of patient (*see* p. 15).

(4) Inspect heart shadow for size, shape and position (*see* pp. 16–19).

(5) Inspect tracheal transradiancy for position and width of lumen (*see* p. 19).

(6) Inspect hilar shadows for size, shape and position (*see* p. 20).

(7) Scan the lung vessels, and thus note any small shadow that is not a vessel. Check distribution and size, upper and lower, right and left (*see* pp. 22–23).

(8) Check that the transradiancy of the two sides is the same.

(9) Identify, if visible, the horizontal fissure and check position.

These basic observations can be done in less than a minute and may be invaluable in coming to any conclusions. If the basic anatomical features appear normal and no additional shadows are seen, this constitutes the normal chest. If some variation is seen in the basic anatomy, then pause to consider whether it represents a normal variation (*see* below), or is an indication of some pathological lesion.

Even when gross abnormal shadowing is seen, the basic anatomy may assist in coming to the final conclusions. For example, a much raised dome towards a shadow will suggest an infarct rather than a bacterial pneumonia, or if the trachea is displaced towards an area of homogeneous opacity, it will indicate a reduction in lung volume, perhaps from collapse.

ANATOMICAL AND PHYSIOLOGICAL VARIATIONS

The misinterpretation of a shadow in the radiograph can lead to gross errors in diagnosis which may prove disastrous. A shadow which is caused by an anatomical or physiological variation may on occasion be interpreted as due to a pathological cause. An example of a physiological variation which may be mistaken for a pathological state is inequality in the range of movement of the right and left domes of the diaphragm, the restriction on one side being mistaken for restriction secondary to some pathological process.

An example of a shadow caused by an anatomical variation which is sometimes mistaken for a pathological lesion is a developmental variation of the anterior end of a rib which may be mistaken for a cavity (Fig. 33); or a breast shadow larger on one side producing a basal haze mistaken for an area of consolidation.

THE DIAPHRAGM

Inspection of the diaphragm shadow in a radiograph should never be hurried or neglected, since it quite often gives valuable clues to the presence of a lesion.

Normally the right cupola or dome lies about 2 cm higher than the left in all phases of respiration. When a discrepancy in the levels of the two domes is noted in an otherwise apparently normal radiograph, an anatomical or physiological cause should first be sought. Only when no such explanation

7

seems reasonable should a more detailed radiological investigation be undertaken, such as a high-penetration view to exclude a shrunken lower lobe, or a lateral view to exclude a tumour, or a view on expiration to exclude local air trapping.

PHYSIOLOGICAL ELEVATION OF THE LEFT DOME

It is common to find the left dome elevated because of an excess of swallowed air in the stomach (Fig. 32). At one hospital it was the custom to take the annual routine radiograph of the nursing staff immediately after a lunch which the unfortunate young women had to eat hurriedly in order to fit in the examination and also be on duty in the ward at the usual time. In a high percentage of radiographs, elevation of the left dome with a large gastric air bubble and fluid level was seen, which was no longer seen when the nurses were subsequently radiographed at a more suitable time. Children are frequently dosed with ginger beer, lemonade, or a cup of tea before a visit to the x-ray department, with the result that the same excess of gastric air is often present, and is sufficient indication of the cause of any slight elevation.

Elevation of the left dome from a gas-distended splenic flexure is rather less common. The distension may be physiological or the result of organic disease, and in either case the transradiancy of the gas-distended gut will give a clue to the probable cause of the elevation.

ELEVATION OF ONE SIDE FROM SPINAL CURVATURE

Severe scoliosis often results in elevation of one dome of the diaphragm. In such cases the cause of the elevation can be presumed to be the spinal curvature. There is no close relationship between the direction of the spinal curve and which dome is elevated, and on deep breathing in such cases both sides move well and equally.

A moderate scoliosis may cause slight elevation of one dome and the scoliosis may pass undetected unless looked for. Slight scoliosis does not usually alter the relative levels of the two domes.

ELEVATION OF ONE SIDE FROM MUSCULAR WEAKNESS

Muscular weakness of one dome, and its consequent elevation, is sometimes caused by a developmental defect, but is more often acquired following damage to the phrenic nerve or to the muscle itself. Damage to the nerve may arise from direct local trauma, pressure from a tumour, an enlarged or scarring mediastinal lymph gland, or the effect of a toxin. Often, however, after full consideration of the case—sometimes even including a thoracotomy at which the thin layer of atrophic muscle is noted—there is no indication of the cause of the condition.

All degrees of weakness are found, ranging from that producing a slight elevation, to one with extreme " eventration ", the left dome then appearing as a thin bow line in the region of the second or third rib (Fig. 2). In a lateral view (Fig. 3), the raised diaphragm appears as an even line with a superior convex curve running from the back of the sternum to the posterior chest wall.

This evenly curved line running right across the thorax will generally differentiate the condition from a hernia of the stomach passing through a moderate defect in the central part of the diaphragm; in the latter case the bow line of the air-distended stomach will only occupy a part of the thorax and will merge in front or behind with a more horizontal line caused by the remains of the diaphragm round the defect. Eventration must also be distinguished from the line formed by the upper margin of herniated gut and surrounding tissue when a gross developmental defect results in the absence of most of the left dome. The bow line in such cases is less well defined and the curve less even.

If the elevation of one dome is considerable and on the left side, it is frequently associated with a great excess of air in the stomach and colon, which condition is secondary to the elevation and not the cause of it. In some cases of gross elevation a barium meal is necessary to exclude a hernia. Sometimes this will show that the stomach is rotated round so that the greater curvature faces upwards and lies beneath the elevated left dome.

If the elevation is on the right side, the right dome and liver will cast a homogeneous shadow in the lower half of the chest, which may suggest a lower-zone tumour or basal effusion (Fig. 4). In a case of doubt, radiographs may be taken after the induction of a small pneumoperitoneum. If the

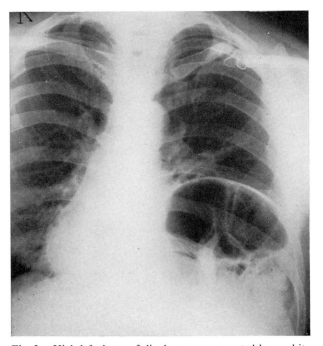

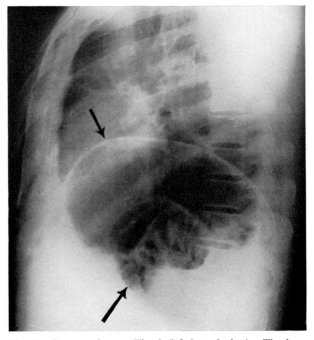

Fig. 2.—High left dome of diaphragm, represented by a white bow line with a superior convex curve reaching to the third rib anteriorly. It may have been caused by damage to the phrenic nerve in an accident 30 years previously (note ununited fracture left clavicle, with wire). Much air distension of the stomach and splenic flexure beneath it. Heart displaced to the right. Lung hypertransradiant due to scoliosis, and shrinkage of part of a segment in the lower zone, cause unknown.

Fig. 3.—Same patient as Fig. 2 (left lateral view). The bow line of the high left dome is marked by the arrow. It extends from the sternum to the posterior margin of the chest in an even line. The air-distended splenic flexure can be seen below it. The right dome, marked by lower arrow, is peaked up anteriorly. Male aged 48 years. Complained of everything turning to wind. Diaphragm plicated with relief of symptoms. Some years later again as above, but asymptomatic.

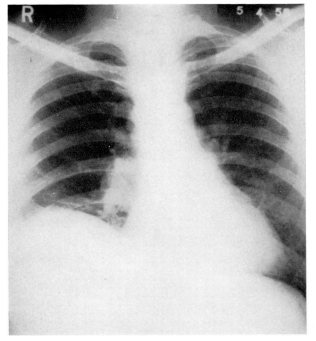

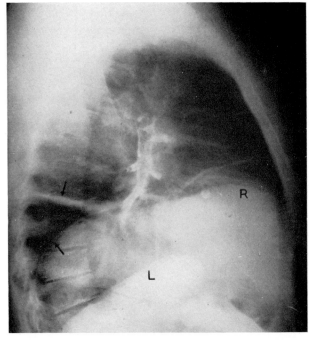

Fig. 4.—High right dome of diaphragm. The cause of this was a phrenic paralysis due to tuberculous glands near the right hilum. The line shadow running horizontally just above it is caused by a blocked bronchus full of secretions in the sub-apical segment of the lower lobe resulting from a tuberculous stenosis of the bronchus. Male aged 45 years. Mass x-ray findings, no symptoms.

Fig. 5.—Same case as Fig. 4 (lateral view, after pneumoperitoneum and bronchography). The letter " R " is printed just below the shadow of the raised right dome, and " L " below the normal left dome. The upper arrow points to the band-like shadow of the blocked bronchus full of secretions in sub-apical segment which was resected. The lower arrow points to the narrow zone of air below the raised right dome.

peritoneal air extends below the right dome, this will be seen as a bow line, 2–3 mm wide, with the transradiant air beneath separating it from the liver shadow (Fig. 5). If, on the other hand, a tumour is present in the thorax, its shadow will lie above the air transradiancy outlining the diaphragm. Old peritoneal adhesions, or poor development of these sub-diaphragmatic peritoneal recesses, may limit the flow of air from the site where it was introduced, so that it may only outline the lower margin of the liver or spleen and not the diaphragm. Careful attention to the shape of the air transradiancy will generally reveal the true state of affairs, especially if the liver and splenic shadows are also sought.

A localized elevation, the result of a localized developmental or acquired weakness of one dome, is not uncommon, particularly in the elderly, and is often neither pathological nor progressive. It is most often seen on the right side, and in the routine anterior view appears as a shallow localized elevation of the normal smooth curve, or as a second shadow superimposed on the main curve (Fig. 6). The innocuous nature of this shadow is usually fairly evident from inspection of the lateral view.

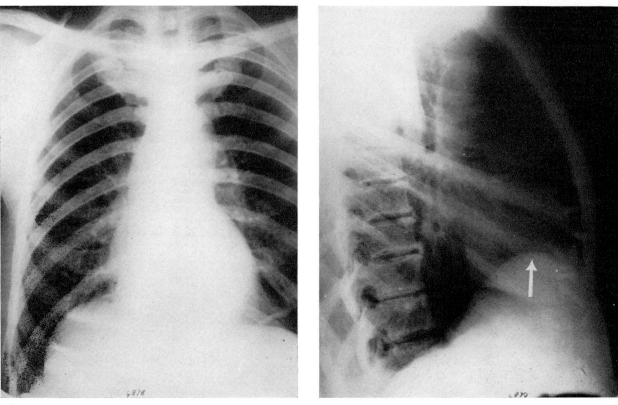

Fig. 6.—Localized elevation of the right dome (anterior view). Prominence of the diaphragm shadow is seen in the medial half below the right lung field. The elevated portion meets the other part at an obtuse angle. Normal male aged 43 years. Asymptomatic.

Fig. 7.—Same case as Fig. 6 (lateral view). Localized elevation of the right dome in the anterior half, marked by arrow. The condition was not progressive, and did not cause any symptoms. It may therefore be considered natural in an elderly adult.

In this view, the normal curve of the diaphragm can be seen extending from the posterior chest wall to well beyond the middle of the thorax, after which an additional hump rises in the anterior third (Fig. 7). The retrosternal position of this elevation which merges smoothly into the line of the rest of the diaphragm will serve to distinguish the condition from a cyst or tumour of the mediastinum, or a small hernia. Such lesions generally meet the diaphragm shadow at a much more abrupt angle (see p. 213). A large pulmonary tumour lying in the posterior recess may give a similar appearance in the anterior view (Fig. 131, p. 75), but its intrapulmonary position will be at once apparent in a lateral view (Fig. 132, p. 75).

A 2–3 cm area of localized weakness of one dome may occur at sites other than the anterior third, and the shadow will then more closely simulate a tumour or hernia of the liver. An artificial pneumo-peritoneum may be of no help since a small peritoneal fold may be carried up through a weakened piece of diaphragm with the portion of liver, and the resulting air transradiancy will be the same whether the diaphragm is intact or whether there is an actual defect (*see also* p. 213).

CHANGES OF LEVEL WITH CHANGES OF POSTURE

Little change in the level of the diaphragm is seen in a normal young adult, whatever posture is taken up for the x-ray examination. On the other hand, an older person, or a weak, ill patient, tends to have a higher diaphragm shadow when lying than when standing; also when the patient lies on one side, that side will be considerably elevated. The latter change is often seen when a lateral view is taken of a patient lying on one side (a common practice in bronchography) or in the less commonly used anterior view taken with the x-ray beam horizontal and the patient lying on one side.

CHANGES IN LEVEL FROM NEARBY PATHOLOGICAL LESIONS

Elevation of one dome without a lung shadow to suggest the cause may be due to pressure from below by a local abdominal mass. For example, an enlarged liver may cause elevation of the right dome or an enlarged spleen elevation of the left dome. Similarly, inflammation in the sub-diaphragmatic region, for instance a sub-phrenic abscess, liver or splenic abscess, a splenic or retroperitoneal haematoma, may cause inhibition of movement and thus elevation of one side in the radiograph on inspiration.

A common lung cause of elevation of one dome is a lower zone pulmonary embolus (with or without infarction). An embolus often causes loss of volume of the lobe so that the main fissure will also be displaced in a lateral view (*see* p. 107). The lateral view may show a small shadow of an associated area of infarction which was invisible in the anterior view. If a major lobar artery is occluded, there will be a zone of oligaemia above the normal or raised dome (*see* p. 160).

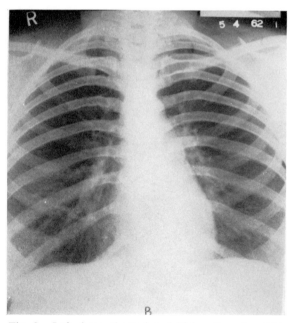

Fig. 8.—Left dome elevated and higher than the right. No excess of air in the stomach, or large spleen felt. Lung appears clear, but lower lobe later seen to be too small. Female aged 36 years, with cough and sputum.

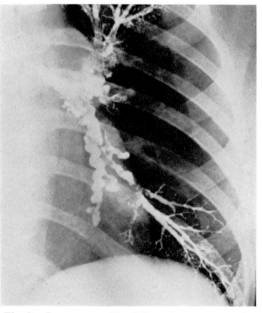

Fig. 9.—Same case as Fig. 8 (bronchogram; anterior view), showing lower-lobe obliterative bronchial lesions. These may have followed an infection in childhood, and because of air trapping may have caused the lower lobe to be underdeveloped or hypoplastic.

A somewhat less common cause of elevation of one dome is relatively poor development (hypoplasia) of a lower lobe (Fig. 8). This may arise from obliterative lesions of many of the airways in the lobe (Fig. 9), so that it is almost entirely aerated by collateral air drift (*see* p. 149). There is thus some relative air trapping, and the blood flow in the lobe is diminished. If the lesions occur in childhood before development is complete, the alveolar number will not increase as much as in a normally functioning lobe; therefore, there will be too few alveoli, of too simple a form, and the lobe will thus be smaller than normal.

Another cause of relative elevation of one dome is depression of the other. This may be seen with a right spontaneous pneumothorax. The right dome may then be at the same level as the left (Fig. 10) or even below it, and if the pneumothorax is shallow it may easily pass undetected in the routine radiograph. In Fig. 10 the line of the visceral pleura could be seen on careful scrutiny, and much more

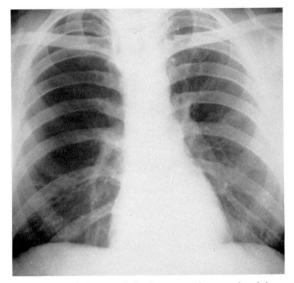

Fig. 10.—Both domes of diaphragm at the same level due to depression of the right from a spontaneous pneumothorax; 14 days later pneumothorax absorbed and right dome 2 cm higher than the left.

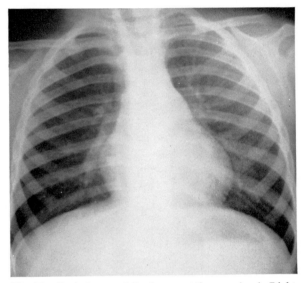

Fig. 11.—Both domes of diaphragm at the same level. Right lung hypertransradiant and vessels small. Check-valve over-inflation from inhaled peanut in right main bronchus. Bronchoscopic removal. Later radiograph normal.

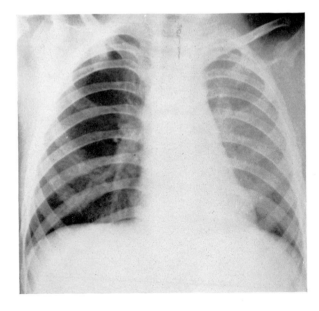

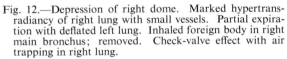

Fig. 12.—Depression of right dome. Marked hypertransradiancy of right lung with small vessels. Partial expiration with deflated left lung. Inhaled foreign body in right main bronchus; removed. Check-valve effect with air trapping in right lung.

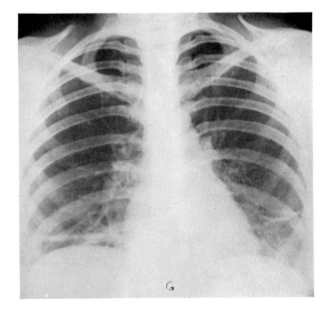

Fig. 13.—Both domes higher than in a previous radiograph. Poor compliance bases. Horizontal long line shadows of vascular lesions. Female aged 34 years. Appearances presenting sign of diffuse lupus erythematosus. E.S.R. 100. L.E. cells in peripheral blood.

clearly in a radiograph taken on expiration. Depression of one dome may occur with local lower lobe emphysema from the check-valve effect of an inhaled foreign body in the bronchus, an adenoma or enlarged glands compressing the bronchus from without. The condition should be suspected by noting a decrease in the vessel size in the lower zone above the depressed dome (Figs. 11 and 12).

Elevation of both domes from lung disease may only be detected if a previous radiograph is available, confirming that at one time the patient could lower the diaphragm more on inspiration. The shadows of the lung disease may be obvious; for example, the nodular and honeycomb shadows of fibrosing alveolitis (Fig. 164). Sometimes, however, the lung fields may appear clear, and yet there may be lack of lung compliance so that the diaphragm is prevented from descending far on inspiration. This may occur in diffuse lupus erythematosus or lymphangitis carcinomatosa. In the former condition, a horizontal band-like shadow may be seen on occasion in the lower zone from a vascular lesion (Fig. 13); in the latter, faint long line or septal line shadows or some fine nodular shadows may be seen on careful inspection with the aid of a magnifying glass.

Bilateral elevation will of course be seen in the later stages of pregnancy, in ascites or with a large abdominal tumour.

Tests of Diaphragm Movement

Diaphragm movements can be studied during fluoroscopy, but in England, where most departments do not have the advantages of an image intensifyer for fluoroscopy, the time taken for the radiologist to become dark adapted may be unjustified, since the range of diaphragm movement can be seen if two radiographs are taken with the films in the same position; for one with the patient holding his breath on deep inspiration, for the other, in deep expiration. The range of movement can then be measured either by superimposing the two radiographs or measuring the distance of each dome from the bottom of the film and noting the difference in the two phases of respiration. In an ill patient, for example one suspected of having a sub-phrenic abscess, the inspiration/expiration radiographs can be taken without moving the patient from bed, which is a kindness and is often more satisfactory than fluoroscopy.

Fluoroscopy can thus be reserved for those patients who do not move their diaphragm adequately in the inspiration/expiration pair of radiographs, but with encouragement can be made to do so while being fluoroscoped. Testing for paradoxical movement on sniffing is also best done by fluoroscopy.

Range of diaphragm movement

Most normal young people will move each dome 3 cm or more, but in the middle aged and elderly the range of movement is often less. This may be partly due to a slower understanding of the instructions or to a lack of conscious control of this particular movement, so that as many as 20 per cent may

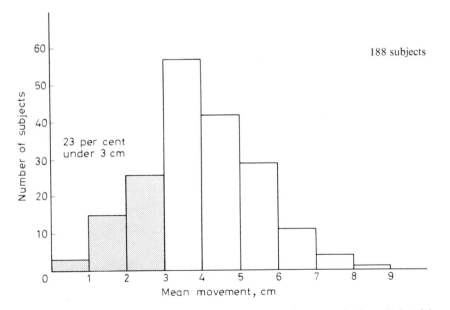

Fig. 14.—Range of diaphragm movement from inspiration to expiration. Industrial workers mainly between 35 and 65 years of age. (Simon and colleagues, 1969.)

move less than 3 cm (Figs. 14 and 15). In addition, they may move much more or much less when retested on another occasion (Fig. 16).

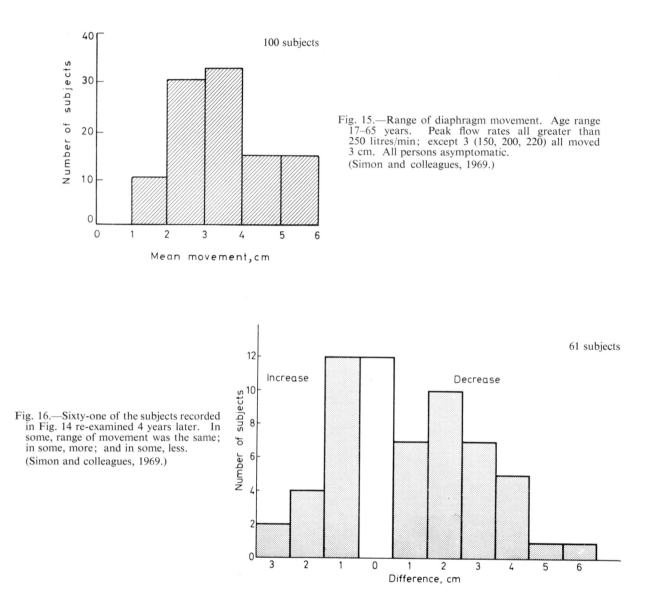

Fig. 15.—Range of diaphragm movement. Age range 17–65 years. Peak flow rates all greater than 250 litres/min; except 3 (150, 200, 220) all moved 3 cm. All persons asymptomatic.
(Simon and colleagues, 1969.)

Fig. 16.—Sixty-one of the subjects recorded in Fig. 14 re-examined 4 years later. In some, range of movement was the same; in some, more; and in some, less.
(Simon and colleagues, 1969.)

Use of diaphragm movement tests in diagnosis

The assumption that the routine radiograph is in full suspended inspiration is justified in most cases. It means that any considerable difference of movement will in fact be detected in this radiograph, since one side will move down further than the other restricted side. The usual right–left difference in level of some 2 cm will thus be altered and fluoroscopy is then unnecessary to prove it. A film on expiration will confirm it and show whether or not the affected side moves at all. Failure to move one dome up and deflate the bases evenly on expiration is a useful test of air trapping, whether in one lung or only in a lower lobe.

Poor movement of both domes is rarely a useful sign. It will usually be present if there is widespread gross emphysema, but then the other signs will also be present (*see* p. 142). Patients with severe airway obstruction, whether due to chronic bronchitis or to asthma, will often show a range of 3 cm or more and a normal radiograph; while some normal persons move their diaphragm very little on such a routine radiological examination.

Finally, many apparently normal persons do not move the right and left domes to the same extent, though the difference is usually less than 1 cm (Fig. 17).

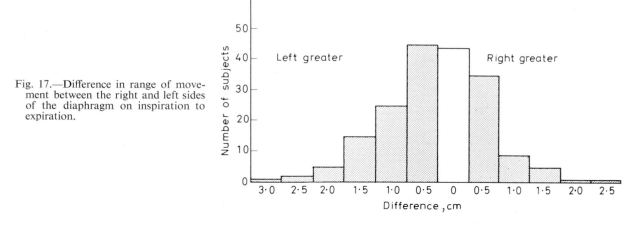

Fig. 17.—Difference in range of movement between the right and left sides of the diaphragm on inspiration to expiration.

In most people, the range of movement is greater in the supine than in the standing position, so that in a case of doubt the patient should be examined in the supine position. The findings are often conflicting, the two sides perhaps moving equally when the patient stands, but one side showing restriction of movement when he lies down; or one side may be immobile when he stands and may perhaps show paradoxical movement when he lies down or (to add to the confusion) may only show paradoxical movement when he sniffs.

Interpretation is not always easy, but reversal only on sniffing indicates that some functioning muscle exists but that it is unable to resist, and least of all overcome, the large rise in intra-abdominal pressure which occurs during sniffing. Sniffing is therefore a valuable test, and should be tried in any doubtful case.

The thickness af the diaphragm

The thickness of the diaphragm, although it cannot be measured in the routine chest radiograph, can together with the thickness of the cardiac end of the stomach be estimated by noting the distance between the top of the air transradiancy in the fundus of the stomach and the top of the diaphragm (Fig. 32). This normally is 5–8 mm. The width of this opaque area will be larger if the top of a sub-pulmonary effusion is mistaken for the top of the diaphragm (Fig. 50). There will be a similar increase in this distance if a portion of the left lobe of the liver comes to lie between the fundus of the stomach and the diaphragm, or if some part of the diaphragm other than that immediately above the stomach is responsible for the shadow in the anterior view. This may occur with a local elevation of the left dome posteriorly, which will be apparent in a lateral view.

In atrophy from paralysis the diaphragm is very thin (Figs. 2 and 3).

THE NORMAL HEART SHADOW

THE SYMMETRY OF THE BONY PARTS

Before examining the heart shadow, the bony parts should be checked for symmetry, since slight rotation of the patient or a scoliosis may cause alteration in its size, shape, or position. A gross scoliosis or gross rotation will render the anterior-view radiograph of little value for the examination of the heart.

The distance of the sternal end of each clavicle from the lateral edge of the vertebral body opposite or over which it lies should be noted, for it will be the same each side if the patient has been radiographed in a straight position. This test is easier to perform than measurement from a presumed thoracic mid-line, the position of which is difficult to fix, or from a spinous process, which may be difficult to see. Slight rotation, so that the left clavicle is only 0·5 cm farther from the lateral vertebral border than the right, may cause considerable apparent displacement of the heart to the left, an increase in the transverse diameter, which may be as much as 1–2 cm, and a bulge of the left border below the aortic knuckle suggestive of enlargement of the pulmonary artery (Fig. 18). Even a slight thoracic scoliosis concave to the left will have a very similar effect on the image of the heart (Fig. 19), so that the general alignment of the vertebral column should also be noted. Rotation or scoliosis in the opposite direction may cause apparent displacement of the heart to the right, and this may expose the left pulmonary artery which may then appear unduly large.

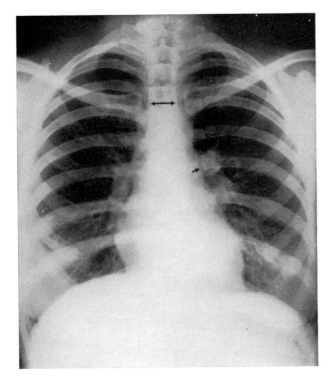 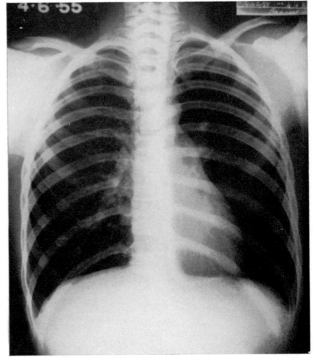

Fig. 18.—Slight rotation of the patient to the left. Horizontal arrow points both ways to the lateral borders of the fourth thoracic vertebra. The sternal end of the left clavicle is farther from the left border than the right is from the right border, indicating slight rotation to the left. The lower arrow indicates a slight prominence of the left border of the central shadow just below the aortic knuckle resulting from the slight rotation. The left hilar vessels are prominent from the same cause. No clinical evidence of intrathoracic disease.

Fig. 19.—Slight scoliosis concave to the left, and slight rotation to the left (normal young adult). Undue prominence of the left heart border below the aortic knuckle. Apparent displacement of the heart to the left. Left hilar vessels are obscured and right hilar vessels appear prominent as they are no longer covered by the heart shadow. There was some relative hypertransradiancy of the left lung which cannot be reproduced. A second radiograph taken with the boy straight showed none of these features.

It is advisable to interpose this examination for symmetry or scoliosis at an early stage, and then to proceed to inspect the heart shadow, hilar shadows, lungs, and the like, and finally to return again to the bony thorax for a more detailed inspection for pathological processes. This advice may seem rather elementary, but adherence to this sequence may well save the patient from many fruitless examinations and consequent inconvenience and anxiety.

THE HEART SIZE

The size of the heart shadow is probably most accurately assessed by measuring the cardiac volume. The method is illustrated in Figs. 20 and 21. The measuring points are not always easy to define, nor has it been proved that the method is superior for most clinical purposes to the much simpler measurement of the transverse diameter (T.D.). This can be measured in the routine anterior-view radiograph taken with the patient sitting or standing at a tube-film distance of not less than 6 feet, and in deep suspended inspiration.

The transverse diameter may give an exaggerated estimate of the true heart size under certain circumstances. For instance, there will be considerable geometric enlargement of the image, the object being some distance from the film, if the tube-film distance is shorter than 5 feet, as may be the case when an ill patient is radiographed supine in bed with a ward unit, or even when standing in the screening stand. There will also be enlargement if the radiograph is taken as an antero-posterior view, since the heart will then be further from the film.

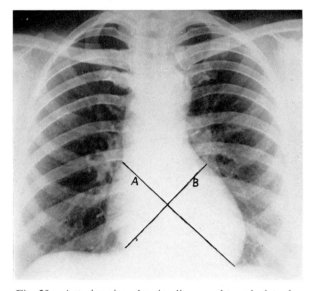

Fig. 20.—Anterior view showing lines used to calculate the cardiac volume. Both lines from cardiophrenic angles; line A to R.A.-S.V.C. junction, and line B to P.A.-left atrial appendage junction.

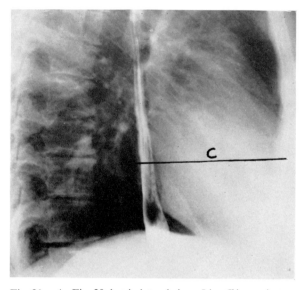

Fig. 21.—As Fig. 20, but in lateral view. Line C is maximum A.P. diameter of heart.

$$\text{Heart volume} = \frac{A \times B \times C \text{ (in cm)} \times K \times M}{\text{B.S.A. (in sq. m)}}$$

where K = 0·63 (ellipsoid factor) and M = magnification factor calculated for individual equipment. B.S.A. determined from height–weight nomogram.

A high position of the diaphragm—whether because the radiograph was taken in expiration (*see* Figs. 353 and 354), or because of elevation from abdominal distension as in pregnancy, ascites, an enlarged liver or spleen or any large intra-abdominal tumour, or because the radiograph was taken with the patient lying down instead of sitting or standing (particularly in the elderly or in babies)—will all cause the heart to lie more horizontally and thus increase the transverse diameter. The high position of the diaphragm will be visible in the radiograph. If it is higher than the anterior end of the fifth rib, it should be suspected of being an adverse factor in relation to the T.D.

These factors in combination may enlarge the image of the heart by as much as 4 cm.

Assuming none of these adverse factors is present, the detection of pathological enlargement from the T.D. is often impossible in the initial radiograph unless, it is gross, owing to the very wide individual variation in the T.D. Neither tables correcting for height and weight, such as those of Hodges and Eyster (1926), nor taking the T.D. as a ratio of the width of the thorax (the cardio–thoracic ratio) are entirely satisfactory.

In some normal persons the T.D. may be 7 cm or less, and the thorax 26 cm, so that the heart T.D. would have to increase by 6 cm before reaching the mythical 50 per cent. While many normal persons have a ratio of more than 50 per cent, figures such as T.D. 14 cm and thorax 23 cm, giving a ratio of 60 per cent, are not uncommon. In other words, slight enlargement of the heart cannot be detected from the initial radiograph. Any heart larger than 15·5 cm is probably a pathologically enlarged heart unless the patient is tall, very muscular, heavy and in an occupation needing much muscular effort.

Slight heart enlargement may, however, be detected in later radiographs if the T.D. increases more than 1·5 cm. In a series of normal persons (medical students, nurses, and so on), radiographed on three occasions at long intervals the difference in T.D. was 1·5 cm or less in 98 per cent (*see* histogram, Fig. 22). Alternatively, any decrease in heart size, unless it is greater than 1·5 cm, may not be significant. In most normal persons the difference between systole and diastole is usually less than 1·0 cm and often less than 0·5 cm, but would be greater on some occasions following an ectopic beat because of the prolonged diastolic pause before the next beat. This may account for some of the day-to-day variations of more than 1·5 cm recorded in Fig. 22. In a high-pressure, forcibly retained inspiration (Valsalva) the heart will decrease in size during the first few beats and then enlarge. Variations of size caused by this factor are probably not uncommon, since the routine procedure in chest radiography is for the patient to be told to take a deep breath in and hold it in, while the exposure may be made by the radiographer either almost immediately after these instructions have been carried out or not until 1–3 seconds have elapsed.

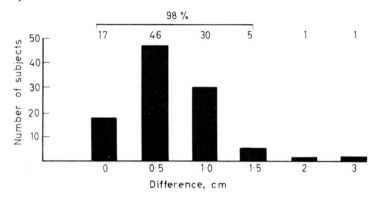

Fig. 22.—Variation in heart size on 3 occasions. There were 100 normal subjects; age range of 18–25 years. (Simon, 1968.)

THE SHAPE OF THE NORMAL HEART

In most normal persons the left border is more rounded and protrudes further out than the right, but in a few individuals the heart is narrow and more vertical and the difference in shape between the right and left borders is less marked. The narrow heart is the result of a low position of the diaphragm. The left border below the aortic knuckle usually shows a lateral concavity.

Occasionally the main trunk, or both the main trunk and the left branch of the pulmonary artery are unduly large, resulting in a prominence of the left border of the central shadow just below the aortic knuckle. In the absence of any clinical evidence of an abnormality, such an x-ray appearance should be considered a normal variation. It is sometimes necessary to prove by fluoroscopy or tomography that the prominence is caused by the artery and not by a tumour.

An unduly high position of the aortic arch, and therefore a high and prominent aortic knuckle, may also be mistaken for a tumour until one of the foregoing simple tests reveals its nature (Fig. 23). Cardiac catheterization or angiocardiography are rarely indicated in these cases from the x-ray appearances alone, especially if the possibility is borne in mind that the explanation of the shadow is an anatomical variation. Very rarely the aortic arch rises to the level of the lower neck region and will give a puzzling shadow to one or other side encroaching on the apex of the lung and simulating a neoplasm. In such cases, if this possibility is born in mind, an aortogram will be indicated to confirm the diagnosis.

Slight asymmetry or scoliosis will produce slight variations in shape, with a tendency to prominence of the left border below the aortic knuckle (*see* Symmetry of the Bony Parts, p. 15). This is often the cause of the so-called " adolescent dilatation of the pulmonary artery ", which is common among such young persons who often stand with a minor scoliosis.

THE POSITION OF THE HEART IN A NORMAL PERSON

The position of the heart should be assessed in relation to its shape. The narrow vertical flask-shaped heart tends to be centrally placed, whilst the larger more horizontal type, which has a relative prominence of the left border, lies with two-thirds of the shadow to the left of the mid-line and one-third to the right. Therefore, if a relatively large but apparently normal heart is placed centrally, this would suggest displacement of the heart to the right, and would not suggest a pathological enlargement of a narrow vertical centrally placed heart. The latter rarely enlarges evenly on both sides, but usually only to the left, and would therefore no longer remain centrally placed and flask shaped with right and left borders similar in outline and equidistant from the mid-line. Similarly if the heart is of average shape but three-quarters of the shadow lies to the left of the mid-line, and only one-quarter to the right, it would suggest enlargement or displacement to the left.

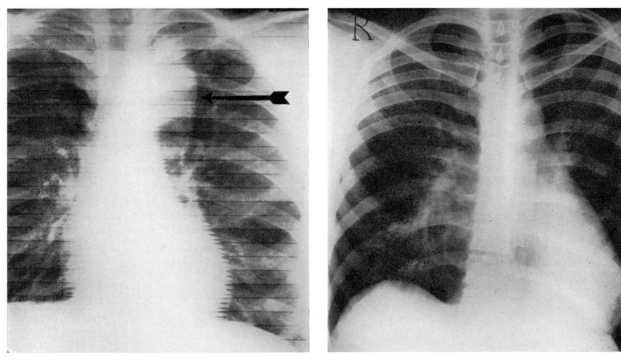

Fig. 23.—High aortic knuckle (kymogram). Found in routine radiograph. Asymptomatic, no abnormal physical signs.

Fig. 24.—Heart displaced to the left by a depressed sternum. Right hilum bared, so appears prominent.

In a normal person without any pulmonary lesion, the heart shadow sometimes seems to be displaced in the radiograph. This is commonly due to unnoticed or uncorrectable rotation of the patient as he stands opposite the cassette, or to thoracic cage asymmetry, particularly that associated with a scoliosis. These factors should be considered first as a possible cause for a displaced heart shadow (by inspection of the bony parts for symmetry, *see* p. 15) before a pulmonary lesion is suspected as a cause of the displacement. In babies, even a very slight rotation is associated with considerable movement of the mediastinal contents to one side or the other.

Kyphosis or a depressed sternum are usually obvious on clinical examination, but if they are forgotten as a possible cause for a displaced heart at the time the radiograph is inspected, they will be obvious when a lateral view is taken. A depressed sternum usually causes displacement of the heart to the left (Fig. 24), although the heart may be occasionally pushed to the right.

Mirror transposition may be mistaken for a heart displaced to the right, but usually the aortic knuckle is also transposed, or the gastric air bubble is noted under the right dome.

When anterior-view radiographs are taken in special circumstances with the x-ray beam horizontal and the patient lying on one side, the heart is displaced towards the lower side to a variable degree.

Whatever the cause of an apparent displacement or a real though normal displacement may be, it will result in the hilar vessels on the opposite side being less covered by the heart shadow and thus appearing unduly prominent. This often results in a fruitless search for a neoplasm, which may cause the patient much anxiety. Hence the need for careful consideration of these factors.

NORMAL TRACHEAL TRANSRADIANCY

The position of the tracheal transradiancy should next be noted. Normally it lies centrally but with a slight bias of the lower third towards the right. Its position must be assessed in relation to the orientation of the patient (indicated by the position of the sternal ends of the clavicles in relation to the vertebral body over or opposite which they lie), and the presence or absence of any scoliosis. Rotation of the patient so that the left clavicle is displaced only 2–3 mm to the left in relation to the vertebral shadow, or a mild scoliosis concave to the left will result in displacement of the tracheal transradiancy to the left. Rotation of the patient the other way or a scoliosis concave to the right will result in an even greater apparent displacement of the tracheal transradiancy to the right.

If there is an actual displacement of the trachea to the right due to some pathological cause, and if in addition there is some rotation of the patient to the left when he is radiographed, then the two factors may balance, and the trachea appear to be central. In such a case the real tracheal deviation to the right will be detected, in spite of its apparent central position, if the orientation of the clavicles is noted.

THE HILAR OR ROOT SHADOWS

The size, shape and position of the hilar shadows should be carefully noted as part of the routine in the examination of a chest radiograph, whether at a quick glance it appears normal or whether an obvious massive shadow is seen somewhere.

In a normal person the hilar shadows are caused by the arteries and veins with a small contribution from the walls of the major airways. These appear as a narrow line shadow outlining the transradiancies caused by the air in the main or lobar bronchi which can often be seen in a well-exposed radiograph. Encroachment on one of these bronchial air transradiancies may be seen if there is a lesion causing obstruction of the bronchus such as a foreign body or a neoplasm. Since this will cause atelectasis of the lung or lobe, it may serve to distinguish the opacity caused by the collapsed lung from one caused by consolidated lung, when the main bronchial transradiancy will be normal.

The Size of the Hilar Shadows

The size of the normal right hilum is best assessed from the size of the right basal artery which can usually be clearly identified in the routine radiograph and with certainty in a tomogram. As the artery width may taper before it divides into the basal segmental arteries, a convenient measuring point is half way down the artery and from its lateral wall to the clearly defined transradiancy of the intermediate bronchus (*see* Fig. 25). The measurement therefore includes the bronchial wall, but this is

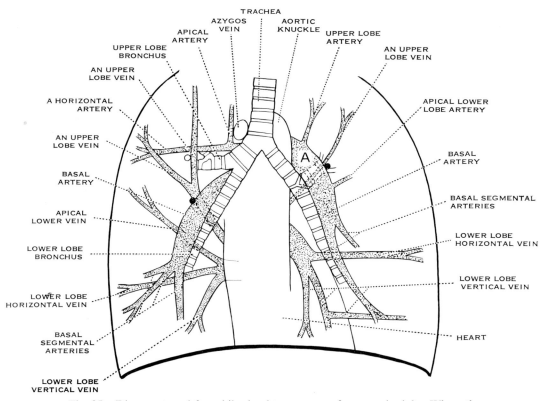

Fig. 25.—Diagram traced from hilar level tomograms of a normal adult. Where the upper-lobe vein crosses the basal artery is marked with a dot, and indicates the centre of the hilum shadow. "A" is measured from the upper-lobe bronchus to the top of the artery shadow. (Hamilton, Hamilton and Simon, 1971.)

only about 2 mm and is fairly constant. In normal middle-aged adults the width of the right artery, including the bronchial wall, varies between 7 and 19 mm (average 13·9 mm). It is similar on the left but the lower lobe bronchial transradiancy is often less easily seen. Another useful measurement is from the transradiancy of the distal end of the left main bronchus to the upper surface of the left pulmonary artery as it arches over the bronchus. This is indicated in Fig. 25 and is referred to as measurement A. In normal adults this is 18–32 mm (average 24 mm).

In widespread emphysema, in pulmonary heart disease or primary heart disease with increased flow or pressure in the pulmonary circuit, the artery may be dilated. In a normal person the basal arteries are much the same size on the two sides. In reduced blood flow to one side, as in Macleod's syndrome (*see* p. 149), the artery on the relatively transradiant side will be smaller than on the normal side. In cases with a thrombus in one basal artery, the artery may be larger on that side.

Apparent enlargement of one hilum may be seen in a normal person if the heart is displaced, for example, by scoliosis or rotation of the patient when the absence of cover of the heart shadow may cause the hilar vessels on one side to appear unduly conspicuous (Figs. 18 and 19). A rather large left main artery as it curves over the bronchus may cast such a large shadow that it is mistaken for a neoplasm and it is then necessary to take a lateral view or even a left lateral tomogram at hilum level to prove there is no abnormal shadow other than the conspicuous normal artery.

Another measurement which can be used is the trans-hilar diameter (joining the two dots shown in Fig. 25), but it does not seem to have any advantage over the basal artery measurement. The range of normal is 10–14·5 cm (average 11·9 cm). These measurements are summarized in Table 1.

TABLE 1

MEASUREMENTS OF HILAR VESSELS IN TOMOGRAMS IN NORMAL PERSONS

	Average	*Range*
Right basal artery	13·8 mm	7–19 mm
Trans-hilar	11·9 mm	10–14·5 mm
Left "A"	24 mm	18–32 mm

THE SHAPE OF THE HILAR SHADOWS

The normal hilum shape is derived from the upper lobe vessels meeting the basal artery. Ignoring any small mid-lateral vessels, it is therefore concave laterally or like a Y lying on its side, thus ≻ (Fig. 93).

This normal shape will not be seen if one limb of the ≻ is missing because of atelectasis of an upper or lower lobe (*see* p. 57), or if additional shadows are present, for instance from enlarged hilar glands when the mid part may become convex laterally. In fact, any shadow not readily identified as a vessel will indicate an abnormal hilum shadow.

THE POSITION OF THE HILAR SHADOWS

The most lateral upper lobe vein should be identified, and where this vessel meets the basal artery (shown diagrammatically in Fig. 25) is a convenient reference point for measuring the trans-hilar diameter and for identifying the level of each hilum. Using this method the centre of the right hilum is opposite the horizontal fissure which meets the sixth rib in the axilla, or is roughly at the level of the third rib anteriorly on deep inspiration. On the left, the centre of the hilum is some 1·0–1·5 cm higher. The centre point will be 2–3 cm higher in upper lobe shrinkage and 1–2 cm lower in lower lobe shrinkage.

The density or radio-opacity of the hilum is normally equal and any increase in density on one side will suggest the shadow of some lesion superimposed on the hilum and will be an indication for a lateral view or even a lateral-view tomogram.

THE LUNG FIELDS

Before a detailed search for pathological shadows is begun, the lung fields should be inspected as a whole and the radiotranslucency of the two sides noted and compared, particular attention being paid to the costophrenic recesses. The vessel pattern should be carefully inspected and compared on the two sides, and the line of the horizontal fissure sought. The presence or absence should be noted of certain parts of the thoracic coverings which may at times cast shadows over the lung fields, such as the scapulae, breasts, nipples, and costal cartilages.

THE RADIOTRANSLUCENCY OR BLACKENING OF THE LUNG FIELDS

The radiotranslucency or blackening of the two sides is the same at the same level in normal people, provided they are positioned straight. If they are rotated, so that the clavicles are slightly to the left, or if there is a scoliosis concave to the left, the left side will appear rather more transradiant or darker than the right. Rotation or scoliosis the other way will result in the right side being the darker side (Fig. 32).

Developmental asymmetry of the thorax may also result in hypertransradiancy of one side. The asymmetry can be detected by inspection of the rib or soft tissue shadows.

THE PULMONARY-VESSEL PATTERN

The arborizing shadows in the lung fields of a normal person (the lung markings) are without doubt in the main due to the pulmonary arteries and pulmonary veins. This can be demonstrated in tomograms taken at hilum level, when the main bronchi, the basal artery and its branches and the venous branches crossing the shadow of the basal artery to reach the left atrium can all be identified as shown diagrammatically in Fig. 25. Further evidence can be obtained by angiography, when first the arteries and then the veins can be seen reinforced by the opacity of the contrast medium.

The pulmonary vessels are of great importance in diagnosis and should be traced or scanned from the periphery to the hilum on each side either by eye or with the aid of a pointer. Any shadow which is not a vessel may thus be detected, and must be considered pathological unless some anatomical variation can be invoked to explain it.

The size of the pulmonary vessels

The size of the pulmonary vessels should be noted, particularly the decrease in size as they pass distally from the hilar regions. Whereas the size of the hilar vessels can be measured with some assurance, the size of the pulmonary vessels can often only be judged subjectively. If the size is uneven in different zones as in upper-lobe diversion or emphysema (*see* pp. 153, 163), then the larger vessels can be used to show the other vessels are small or vice versa. An alternative method is to go through a number of radiographs of normal persons and for each decade select those with the most conspicuous vessels and those with the smallest looking vessels. The patient's radiograph can then be placed between these two control radiographs and thus a decision can be made as to whether the patient's vessels are dilated or too small (hyperaemia or oligaemia). In this matching technique it is surprising how little difference in size of vessels at a comparable level can be seen in the radiograph between those normal persons with the largest and those with the smallest vessels. However, the vessel shadows are much more conspicuous in the radiograph of some subjects than others, mainly because of variations in contrast between the vessels and the surrounding air spaces, and, to a much less extent, due to variations in the actual size of the vessels. They will appear smaller and less conspicuous in a well-exposed radiograph than in a lightly exposed one, but there is also some difference between the appearances of different people even when the radiographic factors are similar.

Usually in normal persons large hilar vessels go with large lung vessels, and small hilar with small lung vessels. Any discrepancy in the balance between the size of the hilar and lung vessels will suggest an abnormality of the pulmonary circulation. However, in the same normal person the pattern is remarkably constant in radiographs taken at different times over a period of many years.

There is also some variability, even in normal persons, in how far out towards the axilla vessels can be traced. In some persons none is seen in the lateral 2 cm, in others vessel shadows can be seen within 5 mm of the pleura, and in some very thin persons even very faint horizontal line shadows of septa can be seen.

The size of the vessels in each zone at a given segmental level is much the same on each side. In some pathological conditions they may be smaller on one side (Fig. 234) or larger in one area (Fig. 263).

In the routine radiograph taken standing up, the upper lobe vessels are either much the same in size or smaller than the lower lobe vessels at a corresponding segmental or subsegmental level. The radiologist should be familiar with this fact and should compare the radiograph of a normal person with that of a patient with mitral stenosis with gross upper lobe blood diversion, so that he can detect abnormal upper-lobe vessel size with some assurance.

It is known from blood flow measurements with isotopes that, when a normal person lies down, the flow between the upper and lower halves becomes more equal, whereas standing up there is more blood flowing to the lower half of the lungs. This change in blood flow is difficult to detect in plain radiographs taken standing and prone, respectively, but can be seen more definitely in tomograms.

It is also known that the cardiac output increases from about 3 to some 30 litres/min on vigorous exercise, but again no change in the vessel size of a normal person can be seen between that in a radiograph taken at rest and one taken immediately after vigorous exercise.

In spite of these difficulties, inspection of the vessel pattern is of great value in predicting the state of the pulmonary circulation as regards pressure and flow, and sometimes pulmonary vascular resistance. Local increase or decrease in vessel size will indicate a local pathological state; for instance, the small vessels in an emphysematous area (Fig. 213).

The number of vessels

The number of vessels in the upper or lower half of each lung (for method of vessel counting, *see* p. 58) is also much the same on the two sides. An exception to this will be found in the lower zones near the heart, where there is a richer pattern on the right side, since the vessels on the left are displaced and obscured by the prominence of the heart shadow.

In the anterior-view radiograph, the close proximity of the larger vessels in the medial segment of the middle lobe together with those of the cardiac segment often results in such a rich pattern that the shadows may be considered pathological. When this type of vascular pattern is seen in the right lower zone, and there is doubt whether it is significant, a lateral-view radiograph should be taken, which in a normal person will show a normal vessel pattern, and confirm the absence of any abnormal shadows. It should be noted that in a normal person such a rich vascular pattern will remain unchanged in serial radiographs taken over a period of years, thus confirming its non-pathological basis.

Occasionally there is not only an apparent increase in the number of vessels near the right heart border but there is also a general haze. This is often due to sternal depression, the upward slope of the soft tissues as one moves out of the depression being almost at right angles to the x-ray beam, and this will increase the depth of soft tissue cover in this area and thus be responsible for the slight opacity. An example of too few vessels on one side is that seen in compensatory over-inflation of one lobe when the other is atelectatic (*see* p. 58).

The vessel pattern should also be traced upwards towards the apices. In a normal person, vessel shadows can be seen extending up to and often well above the clavicles. Failure to see them in one apex might be the first indication of a small bulla or pneumothorax. On the right side two horizontal branches, normally lying either side of the horizontal fissure, may act as a guide to seeing a rather indistinct fissure, or fix its probable position should it be invisible.

On the left a conspicuous horizontal branch, which supplies either the lateral part of the lingula or the apical lower-lobe segment, and which is normally seen extending out from the hilum, should also be identified. It will slope downwards if there is collapse of the lower lobe, the shadow of which may be hidden by the heart shadow.

THE COSTOPHRENIC AND CARDIOPHRENIC ANGLES

The costophrenic angles should be acute, clear and symmetrical in transradiancy. If the diaphragm is abnormally low in position, as in a few normal persons or in emphysema, the costophrenic angles may be obliterated, the extreme axillary portion of the muscle failing to descend as far as the rest of the diaphragm. In fact this relatively high costal attachment may result in the angle becoming obtuse (Fig. 26) and may simulate a small pleural effusion. In case of doubt, a lateral view will confirm the general flattening of the diaphragm, and show that there is no additional shadow in the posterior recess such as would be seen with a pleural effusion.

23

The cardiophrenic angles are normally acute, but that on the left is frequently obscured by a low-density triangular shadow in elderly fat people, due to fat near the apex of the heart (Fig. 27). In some cases it may be necessary to take an additional anterior-view radiograph with greater exposure in order to define the left border of the heart more clearly through the shadow of the pad of fat. It will then be possible to measure the transverse diameter more accurately, or to make sure that the well-defined lateral border of the pad of fat is not caused by the shadow of a collapsed lower lobe.

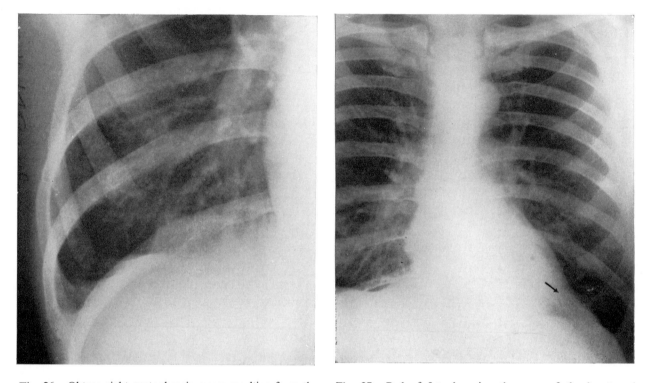

Fig. 26.—Obtuse right costophrenic recess resulting from the low position of the diaphragm on full inspiration. This appearance is seen particularly in patients with severe lower-zone emphysema. It may be present in a patient with no symptoms nor abnormal physical signs (this subject).

Fig. 27.—Pad of fat obscuring the apex of the heart and producing a straight left border (rather obese male aged 45 years). The left border of the heart is visible as a faint shadow 1 cm medially to the edge of the shadow of the pad of fat (*see* arrow).

THE HORIZONTAL FISSURE

The horizontal fissure is visible in a routine anterior-view radiograph in over 80 per cent of normal adults. It is seen as a white hair-line shadow running from roughly the centre of the right hilum to meet the sixth rib in the axilla. Although in most cases it can be seen quite clearly, in some it is seen most convincingly with the aid of a magnifying glass. It is absent or very incomplete in about 10 per cent of people, and may be invisible in the radiograph, even if it is present, in very obese subjects, or in a somewhat under-exposed radiograph, particularly if it is covered by a rib shadow. Although it usually runs straight across the lung field, it may, even in normal persons, slope upwards or downwards at a small angle, or curve downwards towards the outer third. A downward inclination is frequent in elderly persons with a kyphosis. A 10 degree inclination upwards or downwards can be accepted as being within the range of normal. Care must be taken in such cases to ensure it is not displaced as a result of shrinkage of a lobe.

VERTICAL LINE SHADOW AT BASE

Another normal hair-line shadow is sometimes seen running downwards and outwards to meet the diaphragm about 1 cm lateral to the right border of the heart (Fig. 178). This line is not caused by an accessory lobe, but might be caused by an accessory fissure; in most cases it is a part of the main fissure between the middle and lower lobes. For more detail, *see* p. 108.

THE ACCESSORY LOBE OF THE AZYGOS VEIN

A hair line, usually with a slight lateral convexity, running diagonally across the right apex to end in a comma-like expansion near the hilum, is the usual x-ray appearance of an " azygos lobe " (Fig. 28). With a smaller azygos lobe, the line is nearly vertical and close to the shadow of the superior vena cava; with a larger one, it is nearly horizontal, starting from just below the clavicle. The comma-like termination at the hilum can always be seen clearly in a tomogram if not in the plain radiograph.

The hair line is a double layer of visceral and parietal pleura drawn down to the azygos vein which has failed to slide medially clear of the lung as the upper lobe developed. The " comma " shadow is the vein itself lying at the bottom of these pleural folds. The condition is not in itself pathological, and the part of the upper lobe cut off medially by the pleural line, known as " the accessory lobe of the azygos vein ", is not unduly liable to disease.

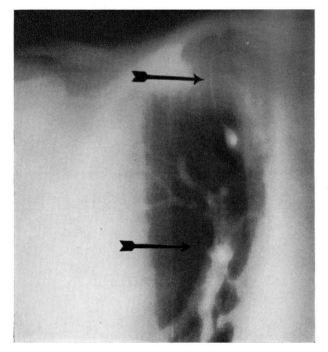

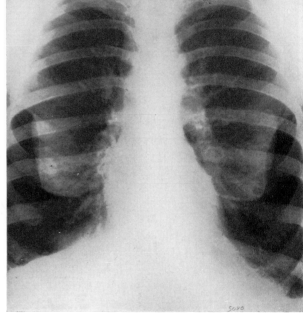

Fig. 28.—Accessory lobe of the azygos vein (tomogram of right upper zone, posterior view). The fold of parietal and visceral pleura cutting off a part of the upper lobe can be seen as a thin line with a lateral convex curve opposite the upper arrow. The " comma-like " shadow of the vein is seen at the lower end of this line, well above the angle between the right main and upper-lobe bronchus. The lower arrow points to the ⤙ shaped shadow of the normal hilar vessels, the stalk of the " Y " being rather indistinct in this case. Upper limb formed by upper-lobe veins, lower by basal artery.

Fig. 29.—Unusual mammary shadow on either side. Anterior-view radiograph of the chest of a female of 66 years. The well-demarcated concave lateral border of the shadow could be traced upwards and outwards beyond the ribs. The diaphragm is low and flattened, and the heart centrally placed. The hilar vessels are normal, but the lung vessels are evenly small. The rather hypertransradiant lung fields are due partly to the thin covering of the patient. Hilar vessels normal.

THE SCAPULAE

Sundry extrathoracic structures, such as the scapulae, breasts, nipples, or muscles, may cast shadows which are superimposed on the lung fields of a normal subject, and these must be recognized and differentiated from shadows caused by intrapulmonary pathological conditions.

The vertebral borders of one or both scapulae may be partly superimposed on the lung field, either because of a faulty technique in positioning the patient or because of their unavoidable relative fixity. Systematic identification of the scapular shadows will avoid errors of interpretation from this cause.

THE BREAST SHADOWS

The breast shadows should be identified where possible. This is usually easy, the shadows being obvious, but in the case of a thin elderly woman with fibrotic atrophic breasts, the unusual homogeneous shadow seen in the lower axillary regions may cause difficulties. Its true nature will be appreciated if it can be traced passing off the lung field to merge with the shadow of the lower axillary fold (Fig. 29). In adolescent girls the breasts are often relatively radio-opaque in spite of their small size and often produce an ill-defined area of clouding in the lower zones, sometimes more marked on one side than the other so that a lateral view may be needed to exclude an underlying consolidation.

If one breast is the seat of disease, has been removed, or is larger or lower than the other, a localized area of opacity or hypertransradiancy may be seen at one base. In a case of doubt, a radiograph taken with the patient lying down may be decisive; if the breasts are small and flat, or very large, insufficient displacement of the shadow may result from this manoeuvre, and a lateral view will be needed to prove the shadow extrathoracic. If the breasts are large and dependent, the lateral view may also be obscure, unless a flannel band is bound round the chest in order to displace the breasts forward and medially and, if possible, clear of the lung fields, or unless the radiograph is taken with the patient lying down. Even after these precautions, a tomogram may sometimes be necessary to make sure that a basal shadow low down anteriorly is only the breast shadow, or that the breast shadow is not masking an intrathoracic shadow.

THE NIPPLES

If the nipples show at all on the radiograph, both are usually visible as 0·5–1 cm circular shadows, so that identification is easy. In some cases, however, one nipple may be much more distinct than the other, especially if the shadow on one side lies in an intercostal space whilst that on the other is superimposed on a rib. Differentiation from an intrapulmonary shadow may then be necessary, and for this the simplest procedure should be chosen which will serve the purpose. If the breast is fairly large, a film with the patient supine will result in lateral displacement of the nipple, which will often fall clear of the lung field. If the breast is small and flat, displacement will not be possible, but a radio-opaque marker, such as a piece of fuse wire, placed round the nipple will show whether the nipple and the shadow do in fact correspond. Another method is to take a pair of radiographs, the first in inspiration and the second in expiration. The nipple will then be seen farther up in the former than in the latter, whereas a lower-third intrapulmonary shadow would be farther down during inspiration than during expiration. If there is still doubt, and if the shadow is too small to be seen in a lateral view, a tomogram may be necessary.

THE MUSCLES OF THE CHEST WALL

The muscles of the chest wall usually cast some shadow over the lung fields, particularly those forming the lower folds of the axillae, and those passing vertically downwards in front of the apices. The nature of these shadows usually becomes obvious when they are traced out beyond the lung fields. This test should therefore be always applied when a doubtful shadow is seen.

Slight asymmetry of the pectoral muscles on the two sides may result in a faint haze over the outer half of one mid-zone. One muscle may be thicker than the other if it is hypertrophied because of being used more—perhaps during some occupational manoeuvre, or in some left-handed people. More often one side is more radio-opaque because a slight scoliosis, or slight rotation of the patient, causes the bulk of the muscle over the mid-zones to be different on the two sides. As a rule, loss of transradiancy caused by this factor is very poorly demarcated, but sometimes the lower margin of the shadow can be traced laterally as a well-defined line passing off the lung field to merge into the shadow of the lower axillary fold with its typical inferior concave curve. If it is very poorly defined and there is no evidence of rotation or scoliosis, a lateral view may be needed to distinguish it from the shadow caused by an area of consolidation.

Occasionally atrophy or a developmental defect of the pectoralis major or some other group may cause the lung field beneath to appear unduly transradiant. Clinical inspection would of course then show the cause quite easily.

The sternomastoid and scalenus anticus show the familiar low-density shadow with a well-defined lateral margin passing down the medial third of the apex. They are frequently not quite symmetrical. They meet another low-density shadow running just above the clavicles, one of the so-called " companion shadows " (*see* below).

None of these muscle shadows is often mistaken for a pathological lesion, but now and again an apical view or even a tomogram may be necessary to make quite sure of the innocent nature of the shadow.

THE SUBCLAVIAN ARTERY

In some adults the left subclavian artery and surrounding tissues may cause a well-defined 3–5 mm wide band-like shadow to be seen passing horizontally in front of the left apex with an inferior concave curve. Medially this band-like shadow may disappear as it reaches the central vascular shadows, but sometimes the inferior border can be seen curving round, becoming more obviously continuous with the lateral border of the central shadow, and finally passing downwards to meet the aortic knuckle. Enlargement or lateral displacement of the proximal part of the artery (as in co-arctation of the aorta) makes this merging with the lateral upper border of the central shadow more conspicuous. Laterally, the artery shadow disappears when it reaches the edge of the lung transradiancy.

Sometimes the subclavian artery lies higher, so that no transradiant area of lung can be seen above it, and its upper margin merges into the general haze of the lower neck region. In such cases the shadow with its inferior concave margin will simulate a cap of thickened pleura over the apex. Differentiation is made possible by the fact that the pleural shadow would extend a short way down the axilla, whilst the shadow of the artery ends abruptly when it meets the axilla as it passes horizontally.

Often only a part of the artery shadow can be seen, where the density of the artery is reinforced by the faint shadow of the sternomastoid and scalenus anticus muscles. This combination may simulate a pathological shadow in the apex. The abrupt ending at the margin of the muscle, or a faint lateral extension of the shadow beyond this, usually gives the identification, but sometimes an apical view or tomogram may be necessary to exclude an abnormality.

THE " COMPANION SHADOWS "

A 2–3-mm wide companion shadow is often seen running parallel to the upper border of the clavicle. It is caused by the fold of skin and subcutaneous tissue lying rather horizontally above the bone, so that a considerable thickness of tissue meets the x-ray beam horizontally. It is often symmetrical on the two sides and can generally be traced laterally beyond the margins of the transradiant lung fields (Fig. 30); if one clavicle is relatively elevated, however, the companion shadow may be more conspicuous on one side. It may also be denser where it is reinforced by the shadow of the sterno-mastoid, and if there is an abnormal vertical linear shadow in the apex as well, the companion shadow meeting this may be mistaken for the lower margin of a cavity.

A second faint 1–2-mm wide companion shadow is often seen running parallel to the infero-medial concave surface of the second rib in the axilla (Fig. 30). It looks like an area of pleural thickening, but is due to extrapulmonary soft tissues and normal pleura made visible because of the tangential direction of the x-rays in relation to them. It is usually symmetrical on both sides.

A third companion shadow is sometimes seen in very thin subjects due to the thoracic coverings over the lower chest casting a 1–2-mm wide shadow in the lower axilla close to the ribs extending up for 1–2 cm from the costophrenic recess (Fig. 31). It is usually bilateral, but may be more conspicuous on one side if the patient is not orientated straight. It closely simulates the shadow of a very small lower axillary pleural effusion, but it can generally be differentiated from these because of its more obvious continuity with the shadowing which lies beyond the ribs laterally. In a case of doubt

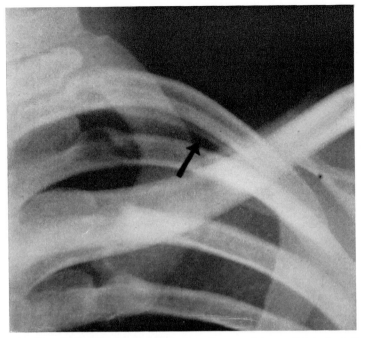

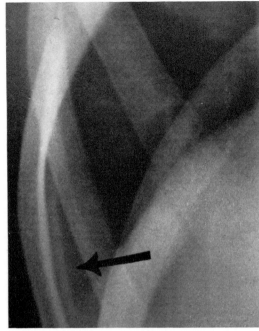

Fig. 30.—Companion shadow seen as a line running parallel to the left second rib (opposite arrow). A 3-mm wide companion shadow is also visible running parallel with the upper border of the clavicle. Similar shadows were seen on the right side. Normal adult male. Routine anterior-view radiograph, subject standing.

Fig. 31.—Companion shadow seen as a line running parallel to the chest wall just above the right costophrenic recess (marked by arrow). In the original radiograph a faint haze could be traced from the line continuous with the extrathoracic soft tissues. Similar line on left. Normal rather thin adult female.

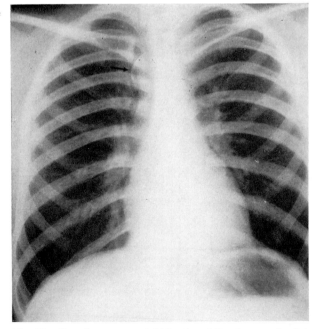

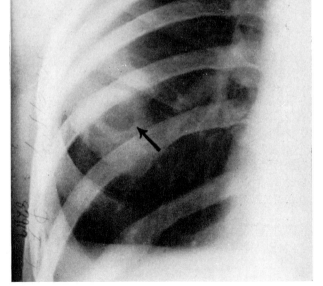

Fig. 32.—Prominent upper right border of the sternum simulating an abnormal mediastinal shadow (marked by arrow). It was caused by slight rotation of the patient to the right. Sternal end of the right clavicle further from vertebral margin than the left, indicating rotation of left shoulder forwards. This has resulted in slight relative hypertransradiancy of the right side. Large gastric air bubble causing elevation of left dome.

Fig. 33.—Bifurcated rib simulating a pulmonary cavity. Arrow points to the circular transradiancy surrounded by bone. Right basal pleural shadow also present with flattening of the right dome of the diaphragm really representing an organizing pleural exudate.

a lateral view may be necessary to show that the posterior recess is clear, thus excluding a small effusion; or an anterior view with the patient lying on that side and the x-ray beam horizontal, when the shadow of an effusion will become wider (Fig. 49).

THE STERNUM

The edge of the manubrium of the sternum is frequently visible just below the sternal ends of the clavicles. If there is slight rotation of the patient, one border of this shadow may be very conspicuous (Fig. 32) and may even suggest the presence of a mediastinal tumour. To avoid misinterpretation it is usually enough to bear in mind the possibility that the shadow may be that of the sternum. Its identity will be confirmed if the lateral border can be traced up as a continuous line into the white line of the articular cortex of the joint with its superior concave curve.

THE RETROSTERNAL AND RETROCARDIAC TRANSRADIANT ZONES

In a lateral view of a normal person, the retrosternal and retrocardiac transradiant areas usually show a similar degree of blackening (Fig. 7). In a very fat person, or if the radiograph is not taken in full inspiration, the retrosternal area may appear relatively opaque. A relative opacity of the retrosternal area may also be seen in the presence of a retrosternal tumour (Fig. 319), and a relative opacity of the retrocardiac area with, for instance, a lower lobe consolidation (Fig. 79).

In addition, in a normal person, owing to the absorption of rays by the scapulae and surrounding muscles, the lower thoracic vertebrae appear darker than those higher up, but this difference in vertebral blackening will be counteracted if the lower vertebrae are shaded by a pathological shadow, as in a lower lobe consolidation (Fig. 79).

A rough measure of the depth of the retrosternal transradiant area can be made by choosing a point on the sternum 3 cm below the sternal joint, and measuring horizontally backwards from this to the front of the ascending aorta. In a normal person it is usually about 2·5 cm (range 1–3·5 cm). In a normal person the lower limit of the dark area is about 7 cm or more above the diaphragm (Fig. 21).

THE COSTAL CARTILAGES AND RIBS

Calcification of the costal cartilages is common even in normal young adults, and some calcification is almost inevitable in the elderly. The first costal cartilages are nearly always calcified after the age of

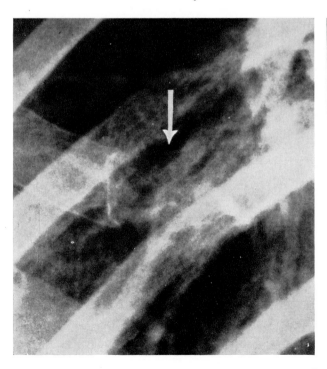

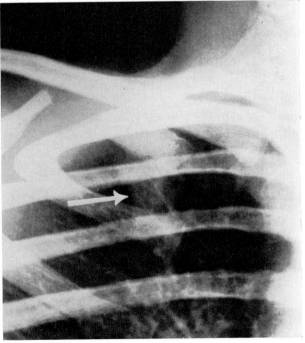

Fig. 34.—Line shadow (below arrow) caused by calcification of the upper margin of the rib cartilage.

Fig. 35.—Ill-defined shadow in right upper zone (opposite arrow) caused by hair plait.

25 years. The calcification is generally rather irregular, giving a series of circular or mottled shadows, and there is often one area which appears as a small pointed extension of the inferior margin of the rib shadow. Occasionally only the upper or lower margin calcifies, giving a short line shadow (Fig. 34).

These shadows are not symmetrical and the pattern varies with different people, so that they form useful identity checks when ensuring that a pair of comparative radiographs are in fact of the same patient.

Shadows of the costal cartilages should be sought and their nature appreciated when inspecting the lung fields for normal variations. They are then unlikely to be mistaken for pathological intrapulmonary foci, but, as in the case of a rib shadow, there is always the possibility that they cover and hide a small abnormal lung shadow. If both cartilage and abnormal focus shadows are present, and are close but not superimposed, it is easy to misinterpret the abnormal focus as belonging to the group of nearby mottled shadows of calcified cartilage, especially if the latter are not very radio-opaque. Tomograms may be indicated in some cases to prove or exclude an underlying lung focus.

Developmental abnormalities of the ribs are common but rarely result in shadows which might be mistaken for pathological lesions. Part of a small cervical rib may be mistaken for an apical lesion, and the circular transradiancy sometimes seen between the end of a bifurcated rib or pair of fused ribs may simulate a cavity (Fig. 33). Careful inspection of the bony parts, which should be a routine, will usually be sufficient to avoid mistakes of this kind.

THE VERTEBRAL COLUMN

An isolated long transverse process of a mid-thoracic vertebra may suggest a fluid level in a cavity, especially when it is superimposed on the mesh of the hilar vessels. Failure to find the lesion in a justifiably taken lateral view will be an indication for a high-penetration anterior view or for fluoroscopy, when the true state of affairs will be clearly seen.

If there is a scoliosis, the edge of the vertebral column on one side will sometimes be visible in the lower part of the chest and may be mistaken for a lesion such as the edge of a collapsed lower lobe, or even a tumour. This mistake should be avoided if the visible part of the vertebral column is inspected at the same time as the ribs. In very severe scoliosis the vertebral column may be superimposed on the whole of one lung (Fig. 357). It is nevertheless often possible to see the lungs clearly by careful positioning of the patient (*see* p. 269 and Fig. 358).

PLAITS OF HAIR, CLOTHING, SKIN TUMOURS AND SUBCUTANEOUS TUMOURS

Plaits of hair (Fig. 35), and even gowns and other clothing, occasionally cast confusing shadows over the upper third of the lungs. Their true nature is usually evident when they can be traced beyond the limits of the thorax.

Skin nodules, such as a mole, a benign tumour or a cystic swelling, may cast circular shadows over the lung. Clinical inspection will often reveal their identity, otherwise their extrathoracic position may not be noted until a tomogram is taken.

DIAPHRAGM CURVE

If the dome of the diaphragm is well curved or very flat, this will be obvious. If there is any doubt, a quick estimate of the curve can be made in the following manner. A line is drawn from the costophrenic to the cardiophrenic recess as in Fig. 246. A vertical from this to the top of the diaphragm will be 1·5 cm or more in a normally curved dome.

CHAPTER 2

HOMOGENEOUS SHADOWS GROUPED ACCORDING TO SHAPE, SIZE, OR DISTRIBUTION

BILATERAL TOTAL HOMOGENEOUS OPACITY

BILATERAL homogeneous opacity of the whole of or most of both lungs is seen in extensive pulmonary oedema. It may be present throughout both lungs in the terminal stages of a failing left ventricle or a large water overload. It was quite a common finding in the post-operative period after cardiac surgery on by-pass. In some cases this may have been due to excessive oxygen enrichment in the respirator circuit; in others the oedema may have been secondary to alveolar wall damage due to some fault during the period of perfusion. However, with improvements in technique in these procedures, this appearance is now uncommon. Widespread pulmonary oedema is occasionally seen in a case of mitral stenosis or acute left ventricular failure (Fig. 36) with almost total opacity of both lungs. Rapid disappearance of the shadow is seen as the patient recovers.

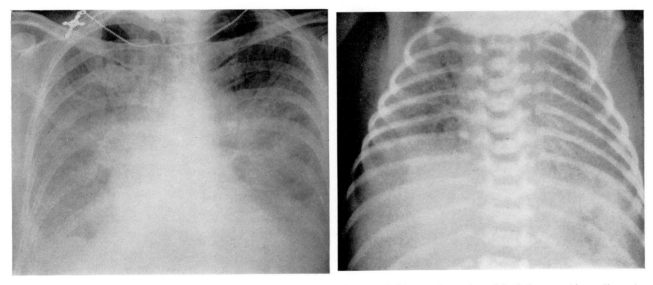

Fig. 36.—Almost total opacity of both lungs from acute pulmonary oedema. Myocardial infarct and acute left ventricular failure. Male aged 62 years. Sudden severe chest pain. E.C.G. indicated recent infarct. Recovery.

Fig. 37.—Widespread opacity of both lungs. Air outlines the proximal bronchi of both lungs. Respiratory distress of a newborn premature infant.

In newborn babies proper aeration of the lungs may be delayed; they will appear opaque, and full inflation may only occur a few hours later. In the respiratory distress syndrome of the newborn premature baby the lungs appear normal at first, and then a ground-glass haze or fine nodular shadows may be seen. A few days later these may increase and finally coalesce to produce total opacity of both lungs save for the transradiancies of some air in the larger bronchi (an air bronchogram) (Fig. 37).

BILATERAL HOMOGENEOUS OPACITY OCCUPYING ONLY THE MAJOR PART OF THE LUNGS

A homogeneous shadow spreading out from the hilum and leaving a rim of transradiant lung along the periphery, the so-called "bat's wing" shadow (Fig. 38), is characteristic of pulmonary oedema whatever the cause. It is a common finding in the end stage of systemic hypertension with uraemia and left

31

ventricular failure. Uraemia itself does not cause pulmonary oedema, but the renal lesion may lead to a fluid overload. Overtransfusion may also lead to pulmonary oedema for the same reason. The bat's wing shadow may be seen with left ventricular failure whatever the cause, and is very occasionally seen with a high pulmonary venous pressure in mitral stenosis. It seems an acute or sudden rise of pulmonary venous pressure is more likely to result in a bat's wing shadow than a chronic and gradual rise of venous pressure. A rare cause is alveolar proteinosis, whatever that may be. The cause of the unusual distribution of the shadow is uncertain. A lateral view will show the opacity extends from back to front, and it is possible the axillary part of the lung escapes because of better respiratory movement here. This will not, however, account for the reverse bat's wing shadow occasionally seen, that is, a peripheral opacity with a core of aerated lung round the hilum. Lymphatic drainage is better at the periphery.

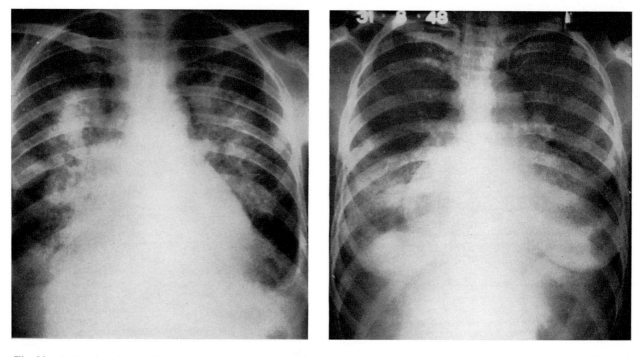
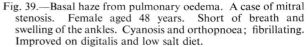

Fig. 38.—Bat's wing shadow from pulmonary oedema. A male aged 27 years with hypertension and left ventricular failure. Blood pressure $\frac{290}{160}$. Albuminuria. Blood urea 50–380 mg per 100 ml. Retinopathy.

Fig. 39.—Basal haze from pulmonary oedema. A case of mitral stenosis. Female aged 48 years. Short of breath and swelling of the ankles. Cyanosis and orthopnoea; fibrillating. Improved on digitalis and low salt diet.

A bilateral homogeneous lower zone haze with a poorly demarcated upper margin (Fig. 39) is rarely due to bilateral pneumonia; it is usually due to pulmonary oedema, particularly in mitral stenosis and myocardial infarction with acute left ventricular failure.

In many cases the shadow of pulmonary oedema is not quite homogeneous as in Fig. 38; in others it is definitely nodular or blotchy (*see* pp. 91 and 93).

UNILATERAL TOTAL HOMOGENEOUS OPACITY

The cause of total opacity of one side of the chest may be obvious from the clinical picture and physical signs, but this is not always the case. In the radiograph the position of the heart and trachea should be observed with particular care, since the patient is usually quite ill and correct positioning is difficult. Displacements must therefore be assessed in relation to the appearance of the bony parts.

Gross displacement to the other side (that is, away from the opacity) indicates a massive pleural effusion (Fig. 40), whilst displacement to the same side (Fig. 41) indicates shrinkage of the lung with airlessness, which is often associated with stenosis and effective occlusion of the main bronchus. If the lesion is on the left side, the air in the stomach will outline the left dome of the diaphragm, which will be considerably raised (Fig. 41).

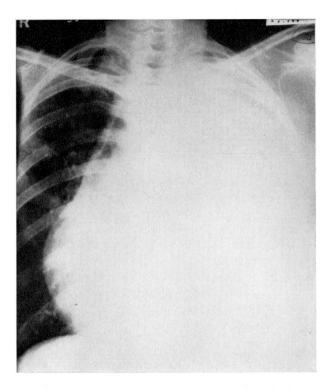

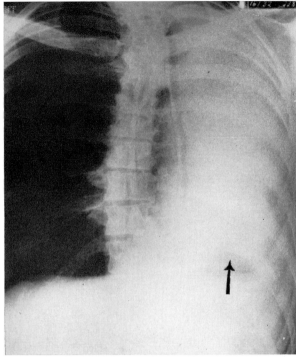

Fig. 40.—Total opacity of left side from massive left pleural effusion. Heart and trachea displaced to the right. Tuberculous infection of the lung. Tubercle bacilli in the fluid on aspiration.

Fig. 41.—Total opacity of left side from atelectasis of the left lung from stenosis of the left main bronchus. Heart and trachea displaced to the left. Arrow points to the gas cap which marks the position of the raised left dome. Carcinoma left bronchus.

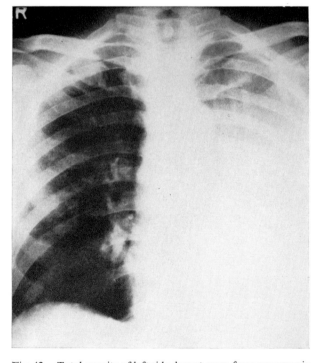

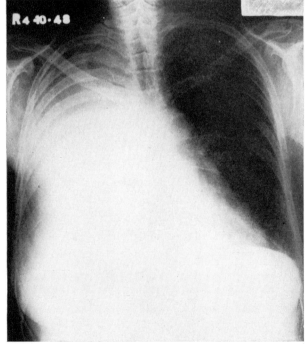

Fig. 42.—Total opacity of left side, less at apex, from pneumonic consolidation of the left lung from pneumococcal infection. No tracheal displacement. Elderly male. Complete resolution.

Fig. 43.—Total opacity of right side from atelectasis of the right lung from stenosis of the right main bronchus, complicated by large right pleural effusion. A month previously the trachea was to the right and is now virtually central.

Acute total pneumonic consolidation on one side is rarely seen nowadays, but if it is seen there is either no displacement of the heart and trachea, or else only slight displacement towards the opaque side (Fig. 42). This feature can rarely be demonstrated with certainty because the patient is usually too ill to be positioned straight.

A hydropneumothorax or haemopneumothorax, if the radiograph is taken with the patient supine, gives a similar picture to that of a massive effusion, except that the displacement of the heart and trachea may be less marked. The clinical picture is usually such that steps to demonstrate the fluid level for purely diagnostic purposes are unnecessary. If the patient cannot sit up or turn on his side (for example, because of other traumatic lesions), the fluid level can still be demonstrated in a lateral view taken with a horizontal x-ray beam.

Sometimes an initial radiograph of a patient shows the x-ray appearances of stenosis with effective occlusion of the main bronchus (similar to those seen in Fig. 41), whilst a subsequent radiograph (Fig. 43) shows the same homogeneous opacity but with the trachea now central and the heart no longer displaced or even both displaced to the opposite side. This indicates the combination of an effusion and occlusion of the main bronchus, in which the shadow of the opaque lung and the fluid cannot be separately distinguished.

When extensive consolidation is present, the development of a small or moderate effusion cannot be detected, even in a well-exposed radiograph, unless some aerated lung is present lying between the two shadows, or unless the consolidation begins to resolve, when the homogeneous shadow of the fluid, usually in the region of the costodiaphragmatic recess, will be seen in contrast to the more patchy clouding in the lung.

Uniform opacity of one side which is often not quite homogeneous because some vessel shadows can be seen superimposed on the haze, is seen on agenesis of a lobe (Fig. 344) or lung. The heart and trachea are displaced towards the opaque side. In partial agenesis the vessels seen are too few in number and take an abnormal course. In total agenesis of one lung, any vessels seen will be those in that part of the normal lung which has herniated across from the opposite side. In this type of abnormality vessels will only be seen in the medial third of the opaque side.

LARGE HOMOGENEOUS SHADOWS OCCUPYING ONLY A PART OF ONE SIDE

A large homogeneous shadow occupying only a part of one lung field may be due to a great variety of causes. When such a shadow is seen for the first time in an anterior-view radiograph, it is usually necessary to take a lateral view to establish its size, shape, and position. It is also necessary to determine, possibly with the help of further radiological investigations, whether the shadow represents a pleural, mediastinal, or intrapulmonary lesion. Distinction between these may be easy, or it may be very difficult and at times impossible. Special attention should be given to the position of the shadow, its relation to nearby normal shadows, particularly the cardiovascular and skeletal shadows, the presence or absence of any displacement of the normal vessels and fissures, and the appearance of the major bronchial transradiancies on tomography. A barium swallow may be necessary to show its relation to the oesophagus, and it may even be necessary to outline the major vessels by angiocardiography.

PLEURAL SHADOWS

A pleural effusion gives a homogeneous shadow, the site of which depends on whether it is free or encysted. The shadow can usually be distinguished from one caused by an intrapulmonary lesion by the anatomical site, by the character of its fairly well-defined margins, particularly when considered in relation to the situation of the shadow, by the position of the nearby fissure, which may be visible and which will not be displaced towards the shadow, or by the absence of any alteration in the pattern of the main blood vessels. The main bronchial transradiancies will also appear normal, should they be demonstrated in tomograms. These criteria are valid even if some air is also present in the pleural space, resulting in a horizontal fluid level demarcating the upper part of the opacity when the patient is radiographed in the upright position or lying with the x-ray beam horizontal.

In some cases it may not be possible to distinguish the x-ray shadow of a pleural effusion encysted medially adjacent to the heart shadow from the shadow of a mediastinal neoplasm, a mediastinal effusion, or even an aortic aneurysm.

The character of the fluid cannot be determined from the radiographs, nor in fact when it is encysted can it be determined from them whether it is still fluid, or whether it has become semi-solid, or even solid and fibrous, as a result of the organization of the cellular exudate.

Moderate-sized free pleural effusion

A moderate-sized free pleural effusion casts a characteristic homogeneous shadow. This lies in the lower part of the lung field; it is of much the same radio-opacity as the heart shadow, and reaches its highest level in the axilla, from which point its poorly defined upper margin runs medially towards the heart shadow with a superior concave curvature (Fig. 44). If the diaphragm is visible, it is often seen

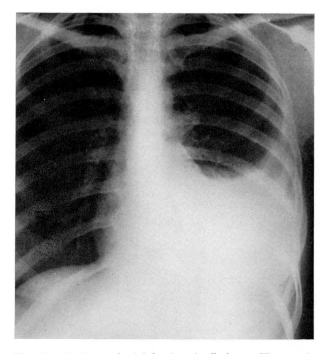

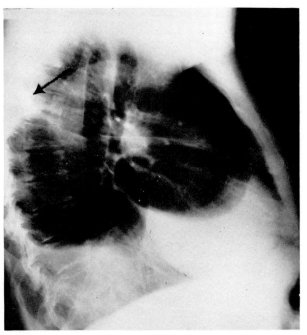

Fig. 44.—Moderate-sized left pleural effusion. The poorly defined superior concave margin is seen, but no apparent displacement of the heart or trachea. The position of the sternal ends of the clavicles indicates slight rotation of the patient to the left, so there is, in fact, slight displacement of the heart and trachea to the right.

Fig. 45.—Moderate right pleural effusion (lateral view). Upper arrow points to fluid in the upper end of the main interlobar fissure, lower arrow to the lower end of this fissure. The upper margin of the opacity of the fluid has a double superior concave curve. The dark transradiant retrosternal region in the upper half contrasts with the opacity of the fluid below and in the region behind the heart shadow below. Right dome invisible, left dome seen below.

to be slightly raised or it may be depressed. There may be some displacement of the heart and trachea to the other side, but this feature cannot be demonstrated with any certainty if the patient is slightly rotated, as is often the case with a sick subject. The position of the shadow of the effusion can often be altered by a change of posture, as shown in a radiograph taken with the patient supine (Fig. 51) or one with him lying on the affected side and the x-ray beam horizontal (Fig. 49). The axilla will be shown with ease if the patient lies on a thick non-opaque (polythene) mattress. Any gross upward shift of the shadow in a radiograph taken with the patient lying compared with one taken sitting will indicate that at least some of the shadow is due to fluid. The shadow will not change if the effusion is old and either encysted or organizing.

The diagnosis of a moderate pleural effusion is usually obvious as a result of the clinical examination, so that the radiograph is as a rule taken only to show the extent and position of the fluid, and the presence or absence of any underlying abnormal lung shadows.

If there is any doubt about the clinical or x-ray diagnosis, a lateral view should be taken which is often characteristic (Fig. 45). At a superficial glance the opacity is very difficult to see at all, but more careful inspection will show that the retrocardiac area is grey compared to the darker retrosternal transradiancy lying just above the heart shadow. Normally the blackening of these two areas is much the same, so it will be obvious from this test that there is a general basal haze. The poorly defined upper margin of this area of clouding runs with a superior concave curvature from the back of the chest to the retrosternal region, and has a peak towards the middle, thus producing a double curve. The middle peak may show a triangular and linear extension pointing upwards and posteriorly if there is an extension upwards of the fluid into the interlobar pleura (Fig. 45).

Small pleural effusion

A small pleural effusion may be difficult to detect on clinical examination, and the diagnosis will be dependent on the radiographs. In the routine anterior-view radiograph the diaphragm may appear to be normal in position, but may show some restriction of movement on the affected side on fluoroscopy. This restriction is not usually great enough to cause sufficient difference in the level between the right and left domes for the condition to be detected in the routine radiograph taken with the breath held at the end of a moderately deep inspiration.

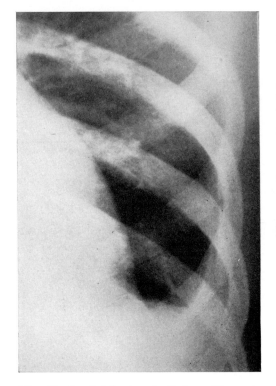

Fig. 46.—Small left pleural effusion. The costophrenic angle is opaque, and a shadow with a well-defined nearly vertical concave margin extends up the axilla for about 3 cm thinning to a line shadow at the upper end. Restriction of movement of the left dome.

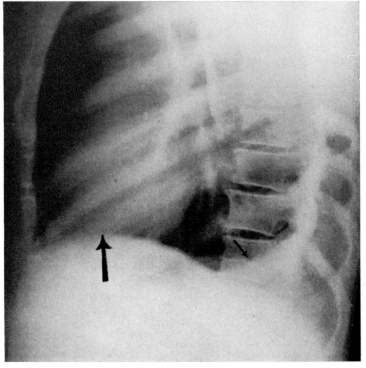

Fig. 47.—Small left pleural effusion (lateral view). Small arrow marks the antero-superior edge of the shadow of the fluid occupying the posterior costophrenic recess. Note how opaque this is in comparison with the dark transradiant retrosternal region above the heart shadow. Vertical arrow marks left dome.

An effusion giving a small homogeneous area of clouding in a costophrenic recess can generally be recognized by its upper margin which is well defined and slightly concave facing towards the hilum (Fig. 46). A small area of pulmonary consolidation in this peripheral situation would give a similar area of clouding, but the upper margin would be less well defined. On rare occasions an infarct or an extrapleural effusion may give an identical shadow, obscuring a costophrenic recess. Inferiorly the shadow of an effusion occludes the recess and merges with a normal diaphragm shadow in contradistinction to the occlusion of the recess which is sometimes seen when the diaphragm is low and flat (Fig. 26).

Sometimes the recess itself is clear but an effusion may be suspected if a 1–2-mm linear shadow due to the pleural exudate is seen extending up the axillary edge of the chest for perhaps 1 cm (Figs. 46 and 48). The linear shadow due to the pleural exudate must not be confused with the soft tissue companion shadow which is occasionally seen in very thin subjects (*see* p. 27 and Fig. 31). In the case of a companion shadow the costophrenic recess remains acute and clear, and the shadow can generally be seen to be symmetrical on the two sides, though if the patient is slightly rotated it may be more distinct on one side than the other.

If there is any doubt as to the cause of the shadow, or if the anterior view is quite normal, but a small effusion is suspected, then a lateral view should be taken. In this, even a small effusion will cast a shadow which will occupy the posterior costodiaphragmatic angle, and end with a fairly well defined slightly concave margin facing towards the hilum (Fig. 47). This is probably the most delicate test for the presence of a small effusion, although in the early stages, before it is limited by adhesions, it may also be detected as a fine band-like axillary shadow in an anterior-view radiograph taken with the patient lying on the affected side with the x-ray beam horizontal (Fig. 49).

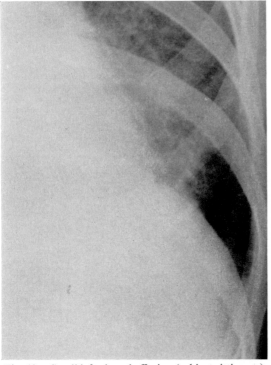

Fig. 48.—Small left pleural effusion (subject sitting up). Line shadow above costophrenic recess almost parallel to the overlying rib shadow.

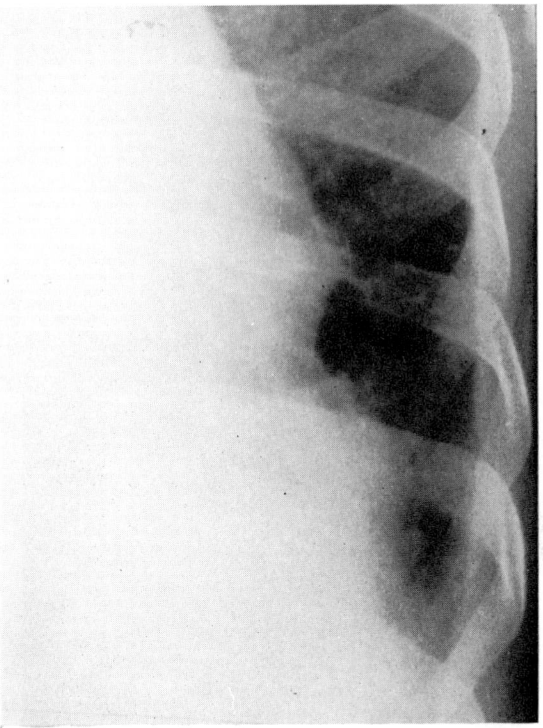

Fig. 49.—Same patient lying on left side, x-ray beam horizontal. Shadow of fluid now wider along axillary border. Mitral stenosis and severe dyspnoea.

Diaphragmatic or sub-pulmonary pleural effusion

Sometimes the fluid collects in the pleural cavity under the lung adjacent to the diaphragm. The upper margin of the shadow of the fluid then runs parallel to the diaphragm and may easily be mistaken for a raised diaphragm. On the left side there will be a 2–3 cm opaque area between the top of the transradiant stomach gas bubble and the transradiant lung above (Fig. 50), instead of an opaque area of only a few millimetres (Figs. 32 and 53). In the lateral view the upper margin of the shadow representing the pleural effusion will also tend to follow the curve of the diaphragm right back to the posterior chest wall, where it will form an acute angle (Fig. 52). The diagnosis will be confirmed if the more usual appearance of a pleural effusion is seen when the patient is radiographed lying down (Fig. 51), though if the fluid is encysted no such change with posture will occur.

a thin line, whilst the lower end will widen out into a triangular shadow with its base merging into the shadow of the diaphragm (Fig. 61).

Generally there is a thin linear extension beyond the shadow of the effusion at one or both ends due to a continuation of the pleural exudate along the line of the fissure, a feature which may be seen most clearly in lateral-view tomograms. These will also confirm that the vessel pattern in the nearby lung is normal, a feature which will distinguish the shadow from that of an atelectatic shrunken middle lobe.

A neoplastic mass adjacent to an interlobar fissure may transgress the pleural boundary and produce an oval shadow with a convex bulge either side of the predicted fissure line; it will then be indistinguishable from the shadow of an interlobar effusion. More often the shadow of a neoplasm is rather more circular or lobulated, and rather less well demarcated than that of an interlobar effusion.

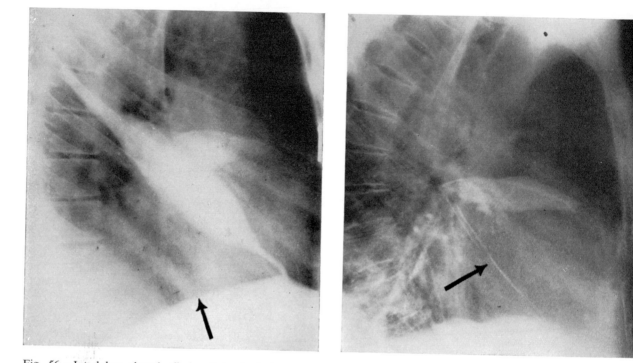

Fig. 56.—Interlobar pleural effusion (lateral view). Arrow points to the right dome of the diaphragm. Spindle-shaped shadow passes upwards and backwards from this in the line of the main fissure, with a forward extension of the shadow into the horizontal fissure. Opacity of the posterior recess is caused by a free pleural effusion which is also present. Idiopathic tuberculous effusion.

Fig. 57.—Interlobar effusion into horizontal fissure seen as a spindle-shaped shadow (lateral view). Arrow points to a line shadow caused by some fluid in the lower half of the main interlobar fissure which meets the right dome 4 cm behind the sternum. The shadow of the interlobar effusion was well demarcated in the anterior view.

Anteriorly encysted pleural effusion

An anteriorly encysted pleural effusion tends to lie rather medially, so that its shadow may merge with that of the heart. In a lateral view it will be seen to lie behind the sternum, and it usually has a well-defined margin, which is posteriorly convex if the effusion is relatively high up, or posteriorly concave if it continues down onto the diaphragm or extends backwards into the horizontal fissure. If it extends into the horizontal fissure, it will have to be distinguished from a lesion of the middle lobe. The normal position of the main fissure, which will probably contain some fluid and therefore be partly visible, and the normal pattern of the middle-lobe vessels and bronchi, shown if necessary in tomograms, will serve to differentiate the two conditions. Differentiation from a retrosternal mediastinal tumour may be difficult. The diaphragm tends to be independent of such a tumour, whereas it is often drawn up towards, and therefore merges into, the shadow of an effusion.

Posteriorly encysted pleural effusion

The large homogeneous shadow produced by a posteriorly encysted pleural effusion may be confusing if seen only in the anterior (or posterior) view (Fig. 58). Its nature will, however, be apparent from a lateral view, in which it will be seen to lie well posteriorly, extending backwards as far as the ribs. It will extend anteriorly for a variable distance, depending on the size of the effusion, and end with a moderately well-defined anterior convex margin (Fig. 59). Unless it is exceptionally large most of the shadow will lie behind the predicted line of the interlobar fissure, which may be visible, so that its anatomical extent and anterior convex margin will differentiate it from a consolidation of the apex of the lower lobe or posterior basal segment.

If it is very large its situation would correspond closely to that of a large lower lobe abscess; in such a case the patient would be too ill for elaborate radiological investigations, such as bronchography or tomography, which would differentiate these two conditions by showing bronchi in the opaque area in a consolidation with abscess. An effusion, however, is much the commoner cause of such a shadow, and should therefore be considered first. A well-exposed posterior and a lateral view can always be obtained, and these radiographs will serve as a guide in selecting the most favourable site for puncture if a diagnostic aspiration is indicated.

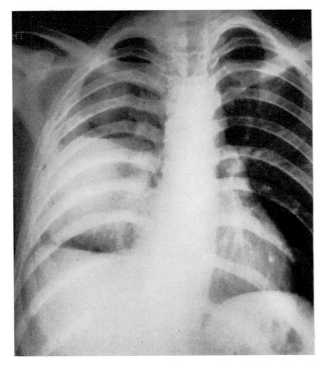

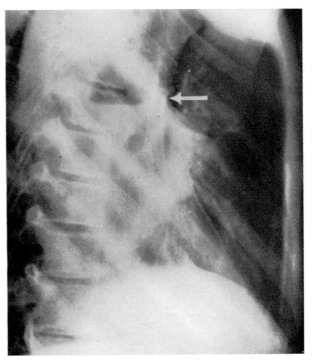

Fig. 58.—Posteriorly encysted fluid (anterior view). The air producing the fluid level is from a diagnostic aspiration. Male aged 59 years. Post-pneumonic streptococcal empyema. Cough, sputum, high fever, and leucocytosis.

Fig. 59.—Same case (lateral view). Arrow marks the anterior limit of the empyema cavity extending forwards beyond the predicted line of the main fissure. The distance between the fluid level and the arrow indicates the thickness of its wall.

A fluid level, the presence of which may lead to a mistaken diagnosis of a lung abscess, is often seen in an encysted effusion, particularly when it is fairly acute and lies posteriorly. It may be the result of a previous diagnostic aspiration with the unintentional introduction of some air, or of a broncho-pleural fistula, or even of a gas-forming organism.

When surgical drainage of the effusion is contemplated, it is useful to mark its lower limit in relation to a rib. This is easily achieved by introducing 5 ml of iodized oil into the pleural space at the time of the diagnostic aspiration. Well-exposed posterior-view and lateral-view radiographs are then taken with the patient sitting up (Figs. 60 and 61), and the lower limit of the opaque oil observed in relation to the posterior part of the particular rib.

Pleural sinograms

Following surgical drainage of an empyema or lung abscess, a sinogram may be needed to outline the sinus track and to show the size of the residual cavity which it is draining, and the relation between

41

the cavity and the sinus and drainage tube. The technique used varies according to the purpose of the investigation in each case.

The size of the residual space or cavity is best shown if the contrast medium is introduced while the patient is lying, and the radiographs taken with the patient still in this position. The contrast medium will then outline the whole of the cavity to which it has access, although it may not show the draining sinus.

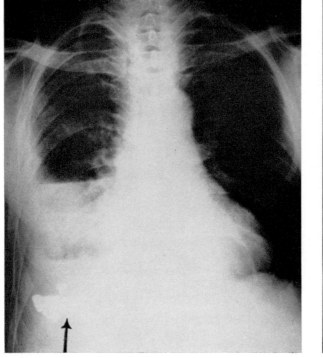

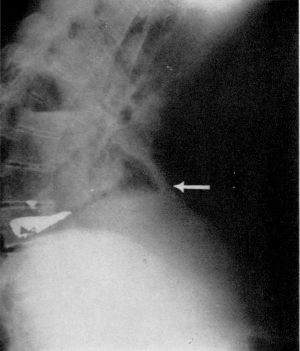

Fig. 60.—Same case. Arrow marks the lower limit of iodized oil introduced at the time of a diagnostic aspiration in order to localize the level of the bottom of the cavity in relation to the ribs.

Fig. 61.—Same case as Fig. 60 (lateral view, patient sitting). Arrow marks an interlobar extension of the fluid. Surgical drainage and rapid recovery.

The relation of the cavity to the sinus track and drainage tube is most readily ascertained from sinograms taken with the patient in an upright position. The contrast medium (usually iodized oil) is injected down the drainage tube actually in use and *in situ*. Since this rubber drainage tube is often of relatively wide bore, it is necessary to have an intermediate conical connecting piece, which will fit any size of drainage tube likely to be used; this is fitted between the tube and the syringe. The space between the tube and the sinus wall should not be tightly packed with wool for fear of an oil embolus, but if the patient lies with the opening of the sinus uppermost, the contrast medium runs in almost by gravity. The syringe is withdrawn and the tube temporarily blocked with a wooden spigot. At this stage the tube may be lightly packed round with wool to stop the medium from running out between it and the sinus wall. The patient then sits up while anterior (or posterior) and the appropriate lateral-view radiographs are taken. These will show whether the sinus track starts at the bottom of the cavity, which will help dependent drainage, or whether it emerges a short way up, so that there is a dependent pocket below the exit. The radiographs will also show whether the tube is of the correct length to encourage natural closure of the space, or whether it is too far in, so that the drainage is not complete, or not in far enough so that there is danger of premature narrowing of the sinus track.

Should a bronchopleural fistula be suspected, an absorbable medium, such as oily propyliodone (Dionosil), may be indicated. The site of the fistula and the state of the nearby bronchi will generally be shown in the sinogram.

Apical pleural opacity

An apical pleural opacity due to a cap of thickened "pleura" or an effusion over the apex is not uncommon, and is generally secondary to an underlying parenchymal tuberculous lesion. The shadow is homogeneous and usually has a well-defined inferior concave margin. If the trachea is deviated towards the shadow, as is usually the case, it must be differentiated from an atelectasis (with bronchostenosis) of an upper lobe, particularly on the right side, but none of the other changes seen in atelectasis will be present, such as alteration in the vascular pattern, fissure displacement, compensatory emphysema, or bronchial occlusion on tomography. If the trachea is not deviated, and there are no clinical clues, such an apical opacity seen for the first time in an elderly male may be indistinguishable from a neoplasm in this region. A neoplasm will be suspected if rib erosion can be seen in the plain radiographs or demonstrated by tomography, and tuberculosis if underlying parenchymal small circular shadows can be seen. Serial x-ray observation will eventually give the correct diagnosis, but whether such a waiting period is justified without exploration must be decided in each case on clinical grounds.

Mediastinal pleural effusion

An encysted effusion of the mediastinal pleura is uncommon. It will result in a homogeneous shadow with a very well-defined lateral convex border projecting into the transradiant lung field (Figs. 62 and 63). Medially it will merge with the heart shadow and will not be separately demarcated from

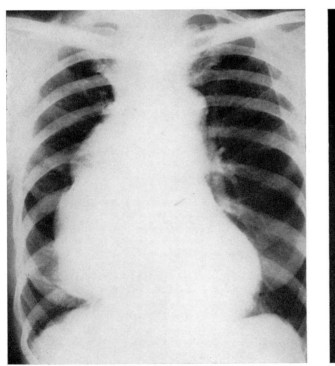

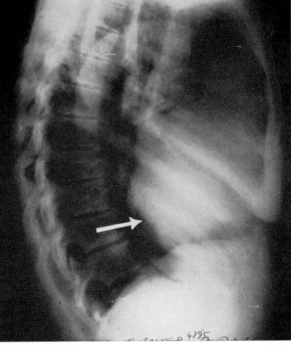

Fig. 62.—Mediastinal pleural effusion on the right side. Female aged 62 years. Recent onset of cough, sputum, and tiredness. Fever 103°F. Miliary shadows in the lung. Some fluid obtained on aspiration; tubercle bacilli in sputum and on culture of fluid.

Fig. 63.—Same case (lateral view). The shadow of the fluid is superimposed on the heart shadow. It reaches the sternum in front. Arrow marks the posterior margin. Diaphragm normal, and posterior recess clear. Resolution after streptomycin and PAS. Well 2 years later.

it. It will therefore be similar to an encysted pericardial effusion or even a tumour of the heart. In a lateral view it will often lie retrosternally and will thus be indistinguishable in the radiographs from a mediastinal space effusion, a mediastinal tumour, or an aneurysm of the ascending aorta. Generally there will be some indication of the cause, such as a pulmonary shadow suggesting it is secondary to a lung lesion, or occlusion of a costophrenic recess to indicate a pleural effusion in the usual site on that side.

Abandoned pneumothorax space

An old abandoned artificial pneumothorax space, now a historical rarity, may fill up with fluid as the air absorbs and result in an encysted pleural effusion (Fig. 64). The x-ray appearances are the same as those just described, but certain sites are more common for an abandoned pneumothorax than for an acute pleurisy with effusion. The apex, for example, is a common site, the homogeneous shadow being well demarcated below with an inferior concave curve. Frequently there is deviation of the trachea towards the shadow. This is usually caused by the inability of the re-expanding lung to come out fully as a result of the healing of lesions with shrinkage of tissue, and other factors, of which organization of the pleural exudate may be one. Another is that pleural adhesions may occur before lung expansion is complete, thus binding the lung down and preventing it expanding fully. Proof of this is found when removal of this tissue by a decortication operation is followed by full expansion of the lung and a return of the trachea to its normal central position. This may also occur following disappearance of the pleural shadow, which is more likely to be due to absorption of fluid than resolution and disappearance of fibrous tissue.

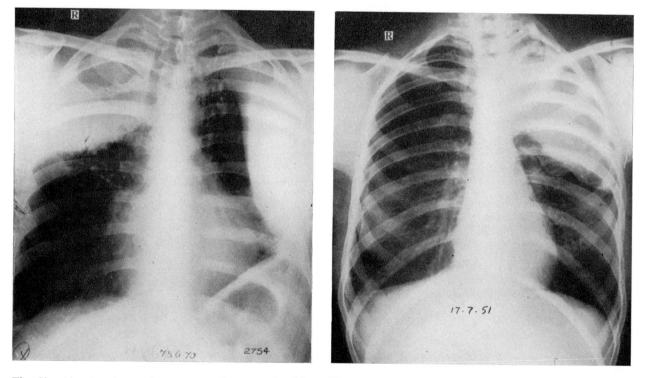

Fig. 64.—Abandoned extrapleural pneumothorax on the right side, with the air replaced by fluid. Regenerating posterior part of the fourth rib. Abandoned intrapleural pneumothorax on the left side with air replaced by fluid. Elevation of the left dome from a phrenic interruption.

Fig. 65.—Plombage on left side with solid lucite balls. Some pressure atrophy of posterior parts of second and third ribs. Operation done for left upper-lobe tuberculous cavity. Cavity closure achieved, sputum previously positive became negative. No recurrence 4 years later. Right artificial pneumothorax.

A somewhat similar shadow is seen in the apical region following an extrapleural pneumothorax if the air is eventually replaced by fluid (Fig. 64). Partial resection of one of the ribs is often necessary during the initial stages of the operation, and the gap in the rib, or the deformity of the rib as it regenerates, as well as the clinical history, will indicate that the shadow is probably due to extrapleural and not intrapleural fluid. If the replacement of the air is with oil as in an oleothorax, the shadow will be of a similar radio-opacity, but if there is some exudate as well, the oil may float above this, and the radio-opacity be sufficiently different to give a horizontal level demarcating the rather more opaque exudate from the lighter oil.

Another common site for the intrapleural fluid following a pneumothorax is down the axilla (Fig. 64). The homogeneous shadow may be a continuation of an apical effusion, or may start just below the clavicle and continue down the axilla sometimes reaching to the diaphragm. It may be quite a narrow band or several centimetres wide, and it generally has a well-defined medial margin which is rather straighter than that seen with an acute axillary encysted effusion.

A third position is in the lower half of the chest, where the fluid is encysted in a thin layer posteriorly, and gives a homogeneous haze over the lower zone with a poorly defined upper margin. It may be difficult to identify such a thin layer of fluid in the plain lateral view, but lateral-view tomograms will show it clearly as a vertical band shadow lying posteriorly just beneath the ribs.

Apical plombage

Another homogeneous shadow over the apex and upper part of a lung field is seen following an extrapleural plombage with solid lucite balls (Fig. 65). The surrounding exudate and fibrous tissue are of much the same radio-opacity as the balls, so that the latter cannot be separately identified. The history will usually indicate the nature of the homogeneous shadow, the lower margin of which either slopes downwards and outwards, or lies more or less horizontal with a slight inferior convex curve.

LOBAR CONSOLIDATION

(LARGE HOMOGENEOUS SHADOW WITHOUT GROSS LOBAR SHRINKAGE)

A large homogeneous shadow occupying the normal position of a lobe, but without evidence of appreciable fissure displacement and therefore of gross shrinkage, may be caused by a massive consolidation of the whole or a large part of a lobe. This in turn may be due to a great variety of lesions, in any of which the alveolar air in a lobe is replaced by fluid or cells: for example, bacterial or viral pneumonia; pulmonary oedema from circulatory failure or from a local arterial or venous occlusion with infarction, noxious gases or biochemical disasters; injury after x-ray or radium therapy; or invasion by neoplastic cells in some forms of carcinoma, particularly adenocarcinoma of a bronchiole with local spread of the cells into the alveoli which are then lined by them (so-called intra-alveolar cell carcinoma or pulmonary adenomatosis, bronchiolar, bronchio-alveolar carcinoma) or by an antigen.

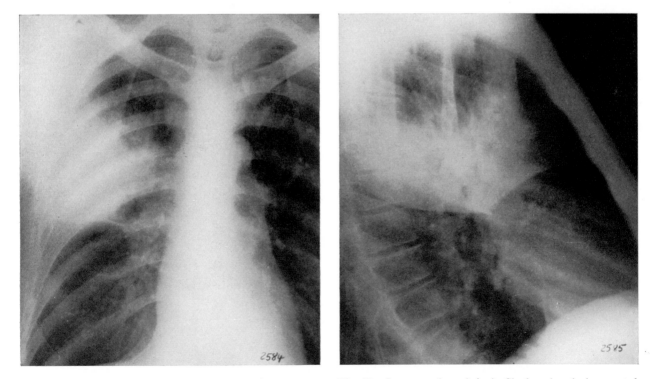

Fig. 66.—Consolidation of the anterior and posterior segments of the right upper lobe and nearby parts of the apical segment. Bacterial pneumonia. The horizontal fissure forming the lower border of the shadow shows a slight inferior concave curvature, thus indicating some shrinkage of the lobe.

Fig. 67.—Same case (lateral view). Shadow sharply demarcated at interlobar fissures, and poorly demarcated where it borders on the apical segment. In this view the slight elevation of the horizontal fissure indicates some shrinkage of the lobe. There was no stenosis of the lobar bronchus, and resolution was rapid.

The x-ray appearances are the same whatever the cause of the consolidation. In most cases the cause is obvious on clinical diagnosis, but in a few cases there are no clues to the diagnosis in the initial stages of the investigations. Sometimes even a bacterial consolidation may cause singularly little disturbance to the patient, whilst a lobar consolidation from some forms of neoplasm may be virtually asymptomatic.

Frequently only a part of the lobe is consolidated, a common finding with the present form of disease and present methods of treatment. The presence of a poorly demarcated edge to the shadow (usually the upper border) where it is adjacent to a small area of still aerated lung is an important feature in the x-ray diagnosis (Fig. 66). The exact site or extent of the still aerated portion, or the margin of the shadow bordering on this will be the same whatever the cause of the consolidation, and will therefore give no clues to the diagnosis. A bronchiolar carcinoma may occupy the same area as a bacterial pneumonia, and have the same ill-defined margin where it borders on still aerated lung, whilst a bacterial pneumonia may be circular and simulate a neoplasm for a short time (Fig. 82). If air-containing bronchi can be seen in the opaque area (an air bronchogram), either in the plain radiograph or in a tomogram (Fig. 89), it will indicate consolidation and not a pleural effusion. Such an air bronchogram is often seen in bacterial consolidation, in a bronchiolar carcinoma, a lymphosarcoma, and more rarely in Hodgkin's disease. It may be seen in extensive lung fibrosis as in the late stage of sarcoidosis (Fig 171) and in radiation damage.

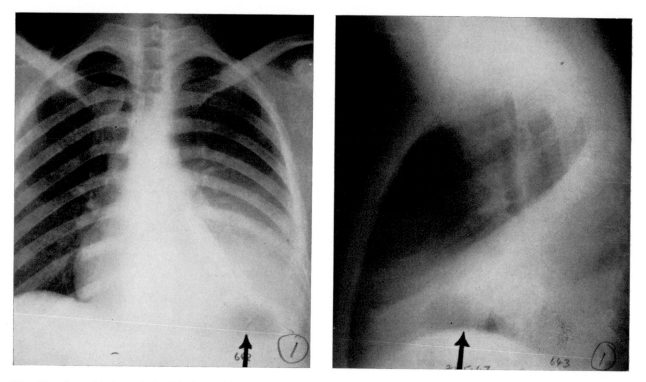

Fig. 68.—Consolidation of the left lower lobe. The upper margin of the shadow is poorly demarcated. The left dome is slightly raised. Bacterial pneumonia. Arrow points to the gas cap of the stomach. Position of sternal ends of clavicles shows that the patient is rotated, which accounts for the apparent displacement of the heart to the right.

Fig. 69.—Same case (lateral view). Arrow points to gas cap, the upper part of which indicates the level of the left dome. The anterior margin of the consolidated lobe is well demarcated by the main fissure which extends in almost a straight line from D4 to meet the diaphragm 4 cm behind the sternum (normal position).

Distinction between a neoplasm invading or pushing the lung tissue aside from one infiltrating and lining the intra-alveolar spaces can only be made on histological examination.

In consolidation with bronchial occlusion the bronchostenosis will be seen in the tomograms, and these will serve further to differentiate the shadow from that of a pleural effusion by demonstrating the alteration of vessel pattern and fissure displacement which are so characteristic of those conditions associated with lobar shrinkage.

Resolution of a consolidation of a lobe is often somewhat uneven, and some areas re-aerate more rapidly than others, with the result that the shadow at this stage is no longer homogeneous.

When the whole lobe is consolidated, the resulting shadow corresponds in size, shape, and position with the expected configuration of the lobe (Fig. 69). The interlobar fissure, which corresponds with the well-demarcated adjacent border of the consolidated lobe, is either not displaced at all or is only slightly displaced in the direction of the shadow. In the latter case the slight shrinkage of the lobe is due to collapse of some alveolar groups. This slight shrinkage of the lobe is in marked contrast to the shadows seen resulting from lobar bronchial obstruction, when the decrease in size is commonly greater and is clearly shown by the considerable displacement of the interlobar fissure. (Compare Fig. 71 showing consolidation of the middle lobe, with Fig. 107 showing atelectasis of the middle lobe from bronchostenosis.)

The trachea is either not displaced at all, or is displaced slightly towards the shadow. The heart is not displaced, but the diaphragm may be raised and show some restriction of movement.

Comparison with lobar atelectasis

The examples of consolidation with very little or no collapse which are shown in Figs. 66–71 should be compared with the shadows seen when there is gross lobar shrinkage or atelectasis, often distal to stenosis of a lobar bronchus and which are illustrated in Figs. 98–114.

It must be admitted that the radiographic picture is not always as clear cut as in many of these illustrations. For instance a bronchial occlusion from a carcinoma may show comparatively little lobar shrinkage if the neoplasm occupies most of the lobe, or if the distal inflammatory changes are severe and the bronchi much dilated and filled with mucus or pus (Fig. 97).

More rarely a chronic pneumonia may proceed to gross lobar shrinkage or collapse without there being any stenosis of the lobar bronchus and without obvious cavitation or fibrosis, so that the shadow remains homogeneous. Such a case is shown in Fig. 88. At first the appearances were similar to Fig. 69 and indicated consolidation, with the antero-superior border passing downwards and forwards in a well-defined straight line. In the course of a few weeks the shadow became smaller, the fissure moving posteriorly and showing a well-marked anterior concave curve. In fact the appearances were identical with those seen with collapse of a left lower lobe distal to a lower-lobe bronchostenosis.

The mechanism of this shrinkage or atelectasis is uncertain. In this particular case bronchoscopy was normal and the larger bronchial air transradiancies were normal on tomography as well as on examination of the resected lobe. There may have been occlusion of a sufficient number of the smaller bronchi to block the access of air and thus cause the collapse. During the early stages of resolution of an acute pneumonia a similar but more limited lobar shrinkage with fissure displacement towards the opaque area is often seen lasting for a few days.

Right upper-lobe consolidation

Consolidation of the whole of the right upper lobe is not very common in adults, but is seen more frequently in young patients. The shadow extends from the apex downwards to end, in the anterior-view radiograph, with a well-defined inferior margin running horizontally to meet the sixth rib in the axilla and thus corresponding to the normal position of the horizontal fissure. In the lateral view the shadow has a well-defined posterior margin running downwards and forwards along the normal line of the main fissure as far as the level of the lower end of the tracheal transradiancy, from which point it has a well-defined inferior margin running directly forwards in a line corresponding to the normal position of the horizontal fissure. (*See* Figs. 66 and 67, which, apart from the transradiant apical segment, show similar x-ray appearances to those of right upper-lobe consolidation.)

Left upper-lobe consolidation

Consolidation of the whole of the left upper lobe is seen in the lateral view as a homogeneous shadow with a well-defined postero-inferior margin corresponding to the normal position of the main fissure. It extends down from the posterior inferior edge of the body of the fourth thoracic vertebra to meet the diaphragm 2–3 cm behind the sternum. Sometimes the lingula is not affected, in which case the shadow has a poorly demarcated lower margin at a level corresponding to the lower end of the tracheal transradiancy.

Right middle-lobe consolidation

Consolidation of the right middle lobe is illustrated in Figs. 70 and 71. In the anterior view the upper border of the shadow is sharply defined as it runs horizontally to meet the sixth rib in the axilla. The shadow occupies the rest of the lung field below this, although if there is some aerated lung in the region of the medial segment, it may be less opaque near the right heart border. In the lateral view it has a

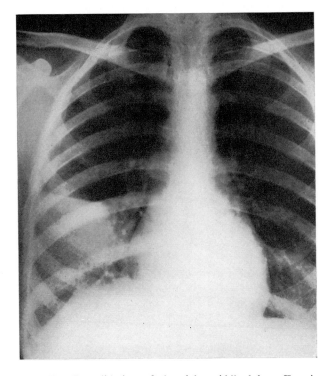 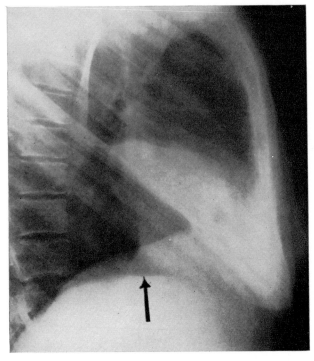

Fig. 70.—Consolidation of the right middle lobe. Female aged 26 years. Low-grade bacterial pneumonia, resolved in 3 weeks. The shadow is sharply demarcated above by the horizontal fissure. Some aerated lung medially. Slight elevation of the right dome. Heart may be slightly to the right, but the position of the sternal ends of the clavicles indicates some rotation of the patient to the right.

Fig. 71.—Same case (lateral view). Arrow marks position of left dome. The shadow of the right dome is seen just above it and is lost where it meets the shadow of the consolidated lobe, the posterior margin of which is formed by the main fissure which is not displaced. The horizontal fissure forming the upper margin slopes downwards, indicating slight shrinkage of the lobe.

triangular shape with the apex near the lower end of the tracheal transradiancy. From here the well-defined upper border runs directly forwards to meet the sternum. If there is slight lung shrinkage this border may be inclined slightly downwards. The postero-inferior border is also sharply defined and runs downwards and forwards to meet the diaphragm 3 cm behind the sternum. The shadow is very different from that seen when there is marked shrinkage of the lobe. Fig. 107, for example, illustrates the small size of the shadow, the greater downward inclination of the superior border, and the forward displacement of the posterior border which corresponds to the displaced main fissure and has a posterior concave curvature, which are all indications of the lobar shrinkage secondary, in this case, to bronchostenosis and atelectasis.

Lower-lobe consolidation

Consolidation of the right lower lobe gives an appearance almost identical to that of the left lower lobe illustrated in Figs. 68 and 69. In the anterior view the upper margin of the shadow is poorly defined and usually lies in the region of the second rib anteriorly, though it may not extend quite as high as this if there is some shrinkage of the lobe, or if the extreme apex of the apical segment of the lower lobe is still aerated. In the lateral view the shadow is well-demarcated antero-superiorly at the line of the interlobar fissure, which lies either in its expected position, or slightly posteriorly to this.

Consolidation with effusion

If a small effusion develops while the lower-lobe consolidation is still present, the shadow may remain homogeneous and show little or no alteration in size, shape, or position. In fact, the shadow of the fluid cannot be separately identified unless some aerated lung is present between the two, or unless the consolidation is beginning to resolve, so that this part of the shadow is no longer homogeneous, or unless the shadow of the effusion extends up the axilla as a line shadow beyond the main basal shadow.

SEGMENTAL CONSOLIDATION

A homogeneous roughly triangular or pyramidal shadow some 3–4 cm long (examples of which are illustrated in Figs. 72–87) is often described as a segmental shadow, and, if the lesion is inflammatory, as a segmental consolidation. These descriptions are facile since the segmental planes interdigitate and are not separated by septa so that the consolidation will either occupy only a part of the segment or more than the segment as it extends into the adjacent alveoli of the other segment. The term in reference to the anatomical site is roughly correct but should not be used to define the exact extent of the lesion.

It is not always possible without clinical help or serial radiographs to decide whether the shadow represents a bacterial or viral inflammatory lesion, an allergic consolidation, a neoplasm or a vascular lesion (infarct) from an embolus or venous thrombosis. The immediate clinical findings may indicate the cause, fever and rapid resolution being characteristic of bacterial pneumonias; persistence of the shadow with onset undated clinically, with perhaps a dull ache or slight haemoptyses, would suggest a neoplasm, confirmation of which may be forthcoming from the sputum cytology. An infarct is often asymptomatic, but in some cases there is a sudden onset of chest pain and a haemoptysis, or there may be calf tenderness, a recent delivery of a child or an operation to suggest the diagnosis. An infarct is commonly followed by a small effusion. The shadow tends to persist for about 3 weeks, and then slowly resolves, though it may disappear rapidly or persist much longer.

In winter when colds are rife, a triangular shadow may be found incidentally, but its rapid resolution will indicate it was an inflammatory lesion.

A similar shadow is also seen in some cases of asthma with bronchopulmonary aspergillosis and eosinophilia, when they represent an allergic consolidation. The diagnosis will be established if there is a positive skin reaction and precipitins to the aspergillus in the serum. The patient may be febrile or almost asymptomatic. The shadows resolve in 2–3 weeks but the lesions starting in the bronchus tend to cause extensive local bronchial damage which may result in residual parallel line or ring shadows, or even a tooth paste shadow if a plug remains in the bronchus. The damage will also cause gross abnormalities in a bronchogram, if it is done (Fig. 333).

A large area of opacity with eosinophilia may result from certain drugs in a sensitive patient; for example PAS, penicillin, nitrofurantoin and others. They are seen in many obscure cases of localized consolidation such as are sometimes found in association with rheumatoid arthritis and periarteritis nodosa.

Upper-lobe segmental consolidation

Consolidation of part of the apical segment of the right upper lobe is uncommon. The resulting triangular shadow occupies roughly the same area as the transradiant zone which in Figs. 66 and 67 lies between the areas of opacity representing the consolidated anterior and posterior segments. In this particular example, the consolidation has spread beyond the segmental boundaries, so that in fact the shadow of a consolidated apical segment would be rather larger than the transradiant zone and, in the lateral view particularly, would extend down to the level of the interlobar fissure.

Consolidation of part of the anterior segment alone is much more common. In the anterior view the shadow is sharply demarcated below by the horizontal fissure, and therefore has a sharply defined margin running straight across the lung field to meet the sixth rib in the axilla. If there is some shrinkage of the consolidated segment, this margin is slightly concave downwards. The upper margin is rather poorly defined, and beyond it the apex and the region medially just below the clavicle remain transradiant. In the lateral view the shadow extends from the middle of the chest to the sternum, and its well-defined lower margin is clearly seen.

Consolidation of the posterior segment of the upper lobe gives a very similar shadow to the anterior segment in the anterior view (Fig. 76). The lower margin is often equally well defined, but it does not reach quite as low as the horizontal fissure, which is seen as a faint linear shadow 2–3 mm below it. In a lateral view the shadow lies posteriorly and has a well-defined margin where it is demarcated by the upper end of the main interlobar fissure (Fig. 77).

Consolidation of the posterior segment on the left side is usually associated with consolidation of the apical segment, and their combined shadow occupies the medial half of the upper zone. The lateral margin of this shadow is usually poorly defined.

The anterior segment of the left upper lobe, on the other hand, is occasionally the only segment to be consolidated. The shadow is then similar to that of the anterior segment of the right upper lobe, already described, except that the lower margin borders on the lingula instead of on the horizontal fissure and is therefore less well defined.

Lingular consolidation

Consolidation of part of the lingula is probably present more often than is realized, since the shadow may be very inconspicuous or obscured by a large breast shadow in the anterior view or by the heart shadow in the lateral view. In the anterior view there may be no more than a faint haze adjacent to the apex of the heart, but sometimes a more definite area of opacity can be seen, as in Fig. 86. The lower part of the lung above the costophrenic recess remains clear but the left border of the heart may become indistinct.

In the lateral view the shadow is superimposed on that of the heart. It is sharply demarcated posteriorly by the line of the interlobar fissure, which is not displaced, and runs in a straight line downwards and forwards (Fig. 87). This straight posterior margin is characteristic and should be compared with that shown in Fig. 114 which, owing to bronchostenosis and shrinkage of the lobe, is posteriorly concave. Anteriorly the shadow of a lingular consolidation reaches to the sterno-diaphragmatic angle, but is poorly demarcated antero-superiorly where it adjoins the anterior segment. The shadow is often difficult to see in a plain left lateral view, but can be clearly seen in left lateral tomograms.

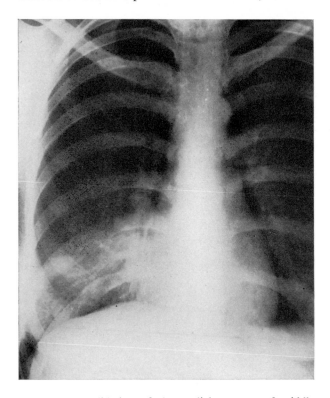 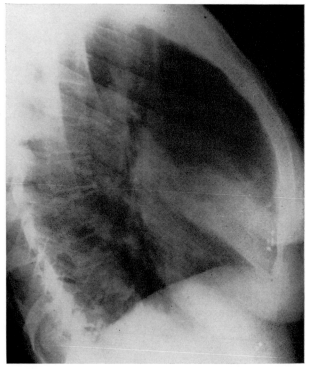

Fig. 72.—Consolidation of the medial segment of middle lobe (5). The costophrenic region is clear, and the diaphragm is slightly elevated. The right heart border is invisible. Upper margin poorly defined. Bacterial pneumonia.

Fig. 73.—Same case (lateral view). Opacity in sterno-diaphragmatic angle. The straight posterior margin corresponds to the expected position of the interlobar fissure. Rapid resolution. Only lower part of segment affected.

Consolidation of the postero-inferior part of the lingula adjacent to the main fissure may be associated with consolidation of the posterior segment of the upper lobe. In the anterior view a triangular shadow is seen with its base in the mid-axilla and its apex at the hilum (Fig. 84). In the lateral view (Fig. 85) the shadows of both segments are sharply demarcated postero-inferiorly by the line of the interlobar fissure. Anteriorly both are poorly defined as they approach the apical segment of the upper lobe and the superior part of the lingula respectively, mainly because the consolidation of the segments is usually incomplete.

Middle-lobe (segmental) consolidation

Consolidation of part of the medial segment of the middle lobe may give no more than a faint area of clouding adjacent to the right heart border in the anterior view (Fig. 72). Often the right heart border becomes blurred or invisible; such a shadow is easily mistaken for a breast or muscle shadow, or may even be overlooked. In the lateral view, however, it stands out quite clearly (Fig. 73). Posteriorly it is sharply demarcated by the lower end of the main fissure which is not displaced. Inferiorly it occupies the sterno-diaphragmatic angle; above it is less clearly demarcated, and does not extend as far towards the hilum nor along the posterior half of the horizontal fissure, as in the case of consolidation of the whole of the middle lobe (compare with Fig. 71). If the breasts are large, or the patient obese so that the shadow is indistinct, confirmation of these characteristic appearances is readily obtained from a right lateral-view tomograph.

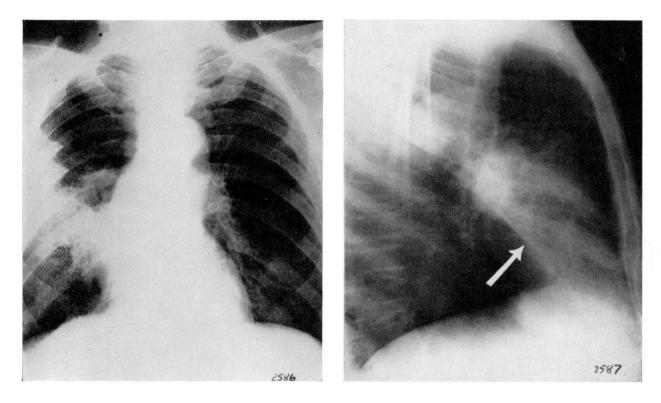

Fig. 74.—Consolidation of the lateral segment of the middle lobe (4) and base of posterior upper. Bacterial pneumonia.

Fig. 75.—Same case (lateral view). Arrow marks line of interlobar fissure. Rapid resolution.

A consolidated lateral segment of the middle lobe gives a more conspicuous shadow than the medial segment in the anterior view, usually being more clearly demarcated above by the line of the horizontal fissure (the case illustrated in Fig. 74 is a rather unusually ill-defined example because the base of the posterior segment is also consolidated). The shadow extends down the axilla almost to the costophrenic recess. An area of normal lung is seen infero-medially in and above the cardio-diaphragmatic angle. In the lateral view (Fig. 75) the shadow is much less conspicuous, but can just be seen either partly superimposed on, or lying just below the hilar vascular shadow. It occupies a rather broad triangular zone clearly demarcated above by the posterior third or half of the horizontal fissure, and behind by the main fissure. Antero-inferiorly it is less well defined owing to the inter-segmental digitations into the medial segment. The sterno-diaphragmatic area, occupied by the normal medial segment, remains clear. Again the shadow and fissure lines can be more clearly demonstrated in right lateral tomograms than in the plain radiographs.

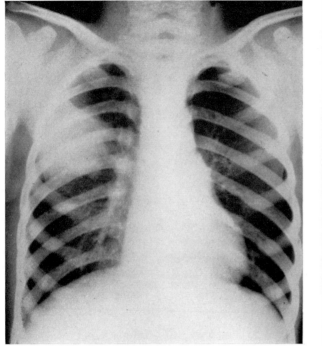

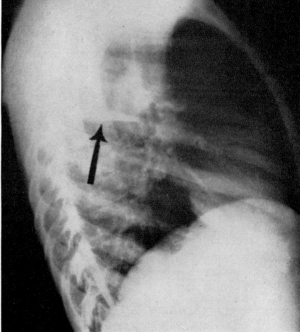

Fig. 76.—Consolidation posterior segment right upper lobe (2). The line of the horizontal fissure is visible 1 cm below the massive shadow. Male aged 11 years. Bacterial pneumonia. Two days cough, abdominal pain, anorexia and vomiting. High fever and rapid pulse.

Fig. 77.—Same case (lateral view). Arrow marks posterior margin of consolidated area. The anterior margin of the shadow is poorly demarcated where it borders on the apical segment. Rapid resolution. Radiographs of lung a fortnight later were normal.

Lower-lobe segmental consolidation

Consolidation of the apical segment of the lower lobe on either side is usually incomplete, but when most of the segment is consolidated a characteristic homogeneous shadow is seen. In the anterior view it is ill defined and spreads out from the region of the hilum into the mid-zone. It may reach as far as the axilla (Fig. 80). In the lateral view the shadow is roughly circular and tends to be partly obscured by the superimposed vertebral, scapular, and lower axillary muscle shadows. Antero-superiorly it is demarcated by the upper third of the main fissure, but the line of this is generally indistinct in the plain lateral view. Antero-inferiorly it curves downwards and backwards (Fig. 81) and is poorly demarcated where it is adjacent to the posterior basal segment. The shadow of the consolidated area and that of the upper end of the main fissure can be seen much more clearly in a lateral-view tomogram than in a plain lateral view.

Consolidation of any of the basal segments is quite common, especially as a result of a so-called " aspiration pneumonia ". Usually only a part of one segment is consolidated, giving a rather small triangular shadow with its apex towards the hilum and its base on the diaphragm. Quite commonly a part of a neighbouring segment is also affected, neither segment being totally consolidated.

Consolidation of part of the anterior basal segment is more commonly seen on the right than on the left side. The shadow lies rather medially in the anterior view. In the lateral view (Fig. 83) it is well demarcated anteriorly where it borders on the lower end of the main fissure. (In Figs. 82 and 83 the lateral basal segment is also partly consolidated.)

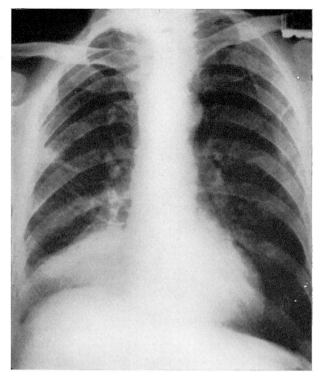

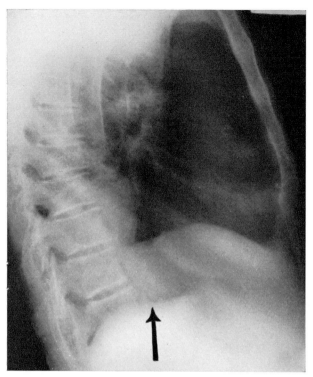

Fig. 78.—Consolidation posterior basal segment right lower lobe (10). Slight elevation of the right dome. Bacterial pneumonia. Note normal hilar vessels and vessel counts.

Fig. 79.—Same case (lateral view). Arrow marks left dome. Shadow of right dome above ends abruptly where it meets the shadow of the consolidated lung posteriorly. In original, main fissure visible and not displaced.

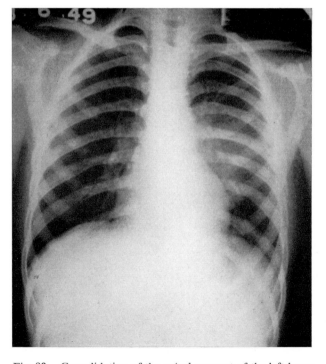

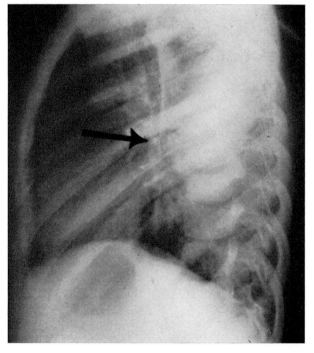

Fig. 80.—Consolidation of the apical segment of the left lower lobe (6). Shadow poorly demarcated. Male aged 9 years. Bacterial pneumonia. Rapid resolution. Lungs clear a fortnight later.

Fig. 81.—Same case (lateral view). Arrow points to anterior margin of shadow, which is well demarcated by the interlobar fissure anteriorly, but poorly demarcated inferiorly where it is adjacent to the posterior basal segment.

In consolidation of part of the lateral basal segment, the shadow lies in the outer half of the lung field in the anterior view, occupying the costophrenic recess. In the lateral view it is triangular in shape and lies in the middle of the lung (rather more posteriorly than the shadow of the anterior basal segment seen in Fig. 83) and barely reaches the interlobar fissure.

Consolidation of part of the posterior basal segment is common on either side, particularly in children. In the anterior view the roughly triangular shadow extends from the hilum almost to the costophrenic recess (Fig. 78), reaches the diaphragm in the medial half, and is poorly demarcated laterally. In the lateral view (Fig. 79) it is poorly demarcated where it borders on the apical segment of the lower lobe above and the other basal segments anteriorly. It extends down to occupy the posterior costophrenic recess.

Localization of the affected segment

In an anterior view a consolidation lying adjacent to the heart in either the middle lobe or lingula will obscure the nearby heart border since there will be no intermediate zone of transradiant air-containing lung to give definition (Figs. 72 and 86). In a lower-lobe consolidation, on the other hand, the heart border will be clearly seen provided the radiograph is sufficiently well exposed.

This maxim cannot be entirely relied on, not only because of the exposure factor, but also because obscuring of the heart border by a middle-lobe consolidation does not preclude the possibility of an additional consolidation of the posterior basal segment behind the heart or even a small pleural effusion, neither of which could be detected in an anterior view.

It is therefore advisable to use a lateral view for the localization of the affected segment. The only disadvantage here is that the shadow of a lower-lobe consolidation will be continuous with that of the posterior half of the adjacent diaphragm, since again there will be no air-containing lung between the two (Figs. 79 and 83), but on the left side, at least, the gas in the stomach will usually suffice to indicate the level of the diaphragm (Fig. 69).

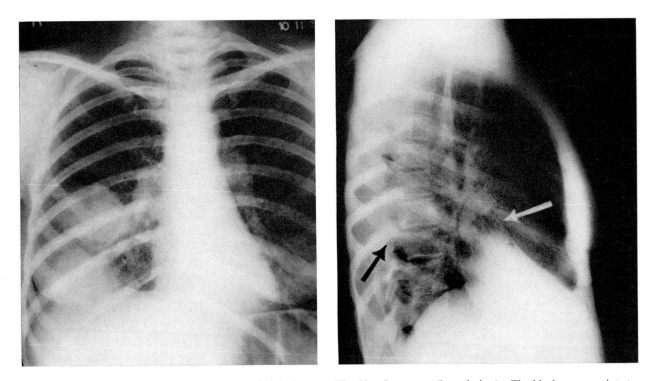

Fig. 82.—Consolidation in the apical segment of right lower lobe (6). Circular shadow mistaken for a neoplasm. Also consolidated anterior and part of lateral basal segment. Bacterial pneumonia with rapid resolution and disappearance of all shadows.

Fig. 83.—Same case (lateral view). The black arrow points to the pneumonia in the right lower lobe. The white arrow points to the interlobar septum with the shadow of the consolidated anterior and lateral basal segments just behind.

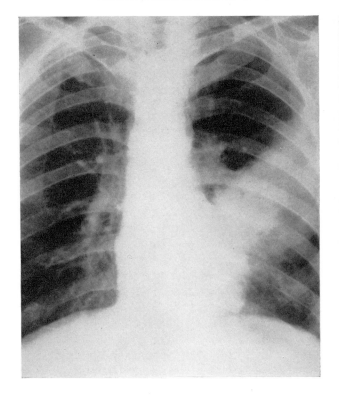

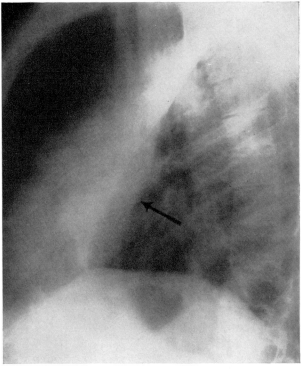

Fig. 84.—Consolidation of the posterior segment of the left upper lobe and part of lingula. Male aged 40 years. Sudden onset of left chest pain, malaise, cough with rusty sputum and leucocytosis. Left dome normal. Rapid resolution.

Fig. 85.—Same case (lateral view). Arrow marks posterior border of heart. Both segments are sharply demarcated posteriorly by the interlobar fissure which is not displaced but poorly demarcated anteriorly because this part of the lung is still aerated.

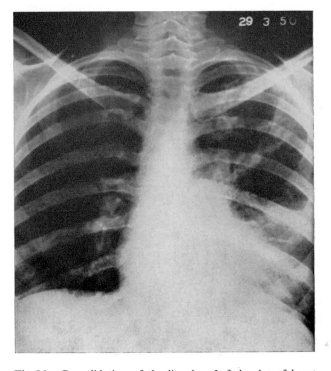

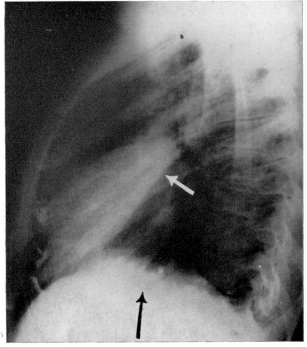

Fig 86.—Consolidation of the lingula. Left border of heart indistinct. Tuberculous pneumonia. Female aged 27 years. Resolution on medical treatment.

Fig. 87.—Same case (lateral view). White arrow marks main fissure which is not displaced; black one marks right dome; left dome just above it.

LOBAR ATELECTASIS (OR COLLAPSE) FROM STENOSIS OF THE LOBAR BRONCHUS OR FROM MANY PERIPHERAL OCCLUSIONS

Stenosis with effective occlusion of a lobar bronchus results in atelectasis (or collapse) of that lobe, and the radiograph then shows a homogeneous shadow with evidence of lobar shrinkage. The occluding lesion may be luminal, such as an inhaled foreign body or plug of mucus; mural in an adenoma, hamartoma or carcinoma; or extrinsic, for instance from enlarged or scarring lymph nodes. Sometimes there are multiple mural inflammatory lesions occluding the bronchi about the fourth or fifth generation down which may be the primary cause of the atelectasis in a chronic pneumonia, or may follow temporary occlusion of a lobar bronchus. In an atelectatic lobe in this instance the first four or five generations may fill in a bronchogram (Fig. 332) in spite of the airless lobe, which is airless because of the more distal occlusions. If scarring of the inflammatory occlusions occurs the atelectasis will be permanent; otherwise if resolution occurs or the proximal block is removed, the lobe may re-expand. Pathologically there are almost invariably other changes present apart from just airlessness of the lobe and consequent apposition of the alveolar and bronchiolar walls. At the very least there is an outpouring of fluid exudate into the alveoli, and usually there are varying degrees of cellular exudate, in fact pneumonic consolidation with lung shrinkage.

In addition, the bronchi go on secreting mucus and are thus distended with secretions which cannot escape because of the proximal occlusions. In a long-standing collapse the histological findings may include irregularity of the bronchi with papillary folding of the epithelium, an increase in the thickness of the interlobular septa, and a decrease in the number of the alveoli. There is also capillary dilatation, although it is known that there is a decreased flow of blood through the collapsed lobe. If there is distal infection the changes of chronic pneumonia will be superimposed. The dilated mucus-distended bronchi will become full of pus and their walls may be eroded.

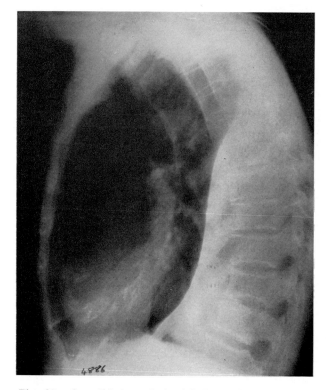

Fig. 88.—Consolidation of the left lower lobe with gross shrinkage. Male aged 48 years. Sudden onset of left chest pain and fever. Physical signs, dullness, diminished breath sounds. At first, shadow corresponded to lower lobe, and it then started to shrink backwards. Bronchoscopy showed pus in lower lobe, but no stenosis.

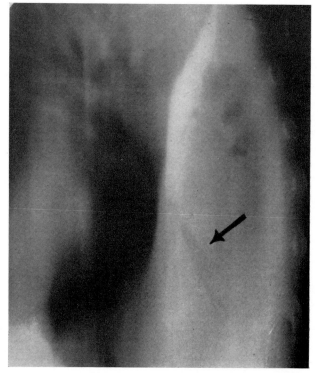

Fig. 89.—Same case (lateral-view tomogram). Arrow marks air-containing bronchi in opaque lobe. Cavities are seen in the apical segment. Two months later resected. No stenosis of larger bronchi. Much dense fibrosis and non-specific inflammatory changes. Cavities in apical segment. No evidence of tuberculosis or neoplasm.

In those cases in which there is no longer stenosis of the lobar bronchus but stenoses of the more peripheral branches, the larger bronchi are filled with air and are usually dilated, so that they give tubular transradiancies (an air bronchogram) within the area of opacity in a well-exposed film or in tomograms (Fig. 89).

The size of the airless shrunken lobe depends to some extent on the duration of the obstruction and on the condition of the lung before the occlusion became effective. The smallest airless lobes are seen when the stenosis is long standing, and when the distal lung changes are either slight or of late onset, coming on after the lung had collapsed—conditions which are most commonly fulfilled in tuberculous endobronchitis and bronchial adenoma. The largest airless lobes are seen associated with a bronchial carcinoma, when much inflammation and retained secretion had already occurred distal to the stenosis before the effective occlusion developed, or when the neoplasm already occupied much of the lobe. In fact the lobar shrinkage may be so slight in such a case that the appearances on the plain radiograph simulate those of consolidation without shrinkage and without bronchostenosis (Fig. 97).

The shape and position of the shadow depend on which lobe is collapsed, the degree of shrinkage and the presence or absence of pleural adhesions. The shrinkage is made obvious by the displaced position of the interlobar fissure, which corresponds to the border of the shadow where it is adjacent to aerated lung. A part of the fissure remote from the collapsed lobe may also be displaced, an example of this being the downward displacement of the horizontal fissure frequently seen with collapse of the right lower lobe (Fig. 121).

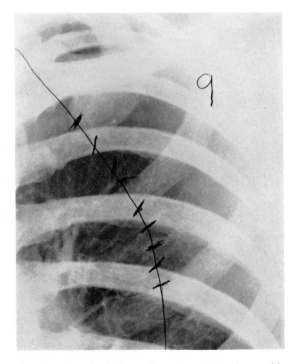

Fig. 90.—A method of vessel counting. Line down mid-lung field. Cross-lines marking vessels (which might not have been visible in the reproduction). Normal person, 9 vessels cross mid-lung line.

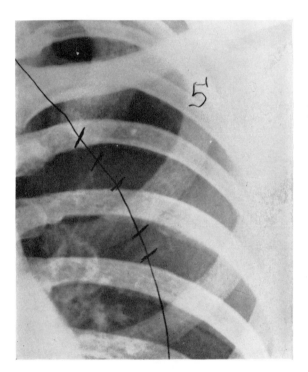

Fig. 91.—Same patient at later date when there is atelectasis of the left lower lobe and compensatory emphysema of upper lobe. Now only 5 vessels cross mid-lung line.

In atelectasis of an upper lobe there may be slight deviation of the trachea towards the affected side. If a lower lobe is collapsed there may be some slight elevation of the diaphragm on that side and displacement of the heart to that side. None of these features is inevitable in all cases. Much more inevitable will be an alteration in the size and appearance of the hilum shadow on that side since vessels in the atelectatic lobe will be invisible because there is no air around them. One lobar vessel and its branches will therefore be missing so that the hilum will be smaller than the opposite normal side, and, because one limb of the ➤ will be missing, it will have an abnormal shape. For instance, in an upper-lobe atelectasis the hilum shadow will be formed by the basal artery and its branches, and because the basal artery will be elevated and slightly rotated the hilum will show a marked lateral convexity (Fig. 93). In lower lobe atelectasis the basal artery will not be seen and the hilum will look far too small (Figs. 115 and 123). Displacement of the trachea is most commonly seen, and most marked, if an upper lobe is affected, and displacement of the heart, if a lower lobe is atelectatic.

The appearance of the neighbouring lobe is altered since it has to occupy more space than it normally would. It will therefore show the x-ray changes of compensatory emphysema. The number of vessels in the upper two-thirds will be half that of the normal side. When doing such a vessel count a line should be drawn parallel to the axillary part of the ribs in the mid-lung field, and a count made of only those vessels which cross that line (Figs. 90 and 91). Since the first vessel dividing at the hilum is no longer the lobar artery but the segmental artery, each vessel is really one generation more distal and thus looks smaller than the apparently corresponding vessel on the normal side.

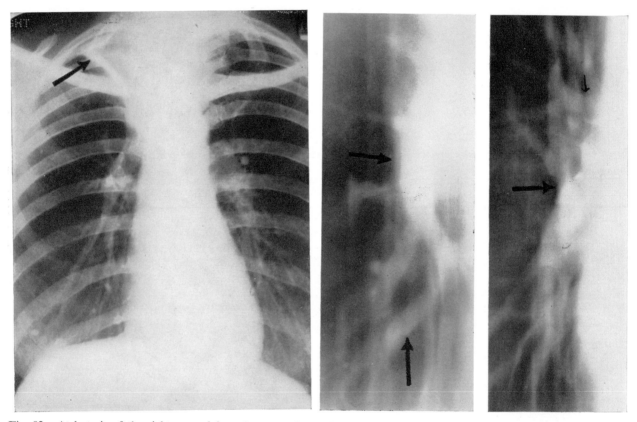

Fig. 92.—Atelectasis of the right upper lobe. Arrow marks lower border of shrunken lobe. Fewer vessels in the lung below than on the left side. Right hilum elevated, convex laterally and smaller than left. Right dome slightly raised. No hypertransradiancy of right side. Tubercle bacilli in sputum. Treated by resection. There was stenosis of the upper-lobe bronchus from healing tuberculous endobronchitis.

Fig. 93.—*Left.* Same case (posterior-view tomogram of right hilar vessels). The slight lateral convexity of the basal artery is shown opposite arrow. Compare with tomogram of a normal person (*right*), in which there is a lateral concavity (opposite horizontal arrow) between the upper-lobe vein above, and the basal artery passing downwards. Vertical arrow (*left*) points to a pulmonary vein.

The lobe is not relatively more transradiant than the opposite normal lung in compensatory emphysema, if care is taken not to mistake the fewer and smaller vessels for increased transradiancy but to compare the actual blackening of the film on the two sides in an area between vessel shadows. The blood flow to the right and left lung will still be equal, but the single lobe on the atelectatic side will have to carry twice the volume of blood that it did before, and this capillary blood increase will counteract any transradiancy from the dilated alveoli. However in some cases, particularly where the atelectasis is associated with bronchiectasis, there is often some bronchiectasis in the other lobe as well which will result in some air trapping and reduced blood flow. There will then be relative hypertransradiancy of the lobe with the compensatory emphysema and two sorts of emphysema—space occupancy (compensatory) and obstructive.

In studying the radiograph in atelectasis of a lobe, two features should be looked for. First, any shadow cast by the airless lobe, and second, the compensatory changes in the other lobe in which the hilum will be too small and of abnormal shape, and the lung vessels will be too few in number and will appear to be too small. In a doubtful case the bronchial occlusion can be shown by tomography (Fig. 96) or bronchography (Figs. 101, 102, 111 and 124).

Right upper-lobe atelectasis

In a typical case of occlusion of the right upper-lobe bronchus the atelectatic upper lobe will be seen as a homogeneous shadow in the apex and subclavicular region with a well-defined inferior concave margin formed by the elevated horizontal fissure, which continues downwards medially to the upper part of the hilum (Fig. 92).

Three variations of this shadow are seen. If there was much previous consolidation distal to the stenosis, the shadow will be relatively larger, and the inferior margin may run almost straight across to meet the third rib in the axilla (Fig. 97). Alternatively if the stenosis is long standing and the distal changes slight, the lobe may shrink to a very small size, so that the lower half lying medially just above the hilum will be very inconspicuous in the radiograph and will simulate a widening of the mediastinal shadow. The upper half of the collapsed lobe will still be seen passing across the apex with an inferior concave margin well above the clavicle. A third, more rare variation is seen in a long-standing stenosis with slight distal changes if the lobe shrinks medially and downwards. The shadow will then lie just above and in front of the hilum (Fig. 94) and, in a lateral view, will reach to the sternum, thus simulating a mediastinal tumour (Fig. 95). However, the small hilum and paucity of lung vessels will reveal the diagnosis.

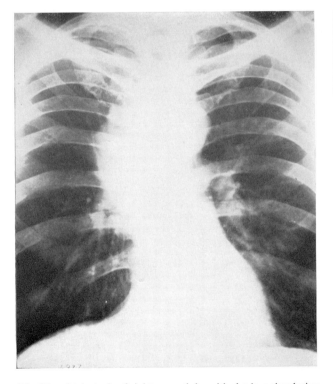

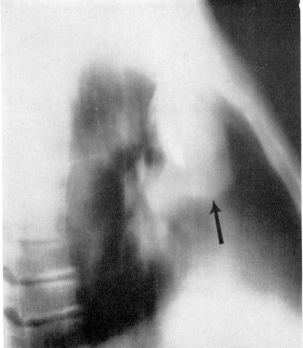

Fig. 94.—Atelectasis of right upper lobe with shadow simulating a tumour. The well-defined lateral convex border of the shadow is seen superimposed on and above the hilum. No hypertransradiancy of right lung, but very many fewer vessels visible than on the left side. Trachea central. Male aged 42 years, no symptoms.

Fig. 95.—Same case (lateral-view tomogram). Arrow marks lower limit of shadow which extends forwards to the sternum. Dense calcification towards hilum. This was a tuberculous gland which was causing stenosis of the upper-lobe bronchus. The lobe was airless, with some dilated mucus-filled bronchi, and some fibrosis.

With all four types of shadow the features of compensatory emphysema as described on page 58, will be seen in the middle and lower lobes. The hilum shadow will be smaller than the opposite normal side (Fig. 92) and the basal artery, which will be elevated, will give the hilum a marked lateral convexity in contrast to the lateral concavity of the normal hilum. The small apical lower artery and vein, although they will occupy much the same site, must not be mistaken for the normal upper-lobe vein, which is larger. These appearances are very clearly seen in tomograms (Fig. 93).

In the upper third of the lung the density of vessels on the right side (that is, the number per unit area) is about half that of the left side when they are counted as described above.

In the case illustrated in Fig. 92, there was no relative hypertransradiancy of the right side.

The inferior concave margin of the atelectatic lobe, incorporating the horizontal fissure, can be seen in the lateral view. Upward displacement of the middle-lobe vessels can be clearly seen in a lateral-view tomogram. The posterior margin represented by the upper end of the main fissure will be displaced forwards about 1 cm and may show a posterior concavity.

Left upper-lobe atelectasis

Left upper-lobe bronchostenosis with atelectasis almost inevitably includes the lingula. In the anterior view the characteristic appearance is a rather faint homogeneous opacity in the upper half of the left lung with a poorly demarcated lower margin (Fig. 98). This opacity may not quite reach to the axilla or the apex if the lobe shrinks towards the hilum leaving the apex free to be occupied by the over-inflated lower lobe. Vascular markings can be seen superimposed on the shadow, but these are spread out so that there are fewer per unit area than in a corresponding area on the right side. They are of course lower-lobe vessels lying behind the collapsed lobe. The altered position of the bronchi, and therefore of the vessels, can be seen in a bronchogram with the apical lower-lobe branches extending up to the apex behind the shadow of the collapsed upper lobe (Figs. 101 and 102). The hilum shadow is abnormal and shows a lateral convexity near its centre due to the rotated basal artery (Fig. 100), with vessels of smaller calibre than normal coming off it at unusual angles. Tomograms (Fig. 100) will show this

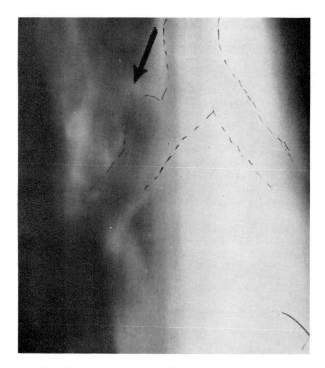

Fig. 96.—Tomogram of right hilum in a case of atelectasis of the right upper lobe, with gross shrinkage of the lobe. Arrow points to occlusion of the upper-lobe bronchus which was due to a small adenoma. Lung distal to this was small and airless with mucus-filled dilated bronchi, and fibrosis.

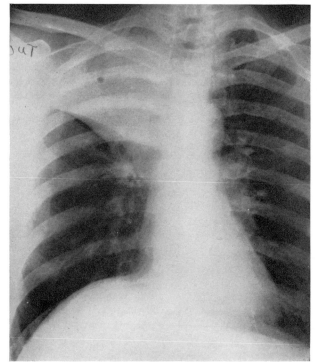

Fig. 97.—Atelectasis of the right upper lobe, with much consolidation and mucous distension of the bronchi distal to a carcinoma occluding the upper-lobe bronchus. Lower margin corresponds to horizontal fissure, which is only slightly raised.

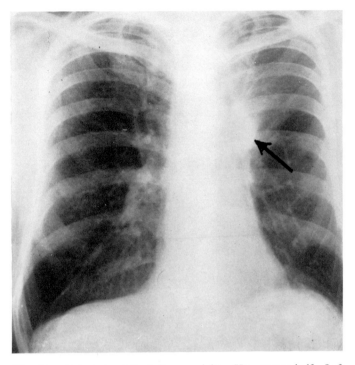

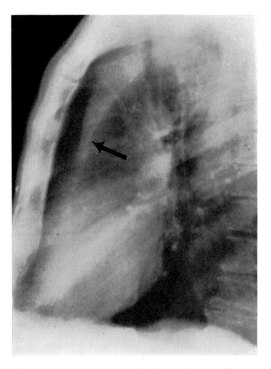

Fig. 98.—Atelectasis of the left upper lobe. Haze upper half. Left hilum much smaller than right, elevated and laterally convex; fewer vessels in left lung. Slight relative elevation of left dome. Carcinoma left upper lobe bronchus.

Fig. 99.—Same case (lateral view). Arrow points to the posterior border of tongue-like shadow. Transradiant area between the front of this and the sternum. No connection of the shadow to hilum can be seen. Male aged 65 years. At resection, shrunken airless upper lobe.

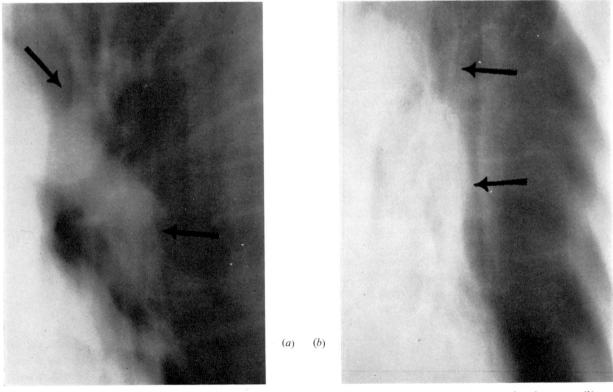

(a)   (b)

Fig. 100.—(a) Normal left hilum (tomogram). Upper arrow to upper lobe artery; lower arrow to basal artery. (b) Atelectasis of left upper lobe. Upper arrow to apical lower vessel, lower arrow to basal artery.

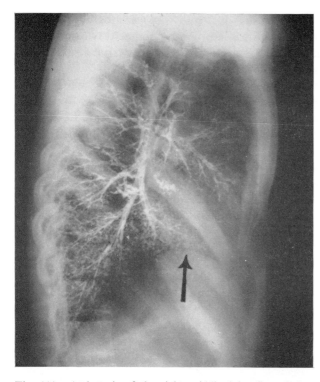

Fig. 111.—Atelectasis of the right middle lobe (lateral-view bronchogram). The deformity of the middle-lobe bronchus can be seen with slight bronchiectasis and much shortening and crowding of the bronchi and no peripheral filling. Arrow marks top of right dome.

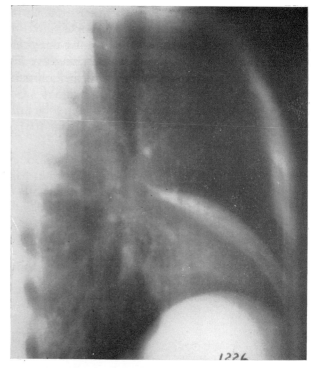

Fig. 112.—Atelectasis of the right middle lobe (same case, lateral-view tomogram). The lobe has shrunk to a very small size, and a calcified gland is seen adjacent to the narrowed bronchus. In the plain film both features were indistinct. Female aged 25 years. Cough and sputum 1 year.

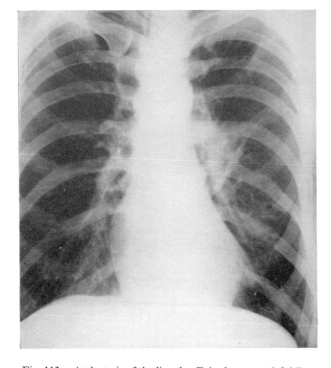

Fig. 113.—Atelectasis of the lingula. Faint haze near left hilum, apex of heart indistinct. Male aged 55 years several haemoptyses. Shadow above hilum in apical lower. Carcinoma of lingular bronchus.

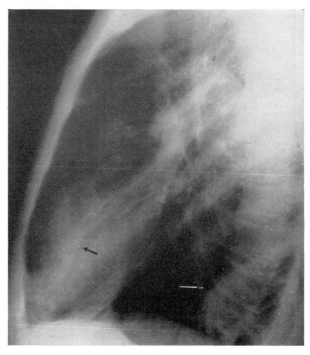

Fig. 114.—Same case (lateral view). Arrow marks posterior concave border of the opaque shrunken lobe. Consolidation of apical segment of lower lobe also present high up posteriorly.

Lingular atelectasis

In lingular bronchostenosis with atelectasis, the shrunken lobe casts such a very faint shadow at the left base adjacent to the heart shadow that it may be difficult to see it at all in a routine anterior view (Fig. 113). In a left lateral view, a well-defined tongue-like shadow may be seen in the lower half of the lung. The anterior edge may either reach the sternum or may be 1–2 cm posterior to it, while the posterior edge, which includes the fissure, has a well-defined posterior concave border lying well forward of the expected line of the interlobar fissure (Fig. 114). The shadow is in fact the same as that seen with atelectasis of the upper lobe, only it does not extend so high up. The condition is not very common, and the shadow may be difficult to see even in the lateral view because of the superimposed heart shadow and, in some women patients, the breast shadows. It will, however, stand out very clearly in left lateral tomograms, which are therefore indicated if this condition is suspected, but not clearly demonstrated in the plain radiographs.

The transradiancy of the lingular bronchus cannot be demonstrated with the same certainty in tomograms as that of the right middle-lobe bronchus, which is more easily positioned parallel to the tomographic layer. Nor can a lesion even a short way down the lingular bronchus always be seen on bronchoscopy. Bronchography may therefore be indicated to prove occlusion, if these other tests are negative (Fig. 331).

Distinction from consolidation without shrinkage is possible if there is marked forward displacement of the main interlobar fissure. Lingular atelectasis is easily distinguished from the rare interlobar effusion, which occurs in the lower part of the main fissure, since the lower margin of the shadow of the effusion would be convex posteriorly and would lie posterior to the predicted position of the fissure.

Left lower-lobe atelectasis

In left lower-lobe bronchostenosis with atelectasis the shrunken airless lobe commonly casts a triangular homogeneous shadow superimposed on the heart shadow, with a well-defined lateral margin passing in a straight line downwards and outwards. This shadow may not be seen in a routine lightly exposed radiograph, but can be clearly seen in a well-exposed radiograph (Fig. 116). If the lobe has shrunk to a very small size it will appear as a narrow paravertebral shadow.

A somewhat similar triangular shadow may be seen with a retrosternal inflammatory or neoplastic mass, but a lateral view will show its anterior position. Another such shadow could be caused by a paravertebral abscess, which is often but not always associated with disc narrowing and vertebral erosion. A neoplastic mass, particularly in Hodgkin's disease, may give a similar shadow, as will hypertrophied marrow tissue in this site in extramedullary haemopoiesis resulting, for instance, from haemolytic anaemia. Occasionally a secondary deposit will develop in the same site and both this and a Hodgkin's deposit may show some erosion of the adjacent vertebral bodies, though this is unusual.

A sequestrated segment is another cause of a shadow behind the heart simulating an atelectatic lower lobe. In this case there are no changes in the hilar or lung vessels. The distinction can also be made in a bronchogram. In a sequestrated segment there may be no communication between its bronchi and the rest of the lung, in which case the opaque area will not show contrast medium in the bronchi within it, and the normal number of segmental divisions will be seen in the nearby normal lobe. Should a fistulous communication develop leading into one of the lower-lobe branches in the adjacent lung, usually as the result of infection and ulceration, then the bronchi in the opaque area will be outlined. These will be in addition to the normal number of lower-lobe segmental branches, and are usually dilated or grossly cystic. In these cases the sequestrated segment is often intralobar. It is not deep in the lung but plastered on the outside of the adjacent lobe, and the abnormal dilated alveoli within it become more normal as they merge with the normal alveolar structure in the rest of the lobe. An extralobar sequestrated segment is separated from the adjacent lobe by pleura, and is more often circular (*see* p. 79). The blood supply is usually from the aorta. Finally, a tortuous descending aorta may give a similar shadow. The absence of any abnormality in the hilar vessels or lung vessels will serve to distinguish all such lesions from an atelectatic lower lobe.

The atelectatic lobe drags the interlobar pleura medially with it, and this forms the lateral border of the triangular shadow. It will tend to pull the axillary pleura inwards and this may result in a small shadow in the costophrenic recess with a medial concave margin just like a small pleural effusion (Fig. 116) (*see* p. 36).

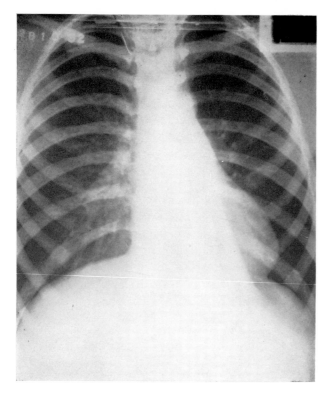

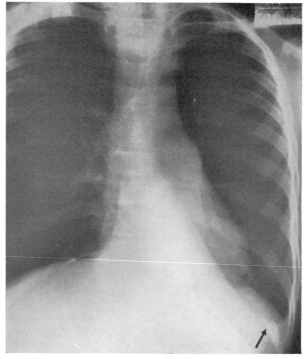

Fig. 115.—Atelectasis of left lower lobe. Shadow behind heart with well-demarcated lateral margin sloping downwards and outwards is the collapsed lobe. Left dome not elevated. Heart to left. Hilum much smaller than right, lung vessels too few and small. Some hypertransradiancy left lung.

Fig. 116.—Atelectasis of left lower lobe (high penetration radiograph). Shadow of collapsed lobe as Fig. 115. Axillary part of pleura pulled medially (above arrow) and the normal but displaced pleura occludes the costophrenic recess. No effusion. Left dome normal level.

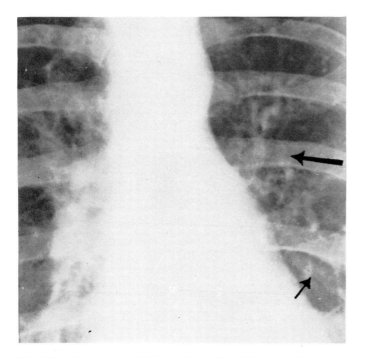

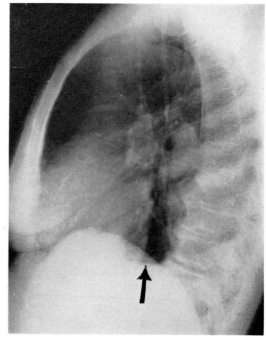

Fig. 117.—Atelectasis of left lower lobe. Small hilar vessels opposite horizontal arrow; they are larger on right. Upward-pointing arrow to anterior end of a rib (not a vessel). No shadow of basal artery.

Fig. 118.—Atelectasis of left lower lobe (lateral view). Lower vertebrae whiter than upper, and this area whiter than retrosternal transradiant area. Shadow of left dome (arrow) does not extend further back.

The hilum may be obscured by the displaced heart shadow (Fig. 115), but in a well-exposed radiograph its small size will be apparent (Fig. 117) and the absence of the shadow of a normal basal artery will be obvious, the downward and medially displaced lingular artery being rather too small to be mistaken for it. The number of vessels in the upper half of the lung should be half that of the opposite normal side and they will appear smaller. Usually all these changes are obvious but sometimes they are not easily seen and a tomogram may be indicated to show them more clearly.

In a lateral view three characteristic changes are often seen (Fig. 118). First, the retrosternal transradiant area instead of being the same is darker or more transradiant than the posterior third behind the heart shadow. Second, the vertebrae just above the diaphragm are whiter than those in the mid-dorsal region due to the collapsed lobe absorbing some of the rays. They should be darker because they are below the opacity caused by the shoulder girdles. Finally, the posterior 2–3 cm of the shadow of the left dome of the diaphragm may be invisible, since the collapsed lobe will be of much the same radio-opacity (Fig. 118).

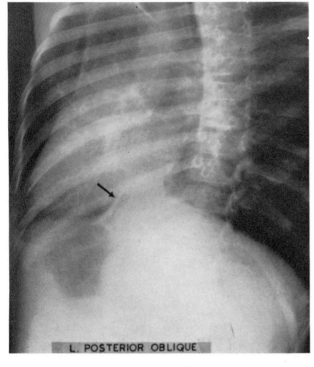

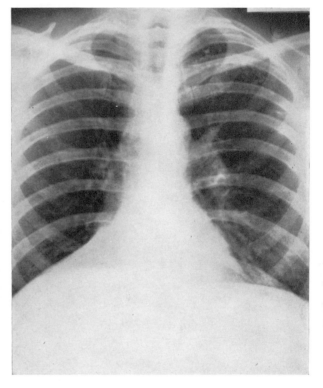

Fig. 119.—Same case as Fig. 116 (left posterior-oblique view). The arrow marks the antero-lateral margin of the collapsed lobe which obscures the adjacent part of the left dome. It was less distinct in the true lateral view and in the left anterior-oblique view.

Fig. 120.—Atelectasis of the right lower lobe. Triangular shadow in cardiophrenic angle. Small hilar vessels. Vessel count less than left; diaphragm normal level and no right lung hypertransradiancy. Adenoma of bronchus. Male aged 43 years; 7 months ago onset of cough, sputum, fever and dyspnoea.

In a left posterior oblique view the collapsed lobe may appear as a triangular shadow with its apex near the lower part of the hilum (Fig. 119). Occasionally if the collapsed lobe is very small and plastered against the vertebrae none of these signs may be seen, but the diagnosis can still be made from a posterior-view tomogram at hilum level which should show the occluded lower-lobe bronchus and the abnormal left hilum vessel anatomy.

Right lower-lobe atelectasis

In right lower-lobe bronchostenosis with atelectasis the shrunken airless lobe may cast a similar triangular shadow superimposed on the right heart and perhaps projecting well beyond it (Fig. 120). If it shrinks to a very small size it will lie entirely behind the heart shadow, and may not be seen in a lightly exposed routine film, but will be seen in a radiograph with more exposure.

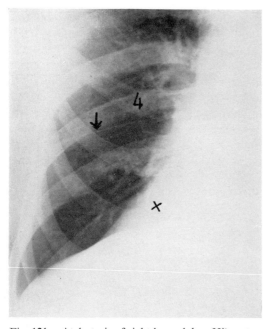

Fig. 121.—Atelectasis of right lower lobe. Hilum too small. Cross on shadow of airless lower lobe. Arrow points to horizontal fissure which is depressed. Vessel count lower half is less than on left. Right heart border distinct. Diaphragm normal level.

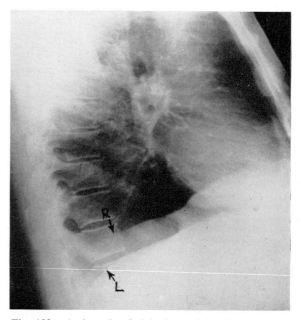

Fig. 122.—Atelectasis of right lower lobe (lateral view). Upward-pointing arrow to left dome. Downward arrow to right dome, shadow of which is invisible posterior to arrow. Lower vertebrae whiter than those above, and this area less transradiant than retrosternal transradiant area. Carcinoma of lower-lobe bronchus; lobe collapsed at thoracotomy.

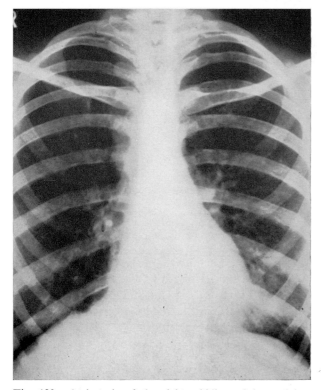

Fig. 123.—Atelectasis of the right middle and lower lobes. Diaphragm normal, heart not displaced. Right hilum too small and no basal artery seen. Two few vessels in right lung, but no hypertransradiancy.

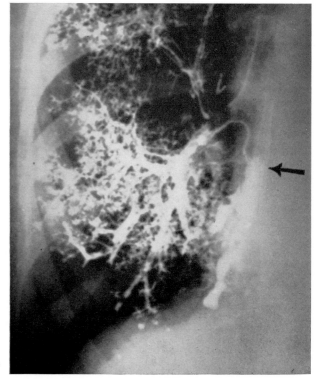

Fig. 124.—Same case (bronchogram). Arrow marks intermediate bronchus, indicating that both middle and lower lobe branches lie within the opaque area covered by the right side of the heart shadow.

The most striking feature will be the small size of the right hilum shadow compared to the left and the absence of the characteristic shadow of the full length of the basal artery. A vessel count done in the manner described on p. 58 will show that there are fewer vessels in the right than in the left lung. If the horizontal fissure is visible it will be depressed and will slope downwards at an angle of between 30 and 60 degrees (Fig. 121). In the lateral view (Fig. 122) the appearances will be the same as those described above in left lower-lobe atelectasis, save that the depressed horizontal fissure may be seen.

Right middle and lower-lobe atelectasis

The appearances are very similar to those of isolated lower-lobe atelectasis. The hilum will be very small and the paucity of vessels more obvious (Fig. 123), and of course no separate line of the depressed horizontal fissure will be seen. The lateral view will be the same as in isolated right (Fig. 122) or left lower-lobe atelectasis (Fig. 118), but the posterior part of the right dome will be invisible in most cases. The occlusion of the intermediate bronchus will be obvious in a tomogram unless there are multiple distal occlusions, in which case these will best be seen in a bronchogram (Fig. 124).

SOME LONG LINE AND BAND-LIKE SHADOWS

The shadow of a segmental atelectasis is naturally smaller than that of a lobar atelectasis and should come under the heading of band-like or even linear shadows (*see* p. 117). They are being considered in this chapter in order to bring the group of atelectases together for aetiological, clinical and pathological convenience.

SEGMENTAL ATELECTASIS (OR COLLAPSE)

Stenosis of a segmental bronchus, even if it is complete, may be present without any abnormal shadow being visible in the plain radiographs, especially if there is no distal inflammation and the segment remains aerated by cross-aeration. Cross-aeration is the means by which air reaches a group of alveoli although the bronchus leading directly to them is occluded. It is assumed that the air reaches them from nearby normally aerated alveoli (Van Allen, Lindskog and Richter, 1931). This collateral air drift may occur *via* the pores of Kohn and Lambert. The mechanism is not very effective across the inter-lobar fissure, but this does not always form a complete barrier. It may be interfered with if there is infection of the segment beyond the stenosis. It is also ineffective at the periphery of the lung if the respiratory excursions are diminished, which is a frequent occurrence in the lower zones for a few days after a major abdominal operation.

Occlusion of a segmental bronchus without airlessness in the lung distal to it is sometimes seen with an inhaled foreign body, but may occur with any of the other causes of bronchostenosis.

Generally the stenosis results in distal inflammation, oedema, alveolar collapse, or bronchiectasis, and these changes will cause a shadow to be seen in the radiograph. If these secondary changes are severe, the appearances may be the same as those seen in consolidation of part of a segment without bronchostenosis. If, on the other hand, the inflammation is slight and has caused little induration of the lung, but is nevertheless sufficient to interfere with cross-aeration, then the segment will shrink and the resulting band-like shadow will be much smaller than that of consolidation when the segment stays its normal size. Sometimes there appears to be such gross shrinkage of the segment that it seems to be represented by a 1–2 mm wide linear shadow. However if this is compared with the actual size of the segment seen at operation or after resection, it will be observed that the shrunken segment is in fact rather larger than the line shadow would suggest. The line shadow represents airless or oedematous alveoli adjacent to the pleura, the rest of the segment being aerated by collateral air drift from the adjacent segment. It is the displacement of the line of the pleura which will indicate shrinkage of the segment and thus suggest a bronchial occlusive lesion.

When a shadow is seen suggesting a segmental atelectasis, serial radiographs at relatively short intervals are useful in differentiating a transient from a persistent lesion. If the lesion persists, tomograms may show transradiancies in the opaque area suggestive of bronchiectasis, or an additional small opacity suggesting a neoplasm. A bronchogram is useful to determine whether a segmental bronchus is obstructed or narrowed, particularly if the lesion is too far distal to be visible on bronchoscopy.

Atelectasis of the right apical and left apico-posterior segments of the upper lobe

Atelectasis of the apical segment of the right upper lobe from stenosis of the bronchus is rare owing to the ease of cross-aeration from the segments on either side of it. Occasionally a narrow band-like or linear shadow is seen in an anterior-view radiograph passing almost vertically upwards from the region of the hilum to the apex, which may indicate this condition. Proof that this represents a collapsed apical segment will generally have to be obtained by means of bronchography which would then show occlusion of the apical bronchus of the upper lobe. The shadow may be invisible in a lateral view.

The left apical segmental bronchus is so closely related to the posterior bronchus that usually both segments are affected. The collapsed lung distal to the stenosis casts a 1-cm band-like shadow with a well-defined posterior margin lying more or less in the line of the upper end of the interlobar fissure. If there is slight forward displacement of the fissure, it is often not sufficiently marked to be detected in the lateral-view radiograph. In the anterior view the collapsed segment is seen as a band-like shadow or ill-defined area of clouding running upwards and outwards from the upper part of the hilum towards the apex.

Atelectasis of the anterior segment of the upper lobes

Atelectasis of the anterior segment of the right upper lobe from stenosis of its segmental bronchus results in a 1–4 mm wide linear shadow or a 0·5–1 cm band-like shadow which runs horizontally with an inferior concave curve. In the anterior view it lies rather higher than the expected position of the horizontal fissure, meeting the fifth rib in the axilla (Fig. 125). In a lateral view a similar band-like shadow is seen running forwards just above the expected position of the horizontal fissure, while the inferior concave curve of the lower margin is particularly well seen (Fig. 126).

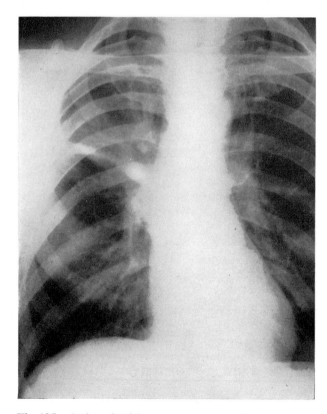

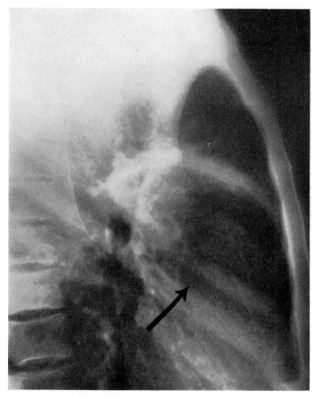

Fig. 125.—Atelectasis of the anterior segment of the right upper lobe. The band-like shadow has an inferior concave margin formed by the raised horizontal fissure, and is seen meeting the fifth rib in the axilla. There is no elevation of the right dome. Male aged 54 years. Two months haemoptysis following a cold. Neoplasm visible on bronchoscopy.

Fig. 126.—Same case (lateral view). Arrow marks line of main fissure clearly seen in the original radiograph. The band-like shadow with the inferior concave lower margin is formed by the airless segment. Specimen showed a 2-cm bronchial carcinoma occluding anterior bronchus. Lung distal to this was airless. Very little other change, except some oedema, and mucus-distended bronchi in the lower half.

Collapse of the anterior segment of the left upper lobe results in a rather shorter band-like shadow lying at a somewhat higher level. The inferior margin borders on the lingula so that it is less well defined, and the segment tends to retract towards the hilum, so that the shadow is shorter than with a lesion of the same segment on the right side.

Frequently, particularly when the stenosis is due to a bronchial carcinoma, both the anterior and posterior segments of the right upper lobe are collapsed (Fig. 128).

Atelectasis of the posterior segment of the right upper lobe

Collapse of the posterior segment of the right upper lobe distal to a stenosis of the segmental bronchus results in a 0·5–1 cm band-like shadow with a well-defined posterior margin against the line of the upper end of the main fissure (Fig. 128). The anterior superior margin is often less well defined. The shadow is more easily seen in a lateral view than an anterior view, and in a lateral-view tomogram than in a plain lateral-view radiograph.

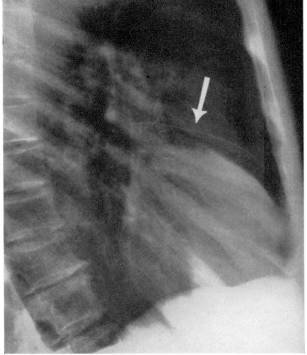

Fig. 127.—Atelectasis of the medial segment of the middle lobe. Arrow points to the line of the horizontal fissure, which has been touched up. Clear area of lung between this and opaque shrunken segment below. Male aged 49 years. Pain in the right chest, and loss of weight.

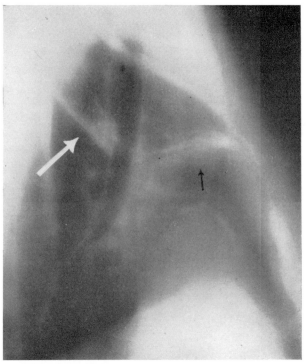

Fig. 128.—Atelectasis of the anterior and posterior segments of right upper lobe (lateral-view tomogram). White arrow points to posterior segment, black arrow to shrunken opaque anterior segment. Confirmation at operation; both bronchi narrowed by tuberculous stenosis.

Atelectasis of the medial or lateral segment of the middle lobe

Collapse of the medial segment of the middle lobe from stenosis of the segmental bronchus is uncommon, but is sometimes seen. In the anterior view there may be no obvious abnormality in the plain radiograph, or there may be slight depression of the horizontal fissure, and a faint haze in the lower zone adjacent to the heart. In the right lateral view a linear or band-like shadow may be seen running downwards and forwards, suggesting atelectasis of the whole of the middle lobe. The diagnosis will be suggested if some aerated lung can be seen between the shadow of the airless part of the lobe and the horizontal fissure (Fig. 127). It may be confirmed on bronchography. At a superficial glance the bronchogram may appear normal with filling of the middle lobe, but on closer inspection it will be seen that there are too few divisions of the middle-lobe bronchus in the lateral-view bronchogram (Fig. 130).

Inspection of the anterior-view bronchogram will show the lateral branch of the apical lower-lobe segment quite clearly, which will indicate the site of the origin of the middle-lobe stem. A lateral division (of the middle lobe) may then be traced downwards and outwards from this, but it will then be obvious that the medial division running close to the right heart border is absent (Fig. 129). Sometimes a short column of the contrast medium will fill the proximal part, and then the obstruction will be clearly shown. The cardiac bronchus comes off the main intermediate-stem bronchus at a lower level than the apical lower-lobe bronchus, so that it will not be mistaken for the medial segmental bronchus of the middle lobe.

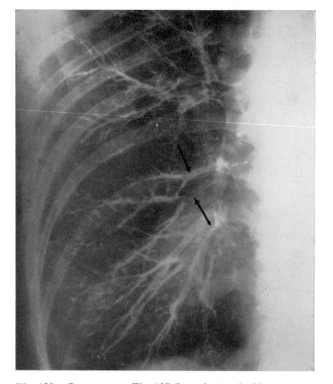

Fig. 129.—Same case as Fig. 127 (bronchogram). Upper arrow marks the lateral branch of apical lower lobe; lower arrow the lateral branch of middle lobe (4). Note absence of filling of medial division (5). The paracardiac division some distance below is the cardiac bronchus.

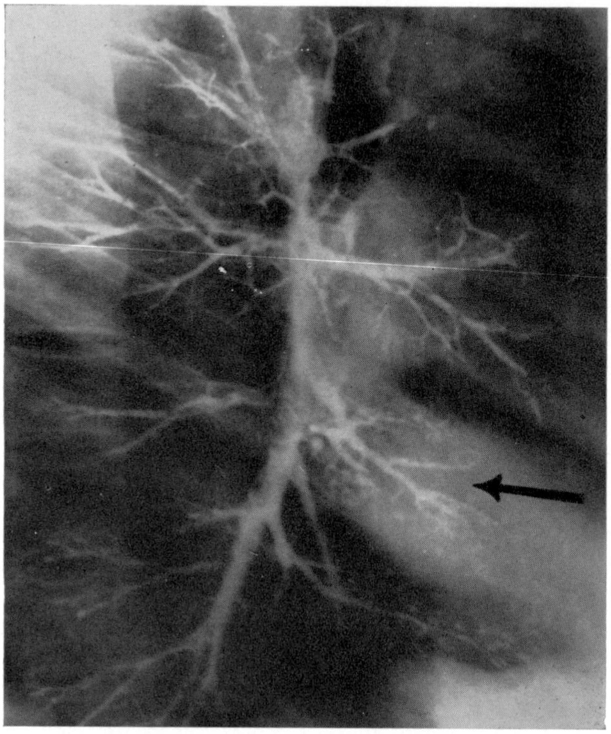

Fig. 130.—Same case (lateral-view bronchogram). Arrow marks lateral bronchus of middle lobe. Medial division not filled. It was occluded by a small carcinoma, and this segment was small and airless. Right middle lobectomy.

Collapse of the lateral segment of the middle lobe may give a similar appearance in the plain radiographs, and in the lateral-view bronchogram, but in the anterior-view bronchogram the medial division will be seen running downwards close to the heart border, and there will be no lateral branch originating at the same level as the lateral branch of the apical lower-lobe bronchus.

Atelectasis of the apical segment of the lower lobe

Occlusion of the bronchus to the apical segment of the lower lobe is not uncommon, however since cross-aeration is often good, the segment may shrink but remain aerated and this can be inferred if there is displacement of the upper end of the main interlobar fissure (*see* p. 106). Occasionally it is opaque and casts a triangular shadow superimposed on the upper part of the hilum in the anterior view and a band-like shadow passing posteriorly across the mid-dorsal vertebrae in a lateral view.

Atelectasis of a basal segment

Collapse of a basal segment in isolation due to stenosis of a basal bronchus is unusual, presumably because it remains well aerated by cross-aeration. Small triangular shadows from such a bronchostenosis are generally the result of bronchiectasis and inflammatory changes rather than collapse. Backward displacement of the line shadow of the lower half of the interlobar fissure with normal transradiancy of the lower lobe will indicate shrinkage of a part or the whole of this lobe. This is discussed more fully on page 106.

CIRCULAR OR OVAL HOMOGENEOUS INTRAPULMONARY SHADOWS

The shadows under this heading range from pin-point size to a size of several centimetres. They may be very well defined, evenly circular or evenly oval or rather lobulated; or they may be poorly defined and perhaps not even regularly circular or oval. Included in the category are single isolated shadows, multiple shadows of similar size and shape, and multiple shadows of dissimilar size and shape.

A Single Large Circular or Oval Well-defined Shadow

A single large circular or oval homogeneous shadow may have been first observed when it was only a few millimetres in size, after which it grew to a much larger size, or it may be first observed when it is already a large isolated homogeneous shadow over 2 cm in size. It may lie anywhere in the thorax, and its spatial position can be determined from plain anterior-view and lateral-view radiographs, though not always its anatomical position.

If it is deep in the lung and remote from the chest wall or mediastinum, its intrapulmonary position is fairly obvious; more often, however, it borders on an interlobar fissure or the peripheral pleural cavity, so that it is not always possible to be certain whether the lesion is in the lung " parenchyma ", or whether it arises from the pleura and pushes the pulmonary tissue aside. If it reaches the chest wall at any point, there is also the possibility that the lesion arises from some structure in this part. An example of this would be a neurilemmoma arising from an intercostal nerve.

If the shadow lies antero-medially and reaches the retrosternal region, or if it lies medially adjacent to the heart shadow, then distinction from a mediastinal lesion may not be easy, and may not in fact be possible, from plain radiographs or fluoroscopy.

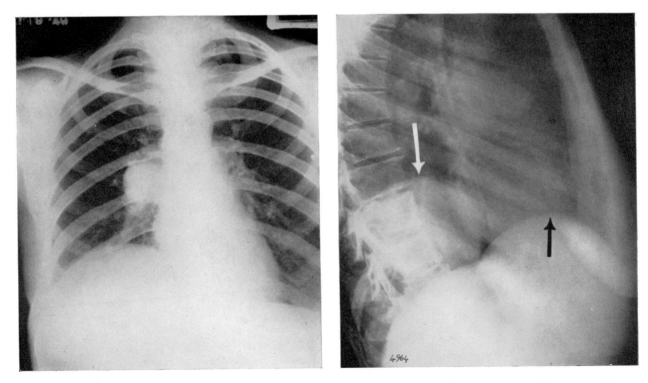

Fig. 131.—Secondary deposit in the right lower lobe simulating a raised right diaphragm. Also deposits in right hilum region. Haemoptysis so chest radiographed. Later found to have a primary osteosarcoma of the pelvis.

Fig. 132.—Same case (lateral view). White arrow points to circular shadow of the tumour. Black arrow to physiological elevation of the anterior third of the right dome. Half the tumour lies above this level. Opacity in front of hilum.

If it lies inferiorly the lower border will merge with the shadow of the diaphragm, and in an anterior-view radiograph the upper border of the tumour may be mistaken for a raised dome of the diaphragm (Fig. 131). A lateral view, however, will reveal its intrapulmonary position, although most of the shadow is at a lower level than the upper border of the right dome anterior to it (Fig. 132). There may be aerated lung right round it, but if it rests on the diaphragm, none will be seen inferiorly.

The diaphragm is often normal, and there is usually no displacement of the heart, trachea, interlobar fissures, or nearby vessels. The presence or absence of local changes in the ribs or vertebrae should be noted.

When a large circular homogeneous shadow is seen, and there are no other obvious abnormal shadows or bone changes, then the list of possibilities is formidable. It may be possible to make a diagnosis on clinical grounds, if for instance a primary neoplasm is found elsewhere, if tubercle bacilli or neoplastic cells are found in the sputum, or if the Casoni test for hydatid disease is positive. Frequently, however, there are no such clues, so that any further evidence obtainable from the radiological appearances will be of help. The presence of other intrapulmonary shadows should be sought, if necessary with the help of tomography, since the demonstration of small satellite shadows, short linear or ring shadows, and perhaps calcifications will suggest tuberculosis whilst small contralateral circular shadows would suggest secondary deposits, and exclude a benign tumour or developmental aberration, which, with the exception of an arterio-venous aneurysm, are generally single. Any large circular shadow may develop near old calcified tuberculous lesions, and more active tuberculous lesions could theoretically coexist with one of the large homogeneous circular shadows of a non-tuberculous origin, but in point of fact neither of these combinations is at all common.

A remote bone erosion would suggest a secondary deposit, so that a careful inspection of the bony parts is indicated. A local bone erosion adjacent to a large oval shadow is sometimes seen with a primary bronchial carcinoma, usually in the apex though sometimes lower. It may be indistinguishable from a primary malignant bone tumour or from a secondary deposit in the bone with a soft tissue extension of the neoplastic mass beyond the limits of the bone and encroaching on the lung field.

In a large number of cases there are neither clinical nor radiological clues as to the nature of the large circular shadow, and a final diagnosis can only be made after serial x-ray examinations, from the cytology of the sputum, at a thoracotomy, or at a subsequent histological examination of the lesion.

The following section deals with the different lesions that may be finally diagnosed in cases in which a large homogeneous oval or circular shadow, similar to that in Figs. 133 and 134, is seen on the radiograph. In each group at least one example has been encountered by the author. Pathological confirmation was obtained in all but the acute infective lesions, for which only clinical and the serial radiographic evidence was available.

Common causes of a large circular or oval homogeneous shadow

Bronchial carcinoma

Bronchial carcinoma is at present by far the most common cause of an isolated fairly well-defined circular shadow in an elderly male who smokes (Figs. 133 and 134). It may be found on mass or incidental radiography of the chest, but more often the radiograph is taken because of the usual symptoms of this condition. The shadow may be well defined, but is rarely quite as well defined as the shadow seen in some cases of bronchial adenoma, an isolated pulmonary secondary deposit, or a hydatid cyst. Quite often the shadow of a bronchial carcinoma has a rather hazy margin without actually appearing to infiltrate out into the surrounding normal lung. Although it may be regularly circular in shape, it is often a little flattened in parts so that it appears like a rather rounded square. It not infrequently shows a localized bulge or may be distinctly lobulated, while sometimes one edge of the circle is less well defined than the rest.

A secondary deposit

A secondary deposit in the lung may be single and grow to a large size. It is usually particularly well defined, perhaps more so than most primary bronchial carcinomas. If the patient is known to have a primary neoplasm, or if one has been removed, perhaps many years ago (sometimes as many as 20), it may be assumed the shadow is a secondary deposit. However, from some sites such as the cervix or uterus, this is unlikely, and the lung lesion in fact turns out to be a primary bronchial carcinoma.

Occasionally no primary neoplasm is found on routine clinical examination, even after the lung shadow has alerted the clinician to this possibility. It is then often assumed that the round shadow in the lung is a primary neoplasm, and then no further radiological search is made. Sometimes after a biopsy or removal of the lung lesion the histological features indicate it is a secondary deposit, and may even be such as to suggest a possible site for the primary tumour. This may indicate the need for an intravenous pyelogram, or barium enema and meal to try to locate a renal or alimentary tract primary neoplasm. If a liver scan is normal, removal of the lung secondary deposit followed by the renal or alimentary tract primary lesion has resulted in long-term survival in some cases.

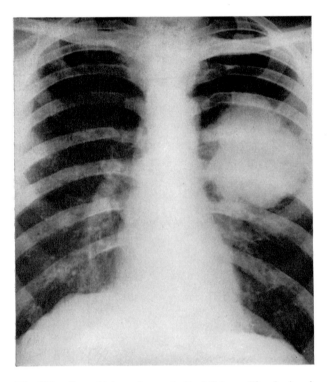

Fig. 133.—Bronchial carcinoma in the left lung. The shadow is quite well defined, roughly oval and slightly lobulated.

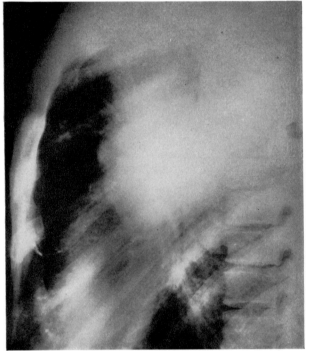

Fig. 134.—Same case (lateral view). Most of the neoplasm lay in the upper lobe, but had transgressed the fissure.

A bronchial adenoma

A bronchial adenoma may occasionally present as a symptomless well-defined 2–3 cm shadow, which is sometimes circular but often elongated, oval, and perhaps slightly lobulated. In some cases the entire shadow represents the neoplasm, but in others the shadow represents a bronchus distended with mucus to a size of 2–3 cm, the neoplasm being much smaller and passing undetected in the radiograph. Generally a bronchial adenoma is visible on bronchoscopy. Haemoptyses are a common presenting symptom, and the picture alters radiologically if the tumour causes stenosis of a proximal bronchus, when atelectasis of a lobe will produce an additional shadow. The picture will also alter both clinically and radiologically if the stenosis is associated with distal inflammatory episodes.

Less common causes of a large circular or oval homogeneous shadow

A leiomyoma

A leiomyoma in the lung is a rare benign tumour arising from bronchial muscle. It may reach a size of 1–2 cm when it may be seen in the radiograph as a well-defined circular shadow. It is usually clinically silent and the diagnosis is only possible after removal and histological examination.

A fibroma

A fibroma usually arises from the visceral pleura and displaces rather than invades adjacent lung tissue. It is not always possible from the radiographic appearances to be certain whether the shadow represents a lesion in the lung or in the pleura, especially if it arises from the interlobar pleura, and thus appears as a circular or oval shadow deep in the thorax. On the other hand, if it lies posteriorly against the ribs, it will be indistinguishable from a neurilemmoma, whilst if it lies at the base it will simulate a parapericardial or pleural cyst, or a liver hernia (*see* pp. 208 and 213).

A fibroma frequently produces a pulmonary osteo-arthropathy. There may be limb pain and stiffness of the joint, or even swelling of the surrounding joints and tissues, or there may be no clinical evidence but only x-ray evidence of the condition. An anterior view of the hand and wrist (Fig. 325) or a posterior view of the knee, ankle, or foot region will show the white line of periosteal new bone quite distinct from the cortex, and often separated from it by a narrow transradiant zone. Similar features may be the presenting symptom of a bronchial carcinoma. In either case, the pain will subside within a few hours or days, and the shadow of the periosteal new bone within a few weeks after removal of the tumour (*see* p. 219).

In spite of the benign histology of these fibromas and the ease with which they appear to be totally removed, there is a strong tendency for them to recur locally with a sarcomatous histology, so that the eventual outlook is grave.

A mixed benign tumour (hamartoma)

A hamartoma is sometimes considered to be a developmental abnormality, but this particular type of benign lung mass only appears in adult life, and may first be observed in old age, and may even grow then. Willis (1967) considers it to be a mixed benign tumour. Opportunities for observing the rate of growth are rare, since the tumour is either removed soon after detection of a shadow in the radiograph, or left *in situ* so that no confirmation of the diagnosis is possible. In one patient, aged 50 years, the lesion grew from 1 cm to 2 cm over a period of three years. It is doubtful whether malignant change ever takes place in this tumour.

In the radiograph it is seen as a circular or oval shadow some 2–3 cm in size, or perhaps a little larger, and it is very well demarcated, a feature which will suggest the diagnosis. In many cases a small spot of calcification can be seen deep in the shadow on tomography (Fig. 135), whilst in a few cases extensive irregular calcification is seen deep in it.

Histologically the tumour is characterized by the presence of cartilage with clefts lined by respiratory epithelium, with perhaps some muscle here and there. It can generally be shelled out of the lung to which it is not closely attached even when lying deep within it.

Sometimes the tumour is endobronchial and for the most part cartilaginous, and will then tend to cause distal collapse or inflammation, which will obscure the small shadow of the tumour.

An arterio-venous aneurysm (fistula)

An arterio-venous aneurysm may be several centimetres across and when it is as large as this it is usually clinically obvious with a thrill or murmur, and with cyanosis resulting from the large volume of blood by-passing the aerating lung surface. Enlarged or aberrant vessels can usually be seen connecting the large shadow to the hilum either in the plain radiographs or more obviously in tomograms (Figs. 136 and 146). In the majority of cases the feeding artery and the draining vein or veins can be seen so clearly in tomograms that an angiogram is unnecessary. Nor should multiple lesions be missed if the tomograms are done carefully and the fistulae are more than 1 cm in size. An example of two separate arterio-venous fistulae shown by tomography is seen in Fig. 146. Very small lesions will not be seen in tomograms and often do not fill in angiograms. Many cases are asymptomatic, but some have cyanosis and dyspnoea or haemoptyses, while the majority have cutaneous or buccal telangiectases.

A fluid-containing cyst

Sometimes a developmental aberration may result in a fluid-containing cyst which will appear as a very well-defined circular or oval homogeneous shadow in the radiograph. Such a cyst may be a retention cyst within the lung, due to an imperforate bronchus, or it may be a cyst with a separate blood supply arising directly from the aorta, in which case it can be considered a sequestrated segment whether it is an isolated cyst or one surrounded by obviously abnormal bronchi and alveoli. Sometimes the cyst lies in the pleura between the lobes, and its interlobar position may only be appreciated at thoracotomy since a diagnostic pneumothorax is not usually considered to be safe or necessary.

If the cyst lies close to the mediastinum it will be indistinguishable from a paratracheal or para-oesophageal mediastinal cyst. All these cysts are probably variations on a common development error, and are clinically silent unless secondary infection occurs. They may then develop a bronchial communication, and the shadow will not remain homogeneous but show air transradiancies and perhaps a fluid level.

The medially placed mediastinal cysts are much more common than the intrapulmonary and inter-lobar cysts. A variable histological picture is found ranging from a lining of non-committal flat epithelium to accessory nodules with a structure indicating a dermoid or portion of lung. A para-oesophageal cyst may have remnants of gastric mucosa, pancreatic tissue, or other elements indicating its foregut origin.

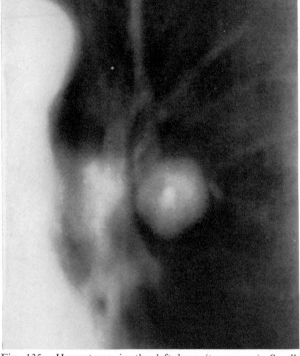

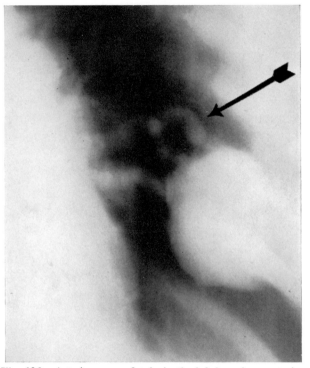

Fig. 135.—Hamartoma in the left lung (tomogram). Small central spot of calcification in well-defined circular shadow. Male aged 51 years. Mass x-ray finding. Tumour enucleated. It contained cartilage, loose connective tissue, fat and clefts with bronchial epithelium.

Fig. 136.—Arterio-venous fistula in the left lung (tomogram). Arrow points to one of three large vessels connecting it to the hilar vessels. Female aged 26 years. Occasional haemoptysis during pregnancy, no cyanosis, systolic bruit audible, haemangioma of lips, nasal mucosa and cheek. Lobectomy performed.

A sequestrated segment

A sequestrated segment may appear as a circular or oval homogeneous shadow some 3–6 cm in size, at either base posteriorly, but more commonly on the left than the right. The shadow is usually well defined and the diaphragm and nearby lung appear normal. It may lie medially and posteriorly outside the lower lobe and will then simulate a posterior mediastinal tumour (*see* p. 112) or it may be fused into the lower lobe, in which case the shadow is triangular rather than circular. The appearances on bronchography are described on page 67. Whether the sequestrated segment is intralobar or extralobar its blood supply is usually from the thoracic aorta, a fact which is not apparent from the plain radiographs. Occasionally its arterial supply is by a large vessel which arises from the abdominal aorta and pierces the diaphragm to reach the lobe, when it may be visible as a short band-like shadow extending from the diaphragm to the main shadow. The blood supply can, if necessary, be shown in an aortogram.

A tuberculous focus

A circular or oval tuberculous focus, whether a blocked cavity or a slowly growing caseous pneumonia, may reach a size of 2–4 cm; at this size it is rarely clinically silent. It is even more rarely isolated, so that tomograms are useful for demonstrating the presence or absence of satellite shadows if none are seen in the plain radiograph—such shadows being uncommon near a circular neoplasm. The presence of calcium in the shadow is not often a very helpful clue, since it is also seen in many dermoids and hamartomas. However, if laminated concentric rings of calcification are found, they will favour the diagnosis of tuberculosis.

An infective lesion

An acute bacterial pneumonia or a lung abscess may appear as a 2–3 cm circular shadow for a day or two in the early stages (Fig. 82). The clinical picture and rapid change in the radiographic appearances will generally be sufficient for the diagnosis, though sometimes if the lesion is sub-acute the diagnosis may remain doubtful for a few days.

A hydatid cyst

A hydatid cyst is more easily diagnosed if the possibility of this condition is borne in mind. It is usually very well defined, oval in shape, with its long axis vertical (Figs. 137 and 138), or when relatively small and some 2–3 cm in size, they are often circular in shape. Large ones may be lobulated. It may lie deep in the lung, or one margin may reach the pleural surface; it is usually in the lower half of the lung. In Britain they are rarely seen until they are 3 cm or more in size. The rate of growth is relatively fast and it may double its size in a few months (hearsay). The most useful clue to the diagnosis is knowing that the patient resided in an area where such a parasite is still common.

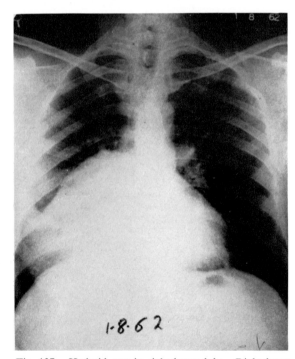

Fig. 137.—Hydatid cyst in right lower lobe. Right heart border invisible, diaphragm normal. Male aged 37 years from Baghdad. Casoni and complement fixation tests + ve.

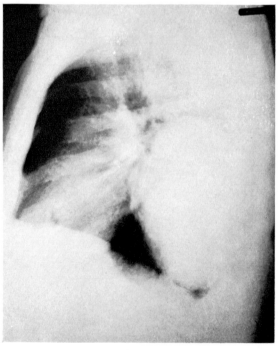

Fig. 138.—Hydatid cyst (same case, lateral view). Oval shadow with long axis vertical in lower lobe. Evacuated, good recovery.

A toruloma

A toruloma (fungus infection—*Cryptococcus neoformans*) is also a cause of a large oval or circular well-defined homogeneous shadow. The lesion may be clinically silent, and only discovered on mass or incidental radiography of the chest. The shadow is generally mistaken for a carcinoma, and the diagnosis in some cases is only made after its removal by lobectomy or pneumonectomy. In other cases there may be a productive cough, and the fungus may then be found in the sputum if it is present in reasonable numbers and if it is sought. Sometimes there is also an intracerebral lesion, and the neurological manifestations of this may predominate.

In one case the radiograph showed a 6-cm oval shadow in the right lower zone, and section of the lung revealed a 6-cm oval well-defined grey soft mass. On histological examination this was found to be due to a form of chronic pneumonia, and contained cryptococci in large numbers lying mainly in the alveoli.

A mycetoma (Aspergillus fumigatus)

Infection of a bronchiectatic space or old tuberculous cavity by *Aspergillus fumigatus* may result in a mycetoma or pink gelatinous mass of mycelia surrounded by the fibrotic cavity wall. If the pre-existing cavity was small it may enlarge from pressure by the growing fungus mass to a final size of several centimetres; if it was already large, the aspergilli may line the wall which will then appear greatly thickened.

In many cases histological examination shows the fungus lying entirely within the cavity, but in a few cases there is some evidence of invasion of nearby lung tissues by it. Clinically some patients are relatively symptom free, while others are quite ill with cough and sputum containing the fungus.

If the mass of aspergilli occupies the whole of the cavity, or if it is an invader of an already solid old infarct, it will cast a well-defined circular or oval homogeneous shadow. If, however, there is a small air space between the central mass of the fungus and the smooth fibrotic wall of the cavity, then a narrow transradiant zone will be seen between the two, giving the " halo " shadow (Fig. 139). (*See also* p. 126). The opacity may well appear circular since the small transradiant band of air may easily be overlooked or only seen in a well-exposed radiograph or in a tomogram.

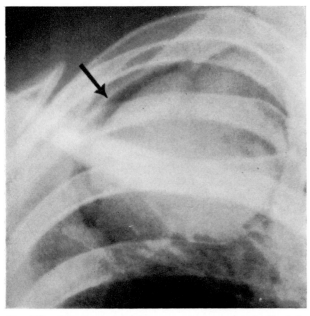

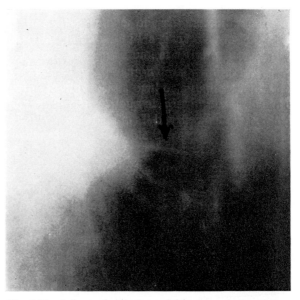

Fig. 139.—Mycetoma in right apex. Arrow points to the halo shadow produced by the small transradiant air space between the wall of the lesion (consisting of fibrous tissue) and the central mass (consisting of aspergilli mycelia). Male aged 48 years. Mass x-ray finding. Aspergilli grown from sputum. Lobectomy performed.

Fig. 140.—Infarct of right lower lobe. Line shadow below arrow, and two others below ended at a vessel shadow which continued on to the hilum (two arteries and one vein). Male aged 45 years. Resected. Pathology: infarct; thrombi in arteries.

An infarct

An infarct may be present and cast a 2–5-cm circular shadow. It is often asymptomatic, though in some cases there may be repeated small haemoptyses over a period of months, suggestive of a bronchial carcinoma. In fact it is not uncommon to find such an infarct in a lobe removed with a provisional diagnosis of carcinoma. Occasionally an infarct will be suspected if a rather large vessel, which can usually be identified as a vein, can be seen connecting the circular shadow to the hilum (Fig. 140). Such a finding would suggest the need for caution before undertaking surgery. Resolution or even a decrease in size of the shadow of an infarct may take some weeks. They are most common in the lower third, but can occur in the upper zone or even the apical region. Other features suggesting an infarct would be the presence of a long horizontal line shadow of a vascular lesion elsewhere (*see* p. 111), either on the same side or on the opposite side, and the presence of phlebitis would be suggestive of the site of an embolus. The infarct is usually the result of thrombo-embolism or a local venous thrombosis *in situ*. Rarely, it is a local manifestation of periarteritis nodosa. The diagnosis may be helped by remembering that such a large circular shadow may be due to a vascular lesion. The haemorrhage may follow trauma.

A syphilitic lesion

A gumma may present as a 2–4-cm circular shadow—some have been removed on a mistaken diagnosis of a neoplasm. They are rather rare and often the diagnosis is uncertain, even after removal. In one of the author's cases, the histology was suggestive of this diagnosis but serological tests were inconclusive.

A non-specific granuloma, and Wegener's granuloma

A granulomatous mass, whose aetiology is uncertain even after removal, or a Wegener's type of granuloma, may also give rise to a large and very obvious circular or oval x-ray shadow.

A paraffin granuloma

A circular or oval 2–3-cm discrete homogeneous shadow may be seen in a patient who has habitually used a paraffin preparation as nasal drops, as a purgative or as a lubricant for an oesophageal tube passed regularly for the treatment of achalasia of the cardia. Why the lesion is sometimes small and discrete, and sometimes more like a lobar consolidation, is unknown. Histologically it has the appearance of a non-specific granuloma containing small droplets of the paraffin oil.

An interlobar pleural effusion

A 2–3-cm circular shadow may suggest a lung shadow in the anterior view (Fig. 141), but a lateral view may show clearly that it lies in the line of an interlobar fissure, and is caused by an encysted pleural effusion (Fig. 142). The line of pleura beyond the shadow will be confirmatory evidence.

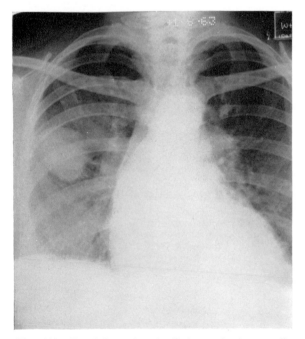

Fig. 141.—Interlobar pleural effusion. A 4-cm well-demarcated circular shadow in right mid zone. Mitral and aortic valve disease.

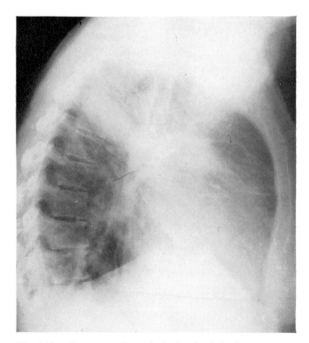

Fig. 142.—Same case (lateral view). Oval shadow at upper end of main fissure and in horizontal fissure. Transient consolidation just previously.

MULTIPLE LARGE CIRCULAR OR OVAL HOMOGENEOUS SHADOWS

Multiple large oval or circular homogeneous shadows (large cannonball shadows) usually indicate secondary deposits (Fig. 143). There may be only two or several and they tend to vary considerably in size. The presence of some smaller shadows, about 5–10 mm in size in other parts of the lungs, is often a characteristic finding.

When the larger shadows are between 2 and 5 cm they are commonly circular, but a particularly large one of 5 cm or more is often oval with a vertical long axis.

A similar appearance may be seen with multiple hydatid cysts. Two hydatids of almost equal size may be seen in either lower zone of the lung, a distribution which would be unlikely to occur with secondary deposits. In Fig. 144 the cyst on the right is circular, and the larger one at the left base is oval with its long axis vertical.

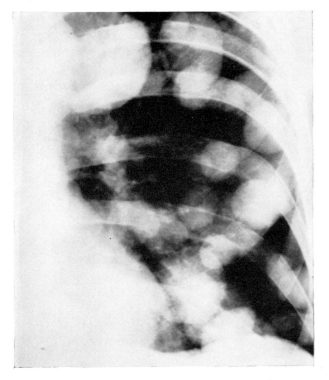

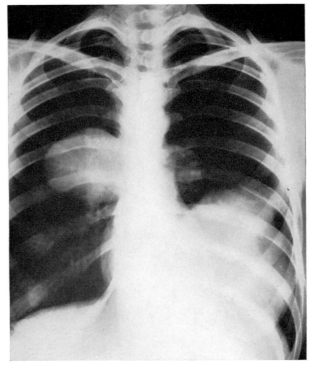

Fig. 143.—Secondary deposits from a carcinoma. Cannonball shadows. These were seen throughout both lungs and varied from 0·5 to 5 cm, most being about 2 cm. All were clearly demarcated and circular in form.

Fig. 144.—Hydatid cysts in the lungs. The cyst in the left lower lobe was infected. The smaller cyst on the right was situated in the posterior part of the upper lobe. Female aged 35 years. Recent left pleurisy. Both cysts removed with good recovery.

Multiple hydatid cysts are usually of the same age and of similar size. Occasionally the growth of one is arrested while the other grows to a larger size. If the two are close to each other and the larger one becomes infected and loses its clear-cut outline, the diagnosis might be in doubt, especially if the smaller well-defined circular shadow is blurred by the nearby inflammatory changes. In such a case, a tomogram would usually show the smaller shadow clearly, and would therefore confirm the diagnosis. Other unfortunately rare escape clauses from a diagnosis of multiple secondary deposits are multiple developmental defects of the hamartomatous type, rheumatoid nodules in the lung with central collagen necrosis and palisading of histiocytes around (with or without a basic coal worker's nodular shadowing) and multiple infarcts.

Another combination of shadows which may very occasionally be seen, is a particularly well-defined shadow lying posteriorly, for example a neurilemmoma, and another rather less-sharply demarcated shadow, probably in the other lung, which may be a bronchial carcinoma or an intrapulmonary secondary deposit from an extrathoracic primary neoplasm. The presence of the long-standing neurilemmoma may be known from a previous radiograph, but more often it is clinically silent and only found as a result of symptoms arising in connection with the malignant neoplasm.

A SINGLE SMALL CIRCULAR HOMOGENEOUS SHADOW

When a small-sized low-density shadow is seen, it is particularly important to make sure if it is in the lung and not an artefact. Unless it can be clearly identified in a lateral view, its position should be fixed by means of tomography. Tomograms would also show any satellite shadows or other abnormal features, such as unsuspected cavitation, calcification, or abnormal vessels in connection with the shadow.

A list of causes of a single small discrete circular low-density homogeneous shadow (between 2 mm and 2 cm in size) will obviously include early examples of all the pathological lesions just quoted for larger shadows, but as detection at this early stage is uncommon, the emphasis will be different.

A tuberculous lesion

Tuberculosis will be by far the most common finding in some countries, but in others it is now less often seen. Three distinct pathological entities have been found, all showing an appearance identical with that in Fig. 145. First there is the small focus of tuberculous pneumonia. This may be found at various stages, at a fairly early exudative and precaseous stage, at a proliferative stage, at a caseous stage—with the ghosts of the lung structure well preserved and therefore presumably capable of resolution—at a stage of total caseation, or at a healing and nearly quiescent stage, with organization well advanced and with much fibrous tissue present. Some foci are laminated, different parts of them being at different stages.

Second, the shadow may be caused by a blocked cavity. The air-containing cavity may have been demonstrated in a previous radiograph, or the diagnosis may be a histological one depending on the nature of the wall of the focus.

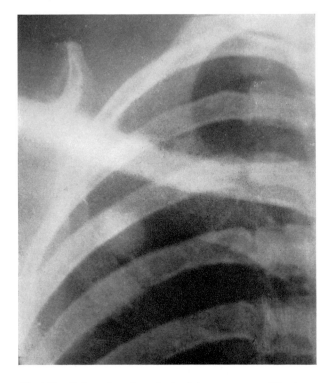

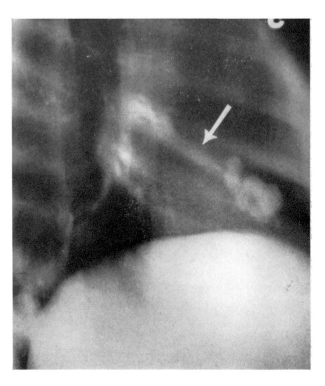

Fig. 145.—Tuberculous focus in the right upper zone. Histology of the lesion was that of a 1-cm circular area of caseous pneumonia. Female aged 35 years. Routine x-ray finding, lesion clinically silent. The shadow increased in size, so lobectomy was done.

Fig. 146.—Arterio-venous fistulae. Lobulated 2 cm shadow in middle lobe with feeding artery and draining vein opposite arrow. Similar appearance in posterior basal segment. Female aged 26 years. Blue all her life. Dyspnoea on exertion, occasional small haemoptsyses. Hb 125 %.

The third pathological entity is an endobronchial tuberculous lesion with peripheral caseous distension of a small bronchus. This may be clearly demonstrable on examination of the specimen, the absence of parenchymal involvement being sometimes indubitable.

Sometimes there is a mixture of all three causes, so that it is impossible to put the case into a clear-cut group. In some cases the shadow is rather elongated and ill defined (smudge shadow).

A neoplasm

All types of neoplasm mentioned in the list of larger opacities are of course at some time in their growth less than 2 cm in size. Differentiation at this early stage from other lesions is often impossible both on the x-ray and the clinical findings. The rate of growth is no safe guide to the diagnosis. When under 2 cm in size, a malignant neoplasm may remain radiologically unchanged for months or years, and after 3 or 4 years suddenly begin to grow rapidly. The rate of increase in size of a tuberculous focus is also very variable. Serial x-ray observation therefore has no place in the diagnosis if removal is contemplated, and the date of operation should not be postponed solely in order to observe whether any changes in the size of the shadow may be detected in further radiographs 1 or 2 months later.

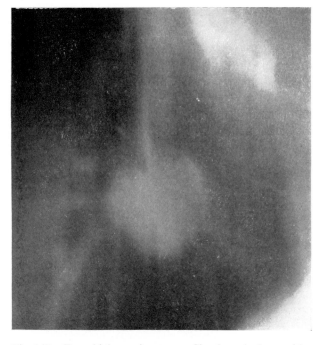

Fig. 147.—Bronchial carcinoma. Circular shadow with notch. The line shadow extending up from the region of the notch was caused by neoplastic cells infiltrating the wall of the bronchus. (Right lateral tomogram.)

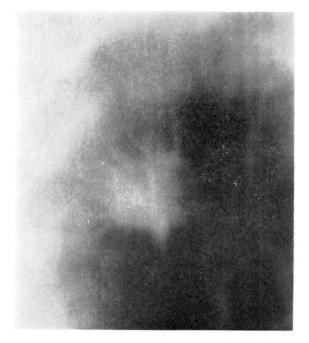

Fig. 148.—Bronchial carcinoma. Circular shadow with radiating line shadows. Some of the lines were caused by fibrous strands, others by dilated lymphatics permeated by neoplastic cells, and sometimes surrounding fibrosis.

Incidentally it is rare to find the shadow of a primary peripheral bronchial neoplasm of less than 1·0 cm in diameter. Certain associated shadows may be seen when the circular shadow is on the borderline between being large or small, that is, between 2 and 4 cm. An example of such associated shadow is small single or multiple satellite shadows due to isolated groups of neoplastic cells or to pre-existing inflammatory lesions; although such satellite shadows are more common in a tuberculous lesion, they do occur with a neoplasm.

A curious notch (Rigler's notch) is occasionally seen in a neoplasm of about 2 cm (Fig. 147). This concave notch faces the hilum and is in the line of the broncho-arterial bundle. It may occur in a tuberculous lesion.

A wide line shadow between the lesion and the hilum formed by fibrous thickening along the broncho-arterial bundle would suggest an inflammatory lesion, but such a change can occur with a neoplasm (Fig. 147).

Another associated abnormality is the presence of a number of 1–2-cm long line shadows radiating out from the circular shadow (Fig. 148). These lines are also seen radiating out from an area of massive fibrosis in a pneumoconiosis (Fig. 192) but in the absence of an industrial history, such line shadows are almost pathognomonic of a bronchial carcinoma.

The pathological basis of such line shadows is very variable, and the following lesions have been observed: blocked and mucus-distended peripheral bronchus; blocked and thrombosed artery or vein; blocked and distended lymphatic with an intense fibrous tissue reaction around it; and any of these lesions with infiltration of neoplastic cells into them. Finally the septa may be thickened or infiltrated with neoplastic cells, or the cells may just stream out in a linear group into the surrounding lung. Several different events are usually found in the same specimen.

A not uncommon finding is a single line shadow between the circular shadow of the carcinoma and the pleura in the axilla. However, such an appearance is also common with a tuberculous lesion (Fig. 193). The line shadow may be caused by a narrow zone of collapsed alveoli together with some indrawn pleura, or by distension with secretions of the peripheral part of the small bronchus occluded by the neoplasm.

A carcinoma may be associated with an infarct (*see* below).

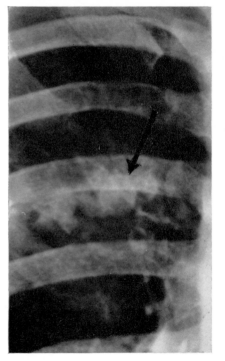
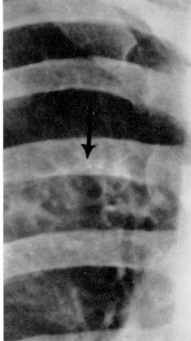
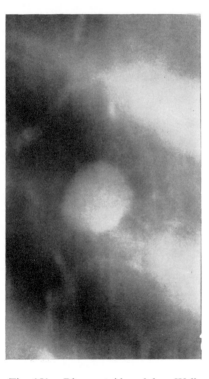

Fig. 149.—A 1-cm circular shadow (below arrow) represents a dilated bronchus full of secretions. Shadow is in the right mid zone. Some less well demarcated 1 cm shadows nearby.

Fig. 150.—Ring shadow (below arrow) at same site when bronchus empty. Female aged 27 years. Asthma and allergic bronchopulmonary aspergillosis with eosinophilia.

Fig. 151.—Rheumatoid nodule. Well-defined 1-cm circular shadow. Asymptomatic, and resected. Necrotic centre with cellular fibrous tissue around, and " palisaded " inner layer. Male aged 55 years with clubbing but no arthritis. Boiler scaler at age of 14–18, so might be Caplan's syndrome.

An infarct

An infarct may present as a somewhat ill-defined 1–2-cm circular shadow (*see also* p. 194). It is often clinically silent, and a thrombo-embolic infarct usually resolves completely in 2–3 weeks, or occasionally leaves a residual line shadow representing the scar. A similar circular shadow of a more chronic infarct may be associated with a bronchial carcinoma. If this is of a main bronchus, it is often invisble in the plain radiograph, but if it is of a more peripheral bronchus, both it and the infarct may be seen either as separate shadows or as adjacent shadows merging into each other. The infarct may be the result of the neoplasm pressing on a vein, or there may be no local mechanical cause. The infarct may be in the same lobe as the neoplasm, or in another lobe; in either case the infarct may be mistaken for a secondary deposit, and lobectomy therefore rejected. Such infarcts are often chronic and the shadow persistent. For the association of a neoplasm with an infarct, see also page 223.

An arterio-venous aneurysm

Even a small arterio-venous aneurysm, giving a circular shadow 0·5–1 cm in size, will, on tomography, show large vessels connecting it to the hilum (Fig. 146), though these may be very inconspicuous in the plain radiographs. This lesion always lies in the mid or lower zones, and not in the apex or sub-clavicular region; it may be clinically silent.

A dilated bronchus full of secretions

A dilated bronchus 2–3 cm in size may fill with secretions, and thus appear as a circular shadow in the lung (Fig. 149). The presence of nearby ring or parallel line shadows will suggest the diagnosis. It is not an uncommon finding in patients with asthma and bronchopulmonary aspergillosis and eosinophilia. The bronchus often empties in due course, and a residual ring shadow is then seen (Fig. 150). Occasionally such a dilated bronchus full of secretions is present distal to a small bronchial neoplasm, and the dilated bronchus may be the predominant shadow.

If the circular shadow is in a lobe which is somewhat hypertransradiant and with small vessels, it will suggest the proximal end of an atretic bronchus (see p. 148).

A rheumatoid nodule

An isolated 1–2-cm well-defined circular shadow may be caused by a rheumatoid nodule (Fig. 151). Histologically the lesion will show a necrotic centre encapsulated with fibrous tissue and palisading of histiocytes around. There may be obvious clinical evidence of rheumatoid arthritis, or there may only be erosions of the metatarsal heads, or a positive Latex test and no radiological changes in the joints.

A Localized Group of Small Circular Shadows or Patchy Clouding

A localized group of well-defined small circular shadows, particularly in an upper zone, would suggest tuberculosis. There are frequently linear and punctate shadows nearby, the presence of which, together perhaps with some dense calcification, would favour this diagnosis. A group of three or four 1-cm circular shadows round a small transradiant area (Fig. 152), with some thin line shadows from the more lateral circular shadows to the pleura in the axilla, is often seen in an acid-fast bacillary infection with " anonymous bacteria" (Runyon, photochromagens, and so on). These are mainly resistant to drugs which will eliminate ordinary tubercle bacilli. In the author's experience, a proliferative focus (a cellular mass replacing the alveoli) and an exudative focus (mainly consisting of fluid in the alveoli) may coexist quite near to each other and give the same kind of shadow on the radiograph. A radiological opinion as to the histology of the lesion causing such a group of small circular shadows is therefore unjustified. Silent chronic pulmonary infarcts may also be multiple and grouped in one zone.

A localized group of rather poorly defined, 3–8-mm, circular shadows may be seen as a result of almost any kind of inflammatory condition, particularly in tuberculosis, or the inflammatory changes distal to a bronchostenosis, often due to a carcinoma of the bronchus invisible in a routine plain radiograph (Fig. 153). It may be seen in the very earliest stages of a bacterial, viral, or aspiration pneumonia, or it may be seen in sensitivity reactions, such as bird fanciers' lung, farmers' lung, or asthmatics with bronchopulmonary aspergillosis and eosinophilia, or in some drug reactions.

When a patient with a bacterial pneumonia shows a group of small ill-defined circular shadows in a lower zone, the appearances are often described as bronchopneumonia. Involvement of the bronchi as well as the lung is often found post mortem in the terminal infection of patients dying of various causes. However, in vivo material shows that patchy areas of consolidation can occur without bronchial inflammation, or with no more than that seen in ordinary lobar pneumonia. The conclusion drawn on an area of patchy clouding in the radiograph should therefore be cautious, and the term patchy consolidation is preferable to bronchopneumonia. It is true that in chronic bronchitics with an inflammatory episode, the radiograph more often shows a patchy rather than a homogeneous shadow, although both patients with pre-existing chronic bronchitis and previously healthy persons may show either

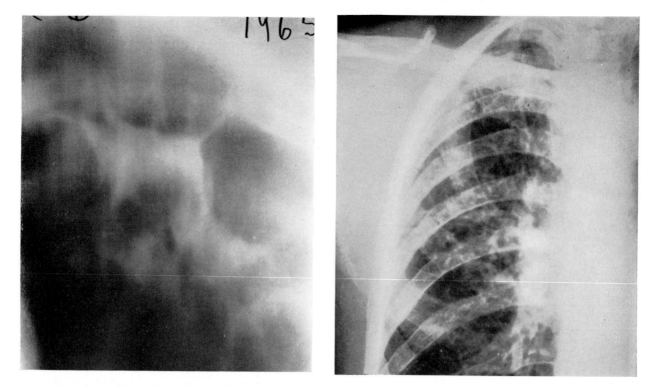

Fig. 152.—Lesions from anonymous microbacteria; 1 cm shadows around a central transradiant zone with line shadows towards the pleura. Male aged 48 years. Sputum: Kansassi + ve. Became negative after chemotherapy.

Fig. 153.—Carcinoma of right upper-lobe bronchus. This was visible on bronchoscopy, but invisible in the radiograph. The small shadows in the right upper zone are caused by distal inflammatory changes. Male aged 58 years. Recent onset of productive cough and fatigue.

type of shadow if they have got an acute pulmonary infection. The increased frequency of patchy shadows in proportion to homogeneous shadows in patients with pneumonia and a previous history of chronic cough and sputum compared to patients with no previous chest complaint, is shown in Table 2.

TABLE 2

NUMBER OF CASES WITH PNEUMONIA SHOWING A SINGLE HOMOGENEOUS SHADOW, MOTTLED SHADOWING, OR AREAS OF PATCHY CLOUDING

	Total	Homogeneous	Mottled	Extent		
				Large	Medium	Small
Emphysema	65	40%	60%	31%	27%	42%
No emphysema	182	74%	26%	34%	35%	31%
Deaths	39	51%	49%	61%	15%	24%

MULTIPLE WIDELY DISSEMINATED SMALL CIRCULAR SHADOWS

Secondary deposits and indolent tuberculosis

Widely disseminated well-demarcated 1–2-cm circular shadows throughout the lungs (the "small cannon-ball" appearance) are characteristic of secondary deposits (Fig. 143). More rarely a similar appearance is seen in a rather indolent form of tuberculosis in which a number of 1–2-cm circular shadows are also seen throughout both lungs (Fig. 154). Distinction between this and secondary deposits may be difficult, as in neither case may there be any clinical clues. A tendency for the shadows to be absent in one lobe is suggestive of tuberculosis, and the distribution of tuberculous foci tends to be less dense per unit area and less even than that of secondary deposits.

No correlation of the " small cannon-ball " appearance in tuberculosis with the morbid anatomy has come to the author's notice so far, but in at least one case a patient has been symptom free and well 5 years after the shadows were first seen; within this period and following chemotherapy and bed rest, some of the shadows have become smaller, some have vanished and many have finally shown a small central calcification.

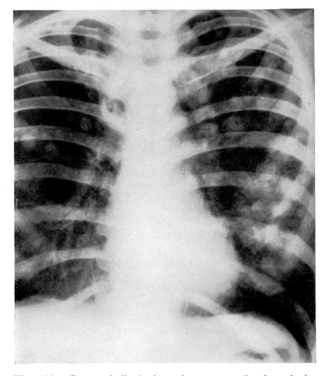

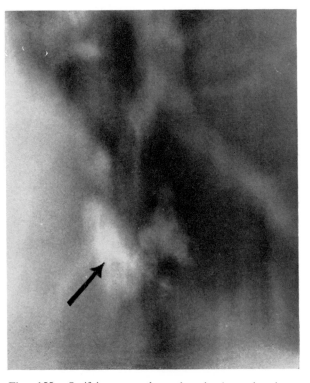

Fig. 154.—Cannon-ball shadows in a case of tuberculosis. Female aged 20 years. Recent cough and sputum which contained tubercle bacilli. Chemotherapy and rest. After 4 years some shrinkage of the shadows. Small central spot of calcium in several of them.

Fig. 155.—Ossifying secondary deposit (posterior-view tomogram left base). Small oval shadow with linear calcification within it, lying behind the left heart border (opposite arrow). Female aged 33 years. Amputation for osteosarcoma of femur 3 years previously. Biopsy proof of bone and lung lesion.

Ossifying secondary deposits

Small calcifications, in fact usually ossifications, are occasionally seen within the "cannon-ball" shadows, particularly when these are caused by secondary deposits from an osteogenic sarcoma (Fig. 155).

Pneumoconiosis and rheumatoid nodules

Several 1–2-cm circular shadows may be seen scattered throughout the lungs of a coal miner with a pneumoconiosis who also has a rheumatoid type of arthritis. They may be sufficiently well defined to suggest secondary deposits but the background of 0·5–1-mm very small circular shadows, together with the occupational history and the evidence of arthritis, will usually indicate the diagnosis. The small background shadows may pass undetected if they are rather inconspicuous, and if the observer's attention is concentrated too much on the larger more sensational shadows. Sometimes, however, they are the predominant feature in the radiograph, or stand out particularly clearly in tomograms. Sometimes the rheumatoid arthritis is obvious, sometimes only really apparent after seeing erosions in radiographs of the bones of the hands or feet.

Much more rarely, similar well-demarcated 2–3-cm roughly circular shadows are seen in a patient with rheumatoid arthritis, but no history of an exposure to an industrial dust hazard or other noxious agent (Fig. 151), and rarely there may be no evidence of joint involvement, but the Latex test is positive, and a rheumatoid type of histology somewhere will confirm the diagnosis.

Histologically such a lesion may show a central necrotic core encapsulated by fibrous tissue with palisading of the cells on its internal aspect.

Fungoid disease

Another cause of the " cannon-ball " type of shadow is histoplasmosis, which in this form is usually only found in patients living in an area where the condition is endemic.

Pleural secondary deposits

Well-defined circular or oval shadows projecting into the lung from its axillary aspect will suggest secondary deposits in the pleura. These may be the only shadows, or there may be a pleural effusion. A large effusion will mask the shadows which nevertheless may still be seen after simple aspiration of some of the fluid. If sufficient fluid cannot be aspirated, the lesions may still be seen after replacement of some of the fluid with air. An anterior-view radiograph is then taken with the x-ray beam horizontal and the patient lying on the opposite side to the fluid, which will then occupy the medial side of the lung field while the air above it will outline the axillary part of the pleura, and thus the lesions (Fig. 156). Such shadows are common in secondary deposits from various primary sites such as the breast or stomach. They may also be seen as local intrathoracic deposits after surgical removal of a thymic tumour, tumour cells probably being seeded into the pleura. Similar shadows may be due to asbestos-induced mesothelioma of the pleura itself.

SINGLE ILL-DEFINED MODERATE-SIZED HOMOGENEOUS SHADOWS

A poorly defined moderate-sized homogeneous shadow smaller than a segment, and without evidence of gross lobar shrinkage, may represent a partial consolidation caused by any of the pneumonias, an infarct, or neoplasm. Such a shadow is seen in asthmatics with bronchopulmonary aspergillosis, consolidation and eosinophilia. These unusual types of consolidation are also seen in some cases of periarteritis nodosa, or diffuse lupus erythematosus. These lesions may be multiple with several such shadows scattered in other lobes.

This poorly defined shadow is sometimes seen associated with other pathological shadows of a different type. Belonging to this category is the 1–2-cm poorly defined area of clouding seen in association with small circular shadows in some cases of coal miners' pneumoconiosis, which Fletcher (1948) called an " ambiguous " shadow—the word being meant to convey the fact that it was not possible to distinguish whether the shadow represented a fibrotic lesion (resulting directly or indirectly from the pneumoconiosis) or an active tuberculous lesion. In either case the very small circular shadows of the basic lesion of the uncomplicated pneumoconiosis are invariably present.

At a later stage in the development of the lesion, the ambiguous shadow becomes rather larger and has a number of linear shadows radiating out from it due to the fibrous scars, the whole lesion being then virtually an area of massive fibrosis (Fig. 192). Throughout all its stages, the larger shadow is always associated with the smaller shadows of the basic lesion. Frequently there is one such large shadow on both sides, giving a " butterfly " appearance.

SINGLE POORLY DEFINED SMALL HOMOGENEOUS SHADOW (THE " SMUDGE SHADOW ")

A poorly defined isolated, small, and rather elongated shadow known as the " smudge shadow " is a variant of the small circular shadow and has a similar list of possible causes. It usually lies in one of the upper zones, and is rather less than 2 cm in size, though it is difficult to measure accurately owing to its poorly defined edges. It is most commonly caused by a tuberculous focus. An ill-defined 1–2 cm shadow or smudge shadow in the lower half of the lung with one aspect against the pleura in the lower axillary region, or against some part of the interlobar pleura in a lateral view, is often due to a small infarct.

MULTIPLE WIDELY DISSEMINATED AMORPHOUS ILL-DEFINED (BLOTCHY) SHADOWS

Secondary deposits

Multiple 1–2 cm amorphous or roughly circular shadows with ill-defined margins, some 1–2 cm in size and which give both lungs an over-all blotchy appearance (Fig. 157), may be seen with multiple secondary deposits, particularly from the prostate, but occasionally from a primary in the breast or stomach, and in pulmonary deposits with one of the reticuloses, usually a lymphosarcoma.

Another form of secondary deposit giving this sort of shadowing is an intra-alveolar spread of a bronchiolar adenocarcinoma. What factors predispose to this type of spread, with a layer of neoplastic cells lining the alveoli, is not known. Occasionally a similar phenomenon may be found from secondary deposits from an extrathoracic adenocarcinoma.

The primary bronchiolar neoplasm and the alveolar spread tend to start insidiously, the chief complaint perhaps being some white frothy sputum, and the radiograph showing an area of clouding suggesting a bacterial pneumonia (*see* p. 45). Some cases are only detected when the lesions are already widespread throughout both lungs.

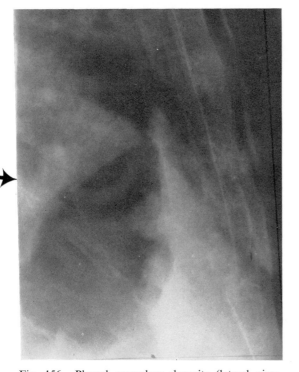

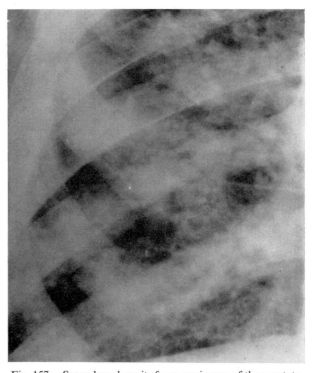

Fig. 156.—Pleural secondary deposits (lateral view, supine, x-ray beam horizontal), 1-cm circular shadows behind the sternum. Arrow points to fluid level after tapping and air replacement. It looks like the edge of the block, but original same width as Fig. 157. In earlier radiograph total opacity left side because of the fluid.

Fig. 157.—Secondary deposits from carcinoma of the prostate. Ill-defined areas of clouding. P.M. Neoplastic deposits and deep lymphatic and perivascular permeation with malignant cells. Also areas of oedema and collapse. Male aged 63 years. No urinary tract symptoms, and chest radiograph for heart lesion. Carcinoma prostate confirmed.

Secondary deposits from a carcinoma of the thyroid are usually of the cannon-ball type, but a less well-defined type of shadow is seen in one form, in which the course is relatively prolonged and benign, and the deposits often disappear after thyroxine or radio-active iodine therapy (Fig. 158).

Pulmonary oedema

In pulmonary oedema, whether the distribution is " bat's wing " (*see* p. 31), diffuse or more localized, the shadowing is rarely homogeneous but blotchy in many or all areas. The opaque blotchy shadows are usually 1–2 cm in size, but may be smaller. The condition may be obvious clinically with signs of heart failure, crepitations in the lungs and frothy sputum. In other cases none of these features is obvious or they are absent, as for instance in pulmonary oedema after cerebral damage from trauma or a haemorrhage, and the radiograph has an important part to play in the diagnosis. In some cases the condition is acute, in others more chronic and the shadows may persist for several days or weeks. The distribution of the blotchy shadows is variable. If the patient happens to lie on the right side all night the shadowing in the radiograph next day may be predominantly on the right (Fig. 160), while if the next night he sleeps on his left side, it may be predominantly on the left. This suggests that the degree of aeration is partly responsible for the blotchy appearance, those alveoli best aerated tending to clear the oedema fluid best; uneven blood distribution may also be a factor. An emphysematous area with poor blood flow (for example, Macleod's syndrome; *see* p. 148) may protect one side entirely from pulmonary oedema.

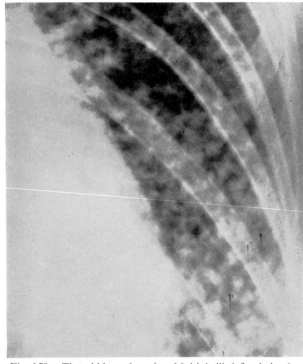

Fig. 158.—Thyroid lung deposits. Multiple ill-defined circular shadows. These were seen throughout both lungs, thinning at the apices. Female aged 37 years. Previous thyroidectomy (innocent). Uptake of [131]I:15 per cent from the lung fields, 6 per cent from the lower neck region. Neck gland biopsy: apparently normal thyroid tissue. Resolution after thyroxine.

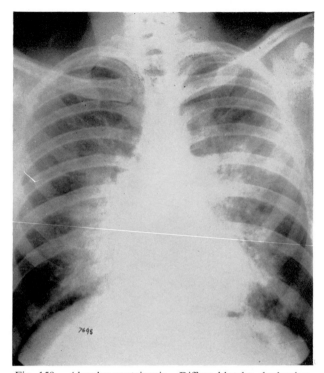

Fig. 159.—Alveolar proteinosis. Diffuse blotchy shadowing perihilar regions. Lung biopsy: eosinophilic alveolar exudate PAS positive, and some alveolar macrophages. Male aged 32 years. Asymptomatic at first, later some dyspnoea. No fever. Normal respiratory function tests. After 3 years' spontaneous recovery, lungs clear.

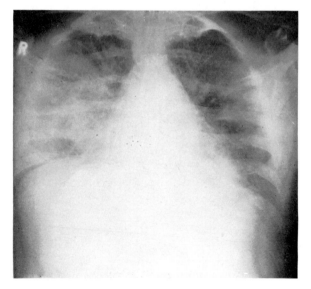

Fig. 160.—Pulmonary oedema of right lung only. Bat's wing distribution. Lay on right side all night. Next night lay on left: right cleared, bat's wing on left.

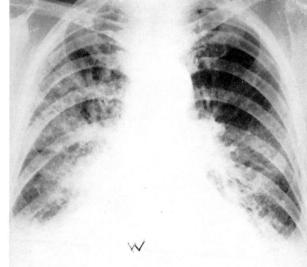

Fig. 161.—Blotchy pulmonary oedema—right lower zone predominance. Male aged 43 years. Acute left ventricular failure from myocardial infarct. Basal crepitations. Resolution after mersalyl and digoxin.

In many cases the shadowing is localized to a part of one lobe (Fig. 161), and in the mistaken belief that the shadows represent inflammatory lesions the patient is treated with antibiotics, whereas digoxin and diuretics would have been more appropriate.

Blotchy shadows may occur in local oedema associated with periarteritis nodosa or are found spreading out from the hila in the condition of alveolar proteinosis described by Rosen, Castleman and Liebow (1958) and illustrated in Fig. 159. Pathologically, a PAS-positive pink-staining exudate is seen in the alveoli.

Blotchy shadows throughout the lungs may be seen after the accidental inhalation of an irritant gas or spray (chemically induced pulmonary oedema or pneumonia) or after the inhalation of vomit, or after drowning with recovery. Similar shadows may be seen in a patient sensitive to some therapeutic drug (examples are PAS, penicillin and nitrofurantoin). They may be caused by the inhalation of paraffin droplets, taken as nasal sprays or as a laxative.

Blotchy shadows or coarse nodular shadows throughout the lungs may be due to haemorrhages into the lungs (lung purpura). This may occur during an acute incident in idiopathic pulmonary haemosiderosis. It is also seen as a result of a blast injury to the lungs or simple trauma.

Unusual immunity mechanisms

Infections of the lung either with an attenuated organism or in a patient in a depressed immunological state, such as agamma-globulinaemia, or a non-specific granulomatous lymph gland lesion in children, may lead to blotchy shadows throughout the lungs because of the unusual relationship between the infecting organism and the patient.

Cystic fibrosis

In cystic fibrosis the local disturbance of mucus secretion makes the lung prone to pulmonary infections, particularly with staphylococci, and these lesions are often patchy and widespread giving the lungs a blotchy appearance. The appearance of such shadows is of grave significance, though several infective incidents may be overcome.

Fungoid lesions

The shadows in a diffuse pulmonary fungoid lesion are often poorly defined, and give the lungs a blotchy appearance. Actinomycosis is one such cause, and the patient may not be very ill at first, while the fungus may only be found in the sputum after a careful search. Histoplasmosis or blastomycosis presenting with this blotchy type of shadow, rather than a miliary type, is found only in regions where such diseases are endemic.

WIDELY DISSEMINATED VERY SMALL CIRCULAR SHADOWS (NODULAR OR MILIARY SHADOWS)

Circular shadows, ranging from pin-point size (perhaps only visible under low magnification) to 5 mm, and scattered fairly uniformly over a considerable area or throughout both lung fields, may be found in a great variety of conditions. A list compiled by Scadding (1952) contains 83 causes. Such a formidable list of possibilities may be much reduced in an individual case partly by the clinical findings and partly by the radiological appearances.

Clinical findings

A case presenting with nodular shadows and fever or constitutional upset will suggest an infection such as miliary tuberculosis, a viral infection and so on.

The presence of a primary neoplasm (in the breast, for example) will suggest secondary deposits, and the murmur of mitral stenosis will suggest haemosiderosis.

An industrial history such as coal mining will suggest a pneumoconiosis. The industrial history should include past as well as present occupations and the duration of the industrial hazard, if this appears relevant. Whereas many years have to be spent in coal mining before nodular pulmonary shadows are likely to appear, quite a short exposure to asbestos may lead to gross fibrosing alveolitis, or an even shorter exposure to beryllium may lead to sarcoid-like lesions in the lungs. Contact with an industrial hazard may only be elicited on careful questioning. In one case of asbestosis the contact consisted of no more than shaking out her sister's clothing after the day's work in an asbestos factory; in another, it was the demolition of a shed with an asbestos lining.

In hobby risks, for instance keeping a bird (budgerigar, pigeon or parrot) as a pet, the contact will not be mentioned by the patient, unless he is specifically questioned about it. Keeping a bird is not sufficient evidence for considering it as a cause of the lung lesion; but it can be presumed to be so if immunological tests such as a skin reaction or a serum precipitin test against the bird's serum are positive. The test will be negative if the patient has cryptogenic fibrosing alevolitis not due to the bird contact.

Repeated haemoptyses in a young adult, or an obscure secondary anaemia in a child, will suggest idiopathic haemosiderosis. In this condition, the lesions tend to progress and the end result may be respiratory failure. Some cases eventually develop a fatal renal lesion. In a few cases the lung lesions become static.

A few small nodular shadows just above the costophrenic angle with some dilatation of the nearby peripheral vessels may be seen in the late stage of some cases of cirrhosis of the liver, and seem to be caused by small lesions in the lungs like the spider naevi sometimes found in the skin. In a patient over 40 years old, dyspnoea and clubbing with nodular shadows, particularly in the lower zones (Fig. 164), will suggest fibrosing alveolitis (Scadding, 1964), sometimes known as diffuse interstitial pulmonary fibrosis; and in one form as acute desquamative pneumonia (Liebow, 1965). Basal crepitations are usually present. There may be a dry cough, while some patients produce sputum, often not until a later stage.

The course is variable. The cases described by Hamman and Rich (1944) ran a relatively acute course, but others described by Scadding (1960) survived for many years, and may have had a different aetiology though a similar histological appearance. The age of onset ranges from childhood to very old, but the common age is between 40 and 65 years. In most cases by the time the patient has dyspnoea, nodular and short line shadows will be seen in the radiograph.

Diabetes insipidus (with a normal sella), or the finding of cyst-like transradiant areas in the bones, either in the routine chest radiograph (Fig. 169) or in additional radiographs taken of the skull, major long bones or pelvis, will suggest xanthomatous granulomas (histiocytosis X) as a cause of the lung shadows.

The presence of scleroderma, or of Raynaud's phenomenon without skin thickening, together with small subcutaneous calcifications (often best seen in a lateral-view radiograph of the finger tips) and perhaps oesophageal inertia (seen during a barium swallow examination done with the patient lying down), will suggest diffuse systemic sclerosis. Mental deficiency with subungual fibromata or adenoma sebaceum, and in many cases small intracranial calcifications in a lateral radiograph of the skull, will suggest that the ill-defined small circular shadows in the lung are due to tuberose sclerosis (mesodermal dysplasia).

Some pathological features related to nodular shadows

In miliary tuberculosis the lesions are discrete, often only 2–3 mm in size and very numerous. It is probable that the nodular shadows seen in the radiograph (Fig. 162) do not represent an individual tubercle, these often being too small or insufficiently opaque to be seen, and it is therefore likely that the shadow seen in the radiograph is due to several small pathological lesions being superimposed. In the early stages before the foci reach a critical size or number per unit area, and again as they are reduced in size by antibiotics, they may be invisible even in a good quality radiograph. Not all the shadows are nodular, and the small ring shadows often seen (Fig. 162) are artefactual and not due to dilated air spaces. This can be shown experimentally. Carstairs (1961) arranged small circular plastic balls spaced like the lesions in miliary tuberculosis. On taking a radiograph of the model nodular shadows were seen, but if the number of layers of the balls was increased, a mixture of nodular and small ring shadows was seen.

In fibrosing alveolitis the nodular and short line shadows are artefactual since the thickening of the alveolar walls is diffuse and not nodular. Carstairs, using sheets of plastic foam of varying pore and wall size, found that as the wall became thicker the x-ray appearance became more nodular. A similar effect may be responsible for the nodular shadows seen in fibrosing alveolitis. In this condition five grades of pathological change can be identified microscopically (Livingstone and colleagues, 1964).

(1) Thickening of the alveolar wall by reticulin or collagen with dilatation of the capillaries.
(2) The changes of (1) with, in addition, cells and exudate in the alveolar spaces.
(3) Fibrosis in the alveolar spaces causing blurring of outline of the alveolar architecture.
(4) Fibrous obliteration of the alveolar spaces.
(5) Cystic spaces varying in size from 3 to 15 mm.

These form the basis for the honeycomb shadows seen in the late stage of fibrosing alveolitis (Fig. 169) whether cryptogenic, related to bird contact, mouldy hay in farming, xanthomatous lesions and so on. The wall of such a space may consist of just collagen and fibrous tissue suggesting it is an alveolar space, or there may be ciliated epithelium and muscle suggesting it is a dilated bronchiolus. Sometimes a single space shows a wall of alveolar tissue in one part and bronchiolar tissue in another part.

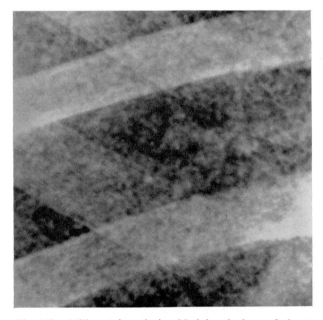

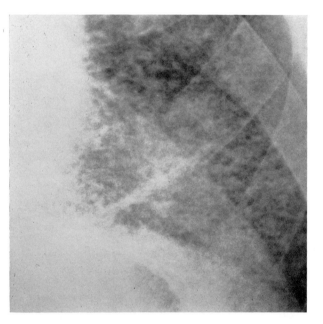

Fig. 162.—Miliary tuberculosis. Nodular shadows of about 3 mm in size in all zones. The apices were equally affected. Many of the nodular shadows appear quite discrete. Male aged 25 years. Fever and weight loss. Sputum: T.B. + ve. Got meningitis and died (pre-chemotherapy era).

Fig. 163.—Fibrosing alveolitis (idiopathic interstitial pulmonary fibrosis). Lower zone haze (both sides) and very small nodular shadows. Male aged 38 years. Increasing dyspnoea and clubbing. Biopsy: alveolar wall thickening with macrophages and fibrous tissue, some organizing exudate.

In grade 2 type of change the alveoli are filled with large " mononuclear " cells which the electron microscope has shown are derived from one of the alveolar lining cells, the pneumonocyte type 2. This is the condition named acute desquamative pneumonia by Liebow. His work was based almost entirely on biopsy material, but if several areas of lung are examined the changes associated with scarring and cyst formation may also be found, suggesting it is probably not a separate disease.

Sometimes honeycomb spaces are associated with other lesions elsewhere. These may be xanthomas and will suggest the cause of the condition. Sometimes small sarcoid lesions or asbestos bodies are seen, suggesting these have caused the fibrosing alveolitis.

In idiopathic haemosiderosis iron is included in macrophages. These accumulate at the centre of the acinus in the alveoli opening into the respiratory bronchiolus and in those at the edge of the acinus. These clumps of iron-containing macrophages are between 0·5 and 5 mm in diameter, and are probably the basis for the very small nodular shadows seen in the radiograph. Surprisingly little fibrosis or tissue reaction is seen.

In mitral stenosis the same histological features may be seen, but there may be alveolar wall oedema as well. The haemosiderin also accumulates adjacent to the septa and may add opacity to the oedematous septum and accentuate the horizontal line shadow.

Radiological features

Certain radiological features may assist in elucidating the cause of nodular shadows in the lungs, or will at any rate limit the number of possibilities. The size, the distribution of the shadows, the number or the density (radio-opacity) of the shadows, and the presence and character of any associated shadows should all be recorded.

Three main types of nodular shadows of tissue density are seen. In the first the shadows are about 2–5 mm in size and are evenly distributed throughout the lungs, including the apices, and many of the nodules appear to be discrete so that one gets the impression that with the aid of a pair of tweezers (fine forceps) it would be possible to grip and pluck out an individual shadow. These appearances are seen particularly in *miliary tuberculosis* (Fig. 162).

The second type consists of nodules which are less easy to distinguish because they are against a background haze or partly lost amongst short line shadows or small ring (honeycomb) shadows, while the distribution is commonly in the lower half of the lungs (Figs. 163 and 164). These appearances are seen in *fibrosing alveolitis*.

The third type of nodular shadow is larger and about 5–10 mm in size. The shadows are either well defined and less numerous than the nodular shadows in miliary tuberculosis, or are ill defined and possibly have a predominantly mid-zone distribution. Alternatively the shadows are pin-point with a mid-zone predominance. On this basis it is possible to divide cases up into those like *miliary tuberculosis* (Fig. 162), those like *fibrosing alveolitis* (Fig. 163) and the rest.

Shadows like miliary tuberculosis

Shadows like miliary tuberculosis (Fig. 162) are also seen in acute histoplasmosis. This diagnosis would be likely if the patient were living in an area in the U.S.A. or Canada where the disease is endemic, and would be most unlikely if they live elsewhere.

In an ill patient with fever, an acute viral pneumonia would be a possibility, though proof of the diagnosis might have to depend either on the clinical course or on the serological tests.

In an asymptomatic person a pneumoconiosis is a possibility if there is a suitable industrial history. In coal workers the size and number of discrete nodular shadows are very variable. The category of the pneumoconiosis can be deduced from the distribution and size of the shadows, as in the Medical Research Council classification (Fletcher, 1948) or that of the International Labour Office (1959). In coal workers there is no evidence that these nodular shadows even when numerous and large (category 3) are the cause of symptoms. However, there is a risk that later the person may develop areas of progressive massive fibrosis as in Fig. 192, and these may cause sufficient loss of lung tissue to give dyspnoea. On the other hand, the finding of nodular shadows like miliary tuberculosis is often more serious in silicosis or china-clay-induced lesions, and even more serious in the case of beryllium.

In sarcoidosis the shadows are very rarely like miliary tuberculosis, though they may be in some cases, or when the larger less well-defined lesions are resolving.

In haemosiderosis from mitral stenosis the shadows may simulate those of miliary tuberculosis, but tend to be rather smaller and are less evenly distributed throughout the lungs, being for the most part concentrated in the middle two-thirds of the lung fields, the apices escaping.

In tropical eosinophilia the shadows may be like miliary tuberculosis, but are often larger and less well defined.

In allergic alveolitis the nodular shadows are often either finer or less well defined than in miliary tuberculosis, but sometimes they are fairly discrete and therefore similar.

In haemorrhage into the lung, and inhalation of blood following a haemoptysis, nodular shadows may be seen like coarse miliary tuberculosis.

Discrete nodular shadows like miliary tuberculosis may be seen in acute pulmonary oedema. The clinical picture will indicate the cause.

In the respiratory distress syndrome of the premature infant nodular discrete shadows like miliary tuberculosis may be seen at one stage (*see* p. 31).

In an infant who is ill from Gaucher's disease there is splenomegaly and there are multiple small bone erosions as well as nodular shadows in the lung like miliary tuberculosis. These are caused by infiltration with the Gaucher's type of cell.

Shadows like cryptogenic fibrosing alveolitis

Shadows like cryptogenic fibrosing alveolitis illustrated in Figs. 163 and 164 are seen in patients with a history of contact with asbestos, a bird, mouldy hay (if a farmer), or some other noxious agents. Alternatively, there may be evidence of a xanthomatous granuloma (histiocytosis X) elsewhere, or of diffuse systemic sclerosis or rheumatoid arthritis (*see* pp. 89 and 94).

In some cases the distribution may be more widespread than in Fig. 164, or may be predominantly in the mid or upper zones.

Compression of lung by upper zone bullae may give an appearance simulating fibrosing alveolitis, but closer inspection of the radiograph will show crowding of small peripheral vessels and not nodular shadows.

Figures 163 and 164 illustrate the appearances seen in many cases of fibrosing alveolitis. In others honeycomb shadows may predominate over the nodular shadows (Fig. 169), or there may be larger areas of patchy clouding with or without upper lobe shrinkage (Fig. 170).

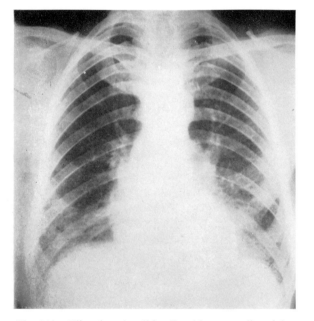

Fig. 164.—Fibrosing alveolitis. Basal haze, small nodular and honeycomb shadows and faint septal line shadows. Male aged 58 years. Dyspnoea and clubbing, basal crepitations. Low DLco. Biopsy: fibrosing alveolitis.

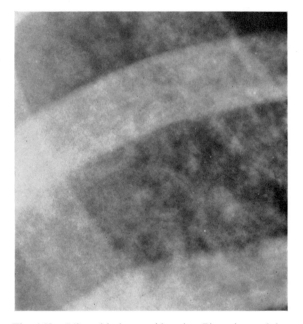

Fig. 165.—Idiopathic haemosiderosis. Pin-point nodular shadows and ordinary nodular shadows. Apices fewer nodules. Female aged 28 years. Small haemoptyses many years. Hb 84%. Biopsy: haemosiderosis.

Nodular shadows not like miliary tuberculosis or fibrosing alveolitis

Discrete 5–10-mm fairly well-defined circular shadows, that is, shadows larger and fewer per unit area than those seen with miliary tuberculosis, will suggest *secondary deposits*. Often the presence of a primary neoplasm is known and this will indicate the diagnosis.

Discrete 5–8-mm rather poorly defined shadows quite unlike miliary tuberculosis, with a predominantly mid zone or upper third distribution, are seen in *sarcoidosis*, and the acino-nodular type of tuberculosis. Differentiation of these two conditions will be possible from the clinical findings.

Discrete ill-defined shadows 2–5 mm in size and fewer in number than miliary tuberculosis are seen in some cases of tuberous sclerosis.

Pin-point shadows, smaller than miliary tuberculosis, or a mixture of nodular and pin-point shadows, will suggest haemosiderosis especially if the patient has mitral stenosis or repeated haemoptyses. The distribution at first tends to be mid zone. If the shadows are very numerous, they may cause a ground-glass appearance. Similar shadows are seen in microlithiasis alveolaris, and the background haze is particularly dense.

The distribution of the shadows

The distribution of the shadows is often of help. For instance, miliary tuberculosis and sarcoidosis tend to involve the apices as well as the rest of the lungs. In many of the pneumoconioses, the shadows are at first predominantly in the mid zones. A predominantly mid-zone distribution is also a feature of haemosiderosis, whether idiopathic or associated with mitral stenosis. A lower half distribution is common in fibrosing alveolitis (Fig. 164), while a predominantly upper half distribution is a feature of bird fanciers' lung. In farmers' lung the distribution is often widespread. A mid-zone perihilar distribution is seen in some cases of pulmonary oedema and alveolar proteinosis.

Many of these lesions, such as haemosiderosis or pneumoconiosis, may start with a mid-zone distribution and eventually spread all over the lungs, so that in the late stage the distribution may be different from that seen in an earlier stage.

The radio-opacity (density) of widely disseminated small shadows

Endogenous particles.—The radio-opacity or density of the small circular shadows should also be noted. In haemosiderosis the radio-opacity may be so great that the radiograph appears under-exposed. Similar very small shadows of high radio-opacity due to endogenous calcification in the alveolar regions of the lungs of unknown aetiology have been described by Sharp and Danino (1953), the condition being known as microlithiasis alveolaris.

Exogenous particles.—Exogenous particles of high atomic number are sometimes inhaled into the lungs and, if they remain there, cast very conspicuous shadows because of their high radio-opacity. A man working in an atmosphere laden with particles of barium, calcium (in the manufacture of talc), iron (particularly in welding, boiler scaling, or haematite mining), or tin (smelting), may have many very radio-opaque shadows varying from pin-point size to 2 mm scattered throughout both lung fields. If the dust or vapour contained only these relatively innocuous atoms of high atomic number, the worker may have no disability at all in spite of the rather sensational shadows seen on the radiograph, but if silica particles were also present, the man may have a coexisting true pneumoconiosis and may suffer severe disability as a result of it. The small shadows of the pneumoconiosis may then be masked in the radiograph by the very radio-opaque pin-point shadows of the exogenous metal particles. In a haematite miner, for example, the relatively innocuous condition of siderosis with iron particles uncomplicated by pneumoconiosis will give similar radiographic appearances to those of the more serious condition in which both lesions are present. The presence of hypertransradiant bullae or bullous areas, or of shadows suggesting areas of massive fibrosis, in addition to the pin-point shadows, would point to the diagnosis of pneumoconiosis.

Iodized oil residues in the lung following bronchography give rise to characteristic dense pin-point spots, or 0·5-mm dense circular shadows, sometimes arranged in small 2-mm rings; there are also true 1-mm ring shadows. Histological examination shows these residues are no longer in the air spaces, but incorporated in the tissues. Not to be confused with these very dense shadows are widely disseminated 1-mm low-density circular shadows which are sometimes seen in the lung following a bronchogram with either iodized oil or propyliodone. They are probably a reaction to the suspending medium, and some of the lesions are small non-specific granulomas. They are not usually progressive or of clinical significance.

Tuberculosis with calcification.—Calcifications, whether these are in tuberculous foci or in some other pathological lesion, are also of considerable radio-opacity. The shadows of multiple calcified foci in a patient with tuberculosis usually show considerable variation in size and shape, some being smooth in outline and circular, and others perhaps oval, linear, Y-shaped or with irregular margins and of no particular shape; they vary from pin-point size to several millimetres. In some shadows the uncalcified part of the initial focus is still visible, so that a low-density halo shadow is seen around the more radio-opaque calcium.

Histoplasmosis.—Shadows of a similar character to this are seen in the late stage of histoplasmosis, but in this condition the shadows are often characteristic and are much more uniform in size and shape, appearing as 1–2-mm circular shadows all more or less of the same size, and at one stage many of them are surrounded with a low-density halo shadow (Fig. 166). These lesions are found mainly in people living in certain areas of the United States of America, and, although cases are sometimes seen in

Britain, it is usually found that the patients have spent some months or years in the areas of America where the disease is endemic. The acute stage, in which the shadows simulate those of miliary tuberculosis, is rarely seen in a patient who has always lived in Britain, and the disease is generally fatal before healing and calcification can occur.

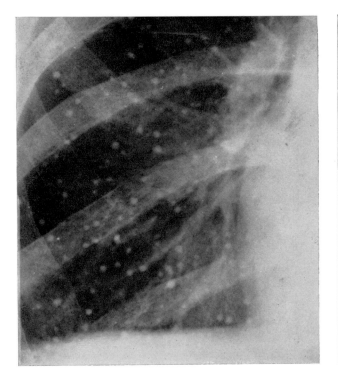

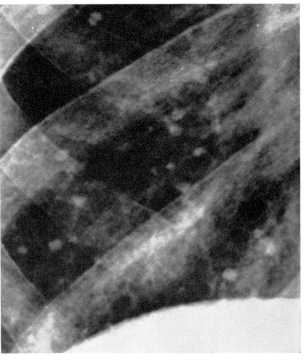

Fig. 166.—Histoplasmosis. Small 2-mm dense circular shadows of equal size. Halo of low-density shadow round many of them. Male aged 43 years. Previous long residence in Canada, and two visits to Detroit. Strongly positive histoplasmin test extract from United States of America.

Fig. 167.—Dense 2–6 mm circular shadows in the left lower zone (similar shadows in the right lower zone). Lung biopsy taken when the left chest explored during operation for mitral stenosis. Histology of hard nodule showed bone with Haversian canals, and marrow spaces with fatty marrow.

Chicken pox pneumonia.—Discrete dense shadows of about 2 mm in size, scattered throughout the lungs may be due to healed lesions of chicken pox pneumonia (Fig. 168). In acute chicken pox with lung involvement in adults, coarse ill-defined nodular shadows may be seen throughout the lungs which resolve with clinical recovery. Dense calcifications may appear some 2 years later reaching a size of 2 mm and then become static (Fig. 168). No pathology of these lesions is yet available.

Ectopic bone.—A few 2–5 mm very radio-opaque well-defined circular shadows of uniform size may be seen scattered in the lower half of the lungs in a patient with mitral stenosis (Fig. 167) and are often found to consist of ectopic bone which may even have Haversian canals. They may also be found following acute rheumatic fever even in the absence of a valvular lesion, and are presumably the result of old rheumatic pulmonary foci. Such shadows develop to full size within a year and then remain static. This transition from a normal lung to the appearance of the small dense circular shadows is seen many years after the initial clinical manifestation of rheumatic fever.

ASSOCIATED SHADOWS

The presence of other shadows in addition to the discrete nodular shadows is often of great help in diagnosis.

Nodular shadows associated with a ground-glass haze

A very fine ground-glass appearance throughout the lungs, seen as a haze with fine pin-point shadows superimposed on it, probably visible only with the aid of a magnifying glass, is seen in the respiratory distress syndrome of the newborn premature baby. In a later stage the nodular shadows may be larger, but unlike miliary tuberculosis are seen against a hazy background. An identical nodular pattern in a newborn infant may be caused by haemorrhage into lung tissue.

Similar nodular shadows may be seen in the Mikity–Wilson syndrome (Wilson and Mikity, 1960). In this condition the shadows change after two or three weeks to diffuse area of opacity and short line shadows with 0·5–1 cm areas of normal lung between them which simulate cystic spaces. In many cases the shadows eventually disappear and the lung appears normal.

Nodular shadows superimposed on a lower zone haze is a common finding in fibrosing alveolitis.

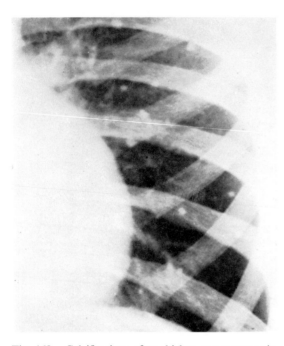

Fig. 168.—Calcifications after chicken pox pneumonia. There are 3–5-mm dense circular shadows in both lungs, mainly mid-half. Aged 9 years. Severe chicken pox 3 years ago. Asymptomatic. (Left base only reproduced.)

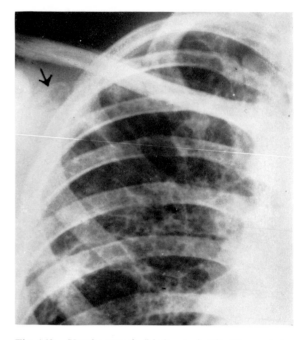

Fig. 169.—Xanthomatosis (histiocytosis X). Linear, hair-line ring up to 2 cm and a few nodular shadows. Erosion scapula (below arrow). Biopsy: eosinophil granuloma. Male aged 12 years. Severe dyspnoea for 9 months, increasing.

Nodular shadows associated with short line shadows

Nodular shadows associated with short line shadows is a common finding in fibrosing alveolitis whatever the cause (Fig. 163). Two sorts of short line shadow are seen; first, very short line shadows mixed up with the nodular shadows, and second, short 1–2-cm horizontal line shadows above the costophrenic recesses due to thickened interlobular septa. A similar appearance is seen in some *pneumoconioses*, particularly asbestosis and in some coal workers' lungs, and tin handlers. They may be seen in some cases of microlithiasis alveolaris.

Short peripheral line shadows rather like septal line shadows and some nodular shadows have been described in patients with the symptoms of severe chronic bronchitis, a condition described as " disease of small airways " by Fraser, Macklen and Thurlbeck (1970).

Nodular shadows associated with long line and septal line shadows

Long 2–4 cm hair-line shadows starting in the periphery of the upper zones and directed towards the hila, but dissociated from the vessels' shadows (Kerley "A" lines, *see* p. 114), when seen with small nodular shadows would suggest *lymphangitis carcinomatosa* (Fig. 189). Sometimes the lines stand out more than the 1–2 mm nodular shadows which may only be seen if carefully sought, if necessary with the aid of a magnifying glass. Sometimes the nodular shadows are most conspicuous and the lines will only be seen if carefully sought. There may or may not be septal line shadows as well.

Nodular shadows associated with small ring (honeycomb) shadows

Well-defined ring shadows with a radius of 3–8 mm and a wall 1–2 mm thick, usually in groups and thus described as honeycomb shadows (Fig. 216), are often seen in association with small or large nodular shadows and are characteristic of the group of lesions described as fibrosing alveolitis, of which pathologically they represent a late stage. They may be seen in the cryptogenic form of fibrosing alveolitis, in asbestos-induced fibrosis, in diffuse systemic sclerosis, or in association with rheumatoid arthritis. They are seen in known allergic alveolitis such as in farmers' lung, bird fanciers' lung, malt workers' lung and so on, and in patients taking pituitary snuff. They are a prominent feature in the late stage of many cases of xanthomatous (histiocytosis X) lung lesions. In this condition the ring shadows are often widespread and may be larger and 1–2 cm in diameter (Fig. 169). Nodular shadows may be conspicuous, or there may only be a few and these only seen if carefully looked for. When there are many ring shadows but few nodular shadows the appearance is sometimes called honeycomb lung. In the late stage of idiopathic haemosiderosis there may even be a honeycomb appearance together with the nodular shadows. This is probably artefactual.

Nodular shadows associated with shrunken upper lobes

Shrunken upper lobes with rather coarse ill-defined nodular shadows below are of course a feature of chronic tuberculosis. A similar appearance is seen in some cases of bird fanciers' lung (Fig. 170). The nodular shadows tend to be smaller than in tuberculosis with shrunken upper lobes, the mantoux reaction is often negative, and in the specimens examined so far there was no evidence of past or present tuberculous lesions. A similar x-ray appearance may be seen very occasionally in cryptogenic fibrosing alveolitis. In allergic aspergillosis lobar shrinkage is common, but nodular shadows are inconspicuous.

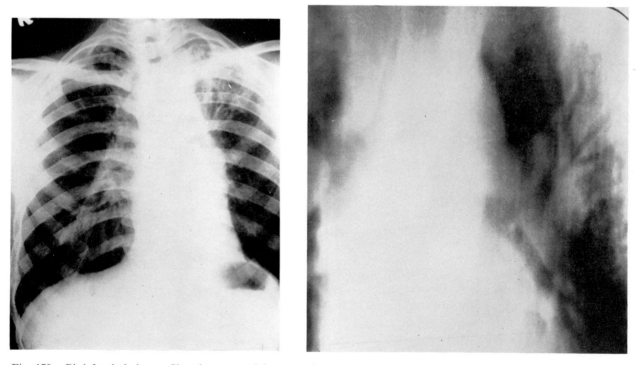

Fig. 170.—Bird fancier's lung. Shrunken upper lobes. Right apical nodular shadows. Male aged 23 years. Keeps pigeons. Skin prick + ve. Serum precipitins + ve. Bronchial challenge + ve. P.M. no tuberculosis. Tubular shadows (of bronchiectases—bronchographic proof) in shrunken left upper lobe.

Fig. 171.—Sarcoidosis (mid-zone tomogram at hilum level). Enlarged hilar glands, diffuse opacity mid zones with air bronchogram. Some nodular shadows (not visible in reproduction). Male aged 42 years. Some dyspnoea. Lung biopsy: sarcoid. Resolution 4 years.

Shrunken upper lobes with a few ill-defined nodular shadows and often some long line shadows in the upper third of the lung may be seen as a late manifestation of sarcoidosis. In such cases, instead of the usual resolution, the lesions have coalesced and become fibrotic.

Nodular shadows associated with large homogeneous shadows

A few nodular shadows with a large homogeneous shadow may be seen in a patient with asthma and bronchopulmonary aspergillosis with eosinophilia. A few residual ill-defined nodular shadows may be seen with a large mid or upper zone homogeneous shadow in the late stage of sarcoidosis in which resolution failed to occur (Fig. 171).

Nodular shadows with a large upper zone circular or oval shadow are seen in some pneumoconioses if they develop an area of progressive massive fibrosis (Fig. 192). Often the large shadows are more or less symmetrical on either side. They may occur in a lower zone. In coal workers these large lesions may be present with very few nodular shadows, and these may only be found if carefully looked for, or there may be many nodular shadows which are clearly seen (*see* p. 114).

Nodular shadows associated with a raised diaphragm

Nodular shadows in fibrosing alveolitis are the result of lesions which will reduce lung compliance, and this may be manifested in the radiograph by a relatively high position of the diaphragm. This feature may be more obvious if earlier radiographs are available showing the diaphragm at a lower level.

In more acute lesions such as miliary tuberculosis or ordinary secondary deposits this is not seen, but it may occur when the nodular shadows and line shadows are due to lymphangitis carcinomatosa.

Nodular shadows associated with abnormalities of the heart shadow

Nodular shadows with cardiac enlargement or a prominent left atrial appendage or pulmonary artery, will suggest that the lesions are secondary to the heart condition, and due either to pulmonary oedema or to haemosiderosis.

Associated hilar gland enlargement

Hilar gland enlargement associated with rather coarse ill-defined mid-zone nodular shadows is a common finding in sarcoidosis. The glands, which are usually present on both sides, are well-demarcated, about 2–3 cm in size, and lying particularly in the angle between the lobar bronchi. Sometimes the hilar regions are much obscured in the plain radiographs by overlying nodular and diffuse shadowing, but they can nevertheless be clearly demonstrated in hilar level posterior-view tomograms (Fig. 348).

Similar nodular shadows and enlarged hilar glands may be seen in tuberculosis, but on the whole they are less symmetrical on the two sides, and tend to lie more medially. In either condition there may also be enlargement of the paratracheal glands.

Enlarged hilar glands and nodular shadows in the lungs may also be seen in Hodgkin's disease and secondary deposits from a carcinoma. In such cases the glands are usually rather less sharply defined.

Associated cavities, bronchiectases or bullae

Cavities or bullae associated with nodular shadows are often best seen in tomograms. Either may be seen in tuberculosis or sarcoidosis, though well-defined rather thick-walled cavities are much more common in tuberculosis. Large ring shadows like cavities may in fact be due to dilated bronchi, particularly in asthma with bronchopulmonary aspergillosis and eosinophilia. The nodular shadows are usually inconspicuous. Bullae associated with nearby stellate or linear scars may complicate the healing stage of any of these diseases. In those few cases of sarcoidosis which do not resolve, the nodular shadowing tends to be replaced by wide bands of opacity with intervening hypertransradiant avascular bullous areas (Fig. 171). Such " emphysematous " areas are local and associated with the scars, general widespread emphysema in fact seldom being a late complication of sarcoidosis. On the other hand, nodular shadows due to xanthomatous lesion may begin to resolve, leaving large areas of vessel narrowing or vessel loss. This may be so obvious that the term " vanishing lung " is appropriate. The diaphragm may become low and flat, so that resolving xanthomatous lesions may truly be the cause of panacinar emphysema in such cases. The xanthomatous granulomata are very erosive, and this may lead to alveolar disintegration and destruction and so to the emphysema.

Guide to interpretation of widely disseminated small shadows

In Table 3 these lesions are grouped according to the variations in their radiographic appearances, and correlated to the more obvious clinical findings. The Table, which is by no means all inclusive, is intended to act as a rough guide to the interpretation of these widely disseminated small homo-geneous circular shadows. It is assumed that, before using the Table, the observer would be familiar with the clinical picture and would have made a careful study of the radiograph, noting in particular the size, number, distribution, shape, and radio-opacity of the shadows. In the many hundreds of such cases seen by the author, of which the pneumoconioses did not form an unduly high proportion, the cause of the shadows was found without undue difficulty in all but a few, although actual bacteriological or histological proof was sometimes lacking. In a few cases, the cause was found only after elaborate, and sometimes possibly unnecessary, investigations, while in only 3 cases has no diagnosis yet been made.

TABLE 3

1. Widely disseminated 2–4 mm nodular shadows (like miliary tuberculosis)

Miliary tuberculosis	Perhaps sputum T.B. + ve. Fever
Acute histoplasmosis	Histoplasmin test + ve. Lives in area
Acute viral pneumonia	Fever, prostration; later viral studies + ve
Gaucher's disease in children	Splenomegaly. Bone lesions
Xanthomatosis (histiocytosis X)	Diabetes inspidus. Bone lesions
Some pneumoconioses	Industrial history (coal, beryllium)
Idiopathic haemosiderosis	Haemoptyses. Often young adult
Haemosiderosis in mitral stenosis	Heart lesion obvious
Periarteritis	Rare, perhaps eosinophilia
Tropical eosinophilia	High eosinophilia in white blood count
Some pituitary disorders	Endocrine lesion obvious
Some inhaled antigens	Immunological tests + ve. Bird contact, mouldy hay

2. Discrete 5–8 mm well-defined shadows

Secondary deposits	Perhaps known primary neoplasm

3. Discrete 5–8 mm poorly defined shadows

Sarcoidosis	Often not ill. Iridocyclitis. Perhaps skin nodule
Acino-nodular tuberculosis	Sputum T.B. + ve
Pulmonary oedema	Cardiac or renal lesion. Water overload
Aspiration	Drowning, blood (haemoptysis)
Fungi	Perhaps sputum + ve
Viral	Obvious chicken pox. Fever

4. Pin-point shadows

Idiopathic haemosiderosis	Haemoptyses, often young adult
Microlithiasis alveolaris	Very radio-opaque
Respiratory distress of newborn	First few days of infancy

5. Ground-glass haze and pin-point shadows

Respiratory distress of newborn	First few days of infancy
Fibrosing alveolitis	Dyspnoea and clubbing. Low DLco

6. Shadows of high radio-opacity (nodular 1–5 mm)

Calcifications in healing lesions	Tuberculous, histoplasmosis. Chicken pox
Endogenous calcification	Microlithiasis alveolaris
Ectopic bone	Rheumatic fever and mitral stenosis
Inhaled material of high atomic weight	Iron, barium, tin and so on. Iodized oil

Nodular shadows associated with other shadows (like fibrosing alveolitis)

7. Associated with short line shadows

Fibrosing alveolitis	Dyspnoea and clubbing. Low DLco
Some pneumoconioses	Industrial history

8. Associated with long line and short line shadows

Lymphangitis carcinomatosa	Perhaps known primary neoplasm

9. Associated with small ring (honeycomb) shadows

Fibrosing alveolitis	Dyspnoea and clubbing. Evidence of xanthomatosis, bird contact

10. Associated with shrunken upper lobes

Tuberculosis	Sputum T.B. + ve
Sarcoidosis	Clinical course
Bird fanciers' lung	Immunological tests + ve
Farmers' lung	Contact with mouldy hay
Fibrosing alveolitis	Cryptogenic. Dyspnoea and clubbing

CHAPTER 3

LINEAR SHADOWS (LINE, BAND-LIKE, TUBULAR AND RING SHADOWS)

A LINE shadow varies in width from a narrow, hardly discernible hair line to a shadow 1–2 mm wide. If it is wider than this it becomes a band-like shadow. If it is about 0·5 cm wide it may be called a " tooth paste " shadow. The band-like shadow may be up to 1–2 cm wide. Both line and band-like shadows vary in length from a few millimetres to several centimetres, and may be straight or slightly curved. If two line shadows run parallel to each other, enclosing a 1–5 mm transradiant zone, the result is a tubular shadow. If the line is curved in a circular or oval fashion, so that it surrounds a central transradiant zone, it forms a ring shadow. All these shadows are essentially linear in type (in contrast, for instance, to triangular, circular, or oval homogeneous opacities) and are therefore grouped together.

LINE SHADOWS

Line shadows, even excluding the vessel shadows, are very common, and are often not given due weight in x-ray diagnosis. They are, however, of considerable importance, whether they represent a normal structure such as the horizontal fissure in a normal or displaced position, or whether they represent a pathological lesion such as an atelectatic segment which may be the first indication of a bronchial carcinoma.

Line shadows are most commonly caused by normal pleura or a small pleural exudate, whether still fluid or organizing and fibrous. The normal horizontal fissure is usually visible in a routine anterior-view radiograph, and the lower half of the main interlobar fissure in the lateral-view radiograph. The pleura over the apex of the lower lobe, or the peripheral axillary pleura, is usually only visible when pathologically widened. A line shadow may also result from a dilated or thickened lymphatic channel, which may be deep in the lung, lying in the interlobular septum, or adjacent to a bronchus. Certain lesions which are more definitely intrapulmonary, such as a fibrotic scar, a zone of atelectatic or oedematous alveoli, or a thrombosed vessel with surrounding alveolar oedema, may also produce line shadows.

HORIZONTAL PLEURAL LINE SHADOW

The horizontal fissure

The normal horizontal fissure is visible as a line shadow in a routine anterior-view radiograph in over 80 per cent of adults, and is a useful landmark especially in the diagnosis of lobar shrinkage. Pathological widening of the horizontal fissure is common in any right-sided pleurisy, in heart failure or in lymphangitis carcinomatosa, and the line shadow is then even easier to identify. In the anterior view it runs horizontally from near the hilum, at about the level of the anterior end of the third rib, to meet the sixth rib in the axilla. It may swing upwards pivoted on its medial end if there is upper-lobe shrinkage, or downwards if there is middle-lobe or lower-lobe shrinkage. In the lateral view, if it is not displaced, it is seen as a horizontal line starting opposite the lower end of the tracheal transradiancy and extending anteriorly as far as the sternum.

Fissure over apical lower lobe

Slightly " thickened " pleura over the apex of the lower lobe, especially if it is lying more or less tangentially to the x-ray beam, is often the cause of a line shadow about 2–5 cm in length running upwards and outwards, either in a straight line or with an inferior concave curve, from near the upper part of one or other hilar shadow towards the axilla in the second interspace (Figs. 172 and 173). If it is on the right side care must be taken to distinguish it from the line shadow which might be caused by the horizontal fissure if it were elevated as a result of some shrinkage of the upper lobe. Distinction will be easy if the horizontal fissure can also be identified in its normal position, as in the case illustrated in Fig. 172. If this is not the case, however, or if the shrinkage of the upper lobe is so great that a line shadow is seen simulating the horizontal fissure though in fact produced by the interlobar pleura between the middle and lower lobe, then great care must be taken in the interpretation of the line shadow and its possible cause. A lateral view may be of considerable help, as it may be possible from this to identify with confidence the normal or raised horizontal fissure lying anteriorly, or the widened upper posterior part of the main fissure lying over the apex of the lower lobe. Sometimes, however, there is so much other abnormal shadowing in the shrunken upper lobe, that differentiation of the cause of the line shadow may not be possible until tomograms or bronchograms show the limits of the various lobes without any doubt, and hence the site of the interlobar pleura responsible for the line shadow.

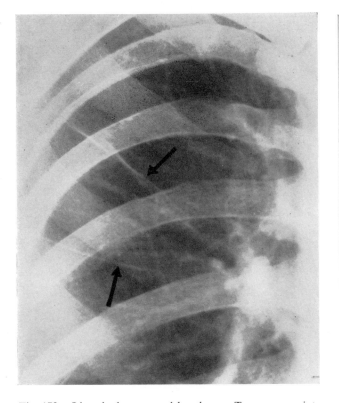

Fig. 172.—Line shadows caused by pleura. Top arrow points to the oedematous pleura over the apex of the right lower lobe. Bottom arrow points to the line of the horizontal fissure.

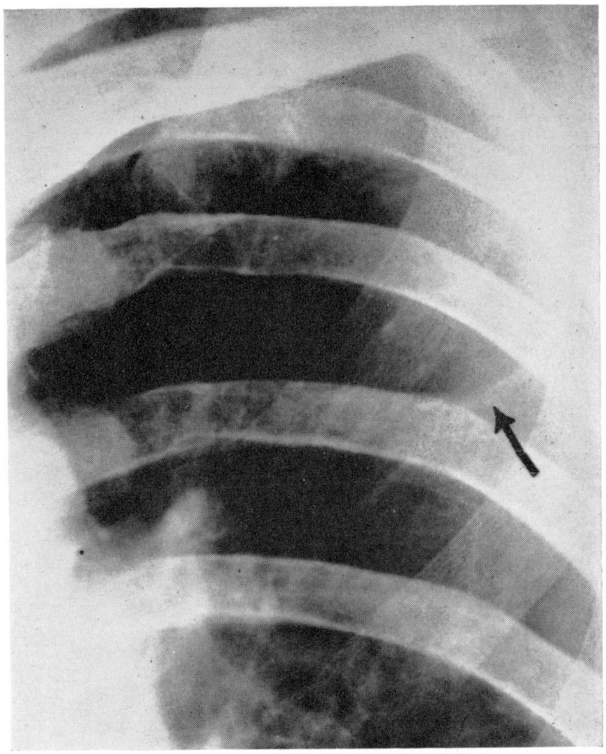

Fig. 173.—Line shadow caused by pleura. Arrow points to pleural exudate producing line over the apex of the left lower lobe. (Confirmed in lateral view.)

Accessory fissure between the apical lower and basal segments

A rather uncommon accessory fissure is that between the apical lower and the basal segments which will best be seen in the lateral view as a line shadow extending horizontally from the region of the lower end of the tracheal transradiancy, across the body of the sixth or seventh thoracic vertebra to end in the posterior chest wall. It can be distinguished from the downward displaced upper end of the main fissure seen with a shrunken apical lower-lobe segment (see below) if the main fissure can be seen in its normal position, sloping downwards and forwards above the horizontal line which will meet it. If the upper end of the main fissure cannot be identified even in a lateral-view tomogram, then the cause of the horizontal line of the accessory fissure can only be confirmed in a bronchogram showing that the apical lower-lobe segment is in its normal position and above the horizontal line shadow. The accessory fissure may form a continuous line with the horizontal fissure right across the chest from the front to the back, as also may be seen with a shrunken apical lower-lobe segment (Fig. 176).

Aerated but shrunken lobe

The chief evidence of an aerated but shrunken lobe is often displacement of the line shadow of the horizontal or main fissure. The line may be slightly accentuated by atelectatic or oedematous alveoli adjacent to the pleura. In right upper-lobe shrinkage the horizontal fissure will be raised, in lower-lobe shrinkage depressed. The line shadow of the fissure may be straight or, more often, will show a slight convex curve in the direction of the shrunken lobe. Forward displacement of the lower end of the main fissure will occur with a shrunken lingula or middle lobe, backward displacement with lower-lobe shrinkage.

Shrinkage of the right apical lower-lobe segment can easily pass undetected, but in the anterior view it can be inferred if a line shadow is seen starting over the upper part of the shadow of the right hilum, then passing downwards and outwards with a superior concave curve (Fig. 174). It ends about half way across the lung field unless it meets the line of the horizontal fissure which will continue on to the axilla. The line seen over the hilum is too high and too medial to represent the horizontal fissure. In

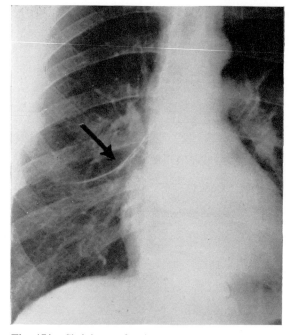

Fig. 174.—Shrinkage of apical segment of right lower lobe. Line shadow (opposite arrow) with a superior concave curve starting over the hilum shadow is the displaced interlobar pleura over it. (*See* Fig. 172 for normal position.)

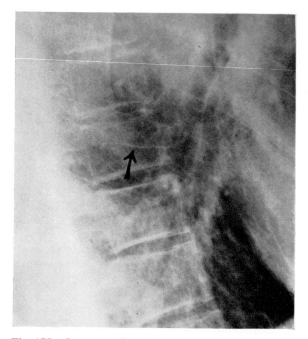

Fig. 175.—Same case (lateral view). Line of pleura over the shrunken apical lower segment (above arrow) crossing D8 is the upper end of the main fissure displaced downwards.

the lateral view a line shadow will be seen passing directly backwards from the region of the lower end of the tracheal translucency, across the shadow of the sixth thoracic vertebra to end in the posterior chest wall (Fig. 175). It is sometimes best seen in a lateral-view tomogram. Occasionally the line continues backward from the horizontal fissure, so that a line passes either straight across or with an inferior concave curve from the front to the back of the lungs (Fig. 176). The shrunken lobe may be confirmed in a bronchogram (Fig. 177). If there is occlusion of the apical lower bronchus this may be seen either in a right lateral tomogram or in a bronchogram. If the lesion is due to a small tumour, the shadow of this may also be seen in a tomogram.

Associated features

If the shrinkage is of a whole lobe and is gross, there may be elevation or depression of the hilar vessels in addition to the line shadow of the displaced interlobar fissure, and the vessels in the adjacent lobe will be spread out from the compensatory over-inflation as with an atelectatic lobe (*see* p. 58). Ring or tubular shadows in the shrunken but aerated lobe will indicate an underlying bronchiectasis.

In some cases the bronchial obliterative lesions with or without dilatation may only be seen in a bronchogram. The vessel shadows within the shrunken lobe will be crowded together and their course in the anterior view radiograph will be distorted, and in the case of a lower lobe shrinkage will show a slight lateral concave curvature instead of running straight downwards and outwards (*see* p. 167). In the lateral view the general course of the vessels will show an anterior concave inclination. In a lower-lobe shrinkage the diaphragm may be elevated on the same side.

Lobar shrinkage with normal aeration (and a normal bronchogram) may be seen as a result of an acute major or minor pulmonary embolus, or radiation damage.

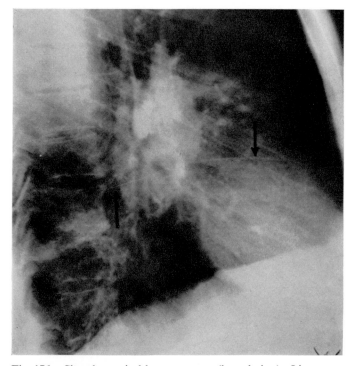

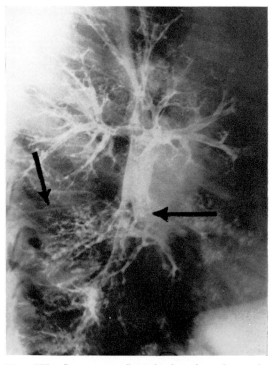

Fig. 176.—Shrunken apical lower segment (lateral view). Line across chest, starting anteriorly as the horizontal fissure (downward-pointing arrow), continuing across D9 (upward-pointing arrow). This is the top of the main fissure displaced down. Appearances in anterior view similar to Fig. 174.

Fig. 177.—Same case (lateral view bronchogram). Downward-pointing arrow to pleural line, with branches of the apical lower bronchus lying beneath. Horizontal arrow to middle-lobe bronchus and its branches which are displaced posteriorly and downwards.

Mechanisms of lobar shrinkage

A lobe may be reduced in volume if lung destructive lesions occur as in tuberculosis, so that when the lesions resolve there is just so much less lung left. Any fibrosis is merely holding the damaged parts together.

In the case of obliterative bronchial lesions occurring in childhood, the lobe may fail to grow fully, so that hypoplasia will be the predominant mechanism responsible for the small size of the lobe (*see* p. 149).

In pulmonary embolism shrinkage of a lobe may well be the result of the drop locally in pulmonary artery pressure and thus a drop in the distending force. There may also be a loss of surfactant, which will increase the retraction force by increasing the alveolar surface tension.

Pleural adhesions following a pneumothorax may prevent full re-expansion of a lobe (*see* p. 44).

VERTICAL PLEURAL LINE SHADOW

The accessory lobe of the azygos vein

A hair-line shadow extending from the top of the apex to a comma-like expansion near the hilum will suggest an accessory lobe of the azygos vein (Fig. 28). It usually lies diagonally across the apex and shows a lateral convexity, but if the amount of upper lobe cut off is smaller or larger, it will be almost vertical or horizontal respectively, and less curved (*see* p. 25).

The main interlobar pleural fissure

A small amount of fluid in the main interlobar fissure results in a clearly visible line shadow in the lateral view extending in a straight line downwards and forwards roughly from the upper posterior border of the fourth thoracic vertebra to meet the diaphragm about 4 cm behind the sternum (Fig. 57). Sometimes the whole length of the fissure can be seen, and sometimes only the lower half.

Vertical line shadow in the lower half of a lung

An almost vertical line shadow starting from near the middle of the right diaphragm and inclined slightly medially so that it points towards the hilum (Fig. 178) is seen in about 5 per cent of normal persons. Should a pleural effusion develop the line becomes wider, and in the lateral view the lower end of the line of the main fissure also widens. In the case shown in Fig. 178, no accessory lobe or accessory fissure was present *post mortem*, and the line was undoubtedly caused by the edge of the main fissure. In another case the patient developed a small area of consolidation in the anterior basal segment, and the shadow of this lay lateral but adjacent to the previously observed line shadow, again suggesting it was a part of the main fissure between the anterior basal segment and the medial segment of the middle lobe. A similar line shadow may be seen when there is an accessory fissure between the basal segments, but in several cases where such a fissure was proved at resection there was not in fact a line shadow in the radiograph.

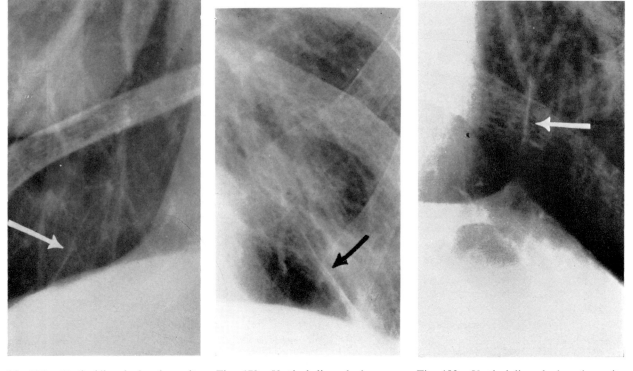

Fig. 178.—Vertical line shadow (opposite arrow) passing upwards and inwards from the diaphragm, and caused by the edge of the interlobar pleura, probably between the medial middle and anterior basal segments. The line was seen to be widened in a similar case with a small interlobar effusion.

Fig. 179.—Vertical line shadow on left (opposite arrow) pointing towards hilum and probably due to the edge of the main fissure between the anterior basal segment and the lingula. At operation: no accessory fissure.

Fig. 180.—Vertical line shadow (opposite arrow) extending up from a triangular peak from the diaphragm shadow. Probably indrawn visceral pleura towards a scar. At operation: no diaphragmatic adhesion.

A similar vertical line shadow is frequently seen on the left side (Fig. 179), especially if there is a trace of fluid in the main fissure between the anterior basal segment and the lingula.

A similar 2–3-cm long line shadow may be seen extending up from the diaphragm on either the right or left side, often running almost vertically or even inclined slightly laterally. This may be due to part of the wall of a bulla, or to diaphragmatic pleura drawn upwards towards a scar in the lung (Fig. 180). Occasionally two or three such lines may be seen.

A much less common vertical line shadow running down the lower half and outer third of the lung, usually the right, sometimes reaching the diaphragm, sometimes stopping short of it, is occasionally seen in an infant. This puzzling shadow may be mistaken for an artefact, such as clothing, but is sometimes the main interlobar fissure lying more or less in an antero-posterior plane, either because the baby is lying rotated to one side, and the effect of this is exaggerated by the free mobility of the intrathoracic contents at this age, or because there is some shrinkage of one lobe.

A broad vertical band-like shadow at one base, extending up from near the diaphragm to the hilum, lying medially superimposed on the heart shadow, is seen—often without symptoms. It appears to be due to a vascular lesion, and is rather elusive, being often invisible in the plain lateral view. A lateral tomogram may show several vessels curving posteriorly in the region of the posterior basal segment, with a zone of opacity around them and some backward displacement of the main fissure. The shadow usually resolves after some weeks.

Vertical line shadow and triangular shadow from diaphragm

An apparent localized peaking up of the diaphragm ending up as a short line shadow (Fig. 180), is often wrongly referred to as a diaphragmatic adhesion. At thoractomy there is no evidence of a diaphragmatic adhesion, and in fact a free pleura is often found. The shadow, which is frequently seen in the elderly or in persons with old shrunken tuberculous lesions of the upper lobes, represents indrawn visceral pleura towards a scar or bulla. The diaphragm itself does not contribute to the abnormal shadow, but cannot be separately identified since there is no air-containing lung between it and the pleural component.

Axillary pleura

A vertical line shadow in one or other axilla in close proximity to the ribs, lying most commonly just above the costophrenic recess is seen with a small exudate between the layers of the pleura, and is often referred to as a line of pleural thickening (Fig. 48). It is common in heart disease when the pulmonary venous pressure is raised.

Diaphragmatic pleura

A dense horizontal line shadow running adjacent to the upper surface of the dome of a diaphragm (Fig. 219) is due to a pleural calcification. Such a line may be the presenting sign of asbestosis. There may be a definite history of exposure to asbestos, or this may only be elicited on careful questioning (*see* p. 94). A similar shadow may be the result of old pleurisy whether tuberculous, from an old haemothorax or a rheumatoid pleurisy. Pleural calcifications from asbestos may occur in other sites (*see* p. 138).

Visceral pleura in pneumothorax

In a pneumothorax, a fine line shadow usually marks the lung edge; in the case of a small shallow spontaneous pneumothorax this line may be more conspicuous than the other features, such as the hypertransradiancy of the air space and the absence of the fine granular appearance usually seen in the outer zone of a normal lung field. The line may be most clearly seen in a radiograph taken during deep suspended expiration. In a pneumothorax, even very fine adhesions may be identified as broad linear shadows.

Mediastinal pleural hernia

A broad, roughly vertical, line shadow, with a lateral convex curvature, extending out for 1–2 cm from the mediastinal vascular shadow, is seen when a so-called " mediastinal hernia of the lung " is present (Fig. 181). Normally the lungs are in contact in the mid-line behind the sternum and in front of the aorta; if one lung, or its pleural space, is distended, however, it may push its boundaries across the mid-line, or alternatively be dragged across as a result of shrinkage of the other lung. It will then occupy an area in the medial part of the contralateral lung field beyond the central shadow which normally covers the point of contact and adjacent lung. The line shadow is caused by the two layers of pleura covering the herniated lung together with the two layers over the adjacent lung seen clear of the central cardiovascular shadow. If the pleura is herniated in a patient with a pneumothorax, the line shadow is caused by the displaced parietal pleura together with the two layers of pleura of the opposite lung contrasted against the air transradiancy of the pneumothorax on the one side. Sometimes a mediastinal hernia of part of one lung across to the contralateral side can be confirmed on tomograms by tracing the visible lung vessels back to the main hilar vessels. If this test fails, the presence of a hernia can sometimes be confirmed in bronchograms. These may be particularly useful in a case of pulmonary agenesis of one side, as the other lung may then occupy most of both sides, while the deformity of the poorly developed part, or absence of its main bronchus, will also be shown.

In most of these pleural conditions the cause of the line shadow is obvious, partly from its position and partly from the length which frequently exceeds 2 cm.

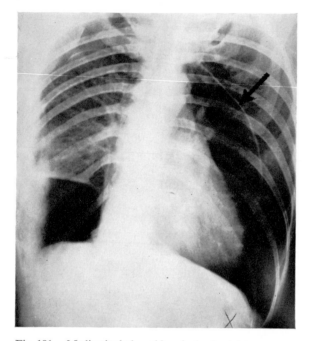

Fig. 181.—Mediastinal pleural hernia due to right pneumo-thorax. Arrow points to the edge of the right pleural cavity, seen as a long line shadow convex laterally. Pleural adhesions are holding the upper part of the right lung against the axilla.

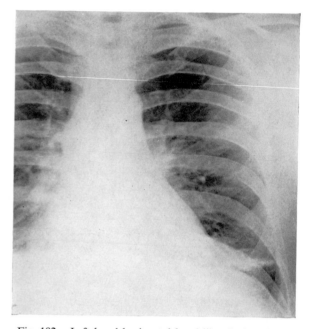

Fig. 182.—Left basal horizontal band-like shadow due to a pulmonary vascular lesion (embolus). Male aged 54 years. Sudden left chest pain. Recovery and dis-appearance of line shadow.

INTRAPULMONARY LINE SHADOWS

Horizontal linear shadow above the diaphragm

A transient shadow some 3–10 cm long and 2–5 mm wide is seen quite frequently lying horizontally 1–3 cm above the diaphragm (Fig. 182). Such a shadow has been described as a Fleischner's line, or as a linear or plate-like atelectasis.

A variant of the horizontal line shadow is a line in the mid zone starting in the mid-lung field and sloping downwards as it passes medially to meet the heart shadow. It lies in the course of the apical lower-lobe vein. In the lateral view such line shadows may be seen traversing a lower lobe. A rather similar line shadow may be seen across the middle lobe or lingula.

Chances to study the morbid anatomical basis for these line shadows are few and far between since the condition is not itself fatal, is often transient and, if the patient happens to die, only a routine post-mortem is done on uninflated lung and the lesion would thus not be detected. In addition, previous radiographs are rarely studied before the lung is examined by the pathologist, so that correlation with the x-ray appearances is not even attempted. In the case examined by Fleischner a zone of airless alveoli (some with fluid in them, some collapsed) was seen, but no relation to a vessel or bronchus was found.   In others a thrombosed vessel with surrounding oedema was identified, while evidence of of scarring and indrawn pleura has also been observed.

When such a line shadow is seen in a radiograph of the chest taken one or two days after an abdominal operation, it may represent an area of lung deflated in the immediate post-operative phase, when the diaphragm may be high and breathing shallow. Secretions in some peripheral bronchi may encourage collapse if collateral air drift is inhibited because of some alveolar oedema and the shallow breathing. In a day or two the diaphragm moves better and the line disappears.

By far the majority of such long line shadows are related to a local vascular lesion. This may be either a small pulmonary artery embolus or thrombosis in a pulmonary vein. The evidence for this is as follows.

(1) Such a long line shadow was found in nearly 50 per cent of cases with a proven embolus in a major pulmonary artery. The long line often precedes the major event by a few days, or both may be seen in the initial radiograph.

(2) Clinical and radiological evidence of a pulmonary infarct may be associated with such a line shadow. Radiologically this may be in the same area as the infarct shadow or in some other area. The line may precede or follow the larger shadow of the infarct. A possible mechanism for a line shadow following an infarct is shown in Fig. 183.

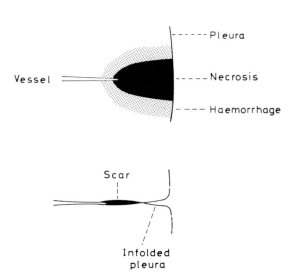

Fig. 183.—Diagram suggesting possible mechanism for indrawn pleura in a healing infarct (after Reid, 1967).

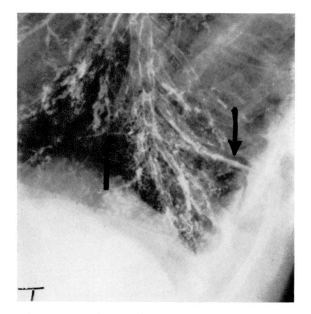

Fig. 184.—Horizontal line shadow of vascular lesion (bronchogram, lateral view). Downward-pointing arrow to line shadow—vessel and pleura. Upward-pointing arrow to line, possibly due to indrawn pleura. Bronchogram normal.

(3) In cases examined by tomography the line started from the pleura and often ended at a vessel shadow. When this vessel was traced towards the hilum it could be identified as an artery in some cases, but more often as a vein. A second, thinner, line shadow was sometimes seen starting from the point of junction of the thicker line with the vessel shadow, proceeding at an angle to meet the pleura again (Fig. 184). This suggests that there is often a pleural component as well as a vascular component responsible for the line, a finding which was confirmed at thoracotomy or in the specimen in some cases. This accounts to some extent for the bizarre anatomical site of many of these long line shadows, which may go right across a lobe from back to front and side to side—representing the plate-like distribution described by Fleischner.

(4) Bronchograms in two cases showed the line was unrelated to a bronchus, and there was no shift of the course of the bronchi to suggest lung shrinkage from local atelectasis.

(5) Angiograms in some cases (done for some other purpose than investigation of the line shadow) showed either an opacified artery ending at the line (Fig. 185) or an opacified vein in the venous phase (Fig. 186).

(6) The clinical course is often in favour of a vascular lesion. Many cases occur 2–3 days after delivery in women, or 7–10 days after a major surgical operation, these being the times major emboli also tend to occur. Only a few cases have haemoptysis or chest pain, and the majority are asymptomatic. They are not related to cough and sputum, which would suggest a bronchial obstructive cause. The shadow may last only a few days or several weeks, after which it may resolve. In a few cases it is permanent. In diseases with a vascular bias such as lupus erythematosus such a long line shadow may be the presenting sign. They are common in disorders of the pulmonary circulation such as the low output state in a patient immediately following myocardial infarction, or in a patient with mitral stenosis shortly after a valvotomy. In most cases, including those with infarct shadows or major artery emboli, there was no close relation between diaphragm elevation and the line shadow.

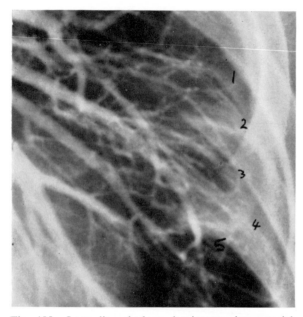

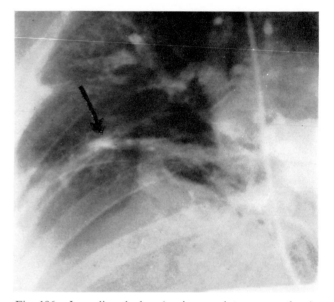

Fig. 185.—Long line shadows (angiogram, late arterial phase). Elsewhere contrast medium has reached the arterioles. Artery blocked by lines 1–3 and 5. Line 4 flooding into small infarct. Unchanged 1 year later.

Fig. 186.—Long line shadow (angiogram, late venous phase). Left atrium opacified. Opposite arrow contrast medium in a vein is blocked opposite line shadow which ran horizontally in lower zone. Case of massive pulmonary embolism.

Pathological features

The pathologist is very familiar with infarct scars. One such scar is shown diagrammatically in Fig. 183, but usually when a scar is found there is no recent radiograph available to relate it to a line shadow. Sometimes conditions are more favourable. The line shadow across the middle lobe illustrated in Fig. 187 was related to a grey line visible in the specimen which had been suitably inflated, and which was obtained as a result of a lobectomy 24 hours after the radiograph. Histological examination showed the line was due to a thrombosed artery with oedematous alveoli and some fibrosis around. There was also a septic infarct in the adjacent lobe.

An uncommon cause of a horizontal line shadow is a blocked bronchus full of secretions without much atelectasis of the lung around (Fig. 5).

A long horizontal line shadow in a lower zone may also be caused by the indented pleura round a bulla (*see* p. 128). In a lateral view a large bulla may be clearly seen against the posterior chest wall, demarcated anteriorly by a thin line shadow. It is the upper part of this line of pleura over the bulla, which, seen tangentially in the anterior view, is responsible for the horizontal line shadow. These lines tend to be of hair-line thickness and thus thinner than the line due to a vascular lesion, although occasionally the wall of a bulla is 2–3 mm wide.

Horizontal line shadow above the costophrenic recess (septal line shadows)

Another small horizontal line shadow is frequently seen lying just above the costophrenic recess (Fig. 188). There may be a single hair line extending horizontally from the axillary pleura for 1–2 cm, but usually there are several parallel line shadows at intervals of about 5–10 mm. Some are truly hair line in width, others some 1–2 mm wide. Some end abruptly medially, others seem to end over or in one of the nearby vessel shadows, and can thus in a sense be traced right back to the hilum.

These lines (Kerley " B " lines) are caused by a variety of pathological changes. Essentially they represent thickened interlobular septa, the thickening being due partly to an engorged lymphatic within the septum, although this in fact will only account for a small part of the increase in width, and partly to gross oedema of the septum. Sometimes it becomes almost a fibrotic thickening, a difference which accounts for the varying rate of disappearance of these line shadows after a successful valvotomy for mitral stenosis. In mitral stenosis the shadow of the oedematous septum will be further reinforced in some cases by extensive haemosiderin deposits in alveoli lying in the neighbourhood of the septum. The balance of these pathological changes will vary from case to case.

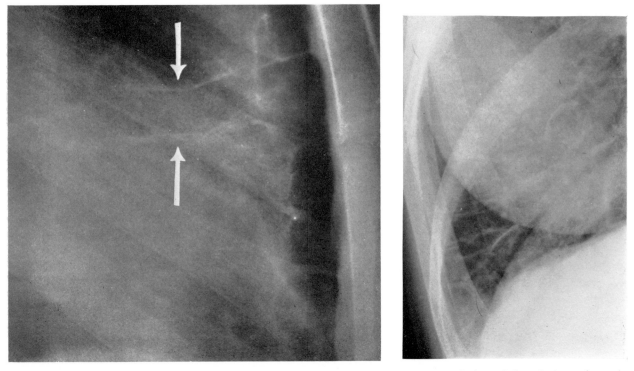

Fig. 187.—Horizontal line shadows (opposite arrows—lateral view) extending across the middle lobe. Male aged 34 years. Several haemoptyses. Cavitated infarct right lower lobe. Middle and lower lobectomy. Line shadow across middle lobe from thrombosed artery and oedema of surrounding alveoli, with some fibrosis.

Fig. 188.—Horizontal line shadows above the right costophrenic recess. Some continue on as vessel shadows, some have free end medially (Kerley " B " lines). Mitral stenosis. Disappearance of lines after valvotomy.

Such lines are commonly seen when the pulmonary venous pressure is raised, as in mitral stenosis or in acute left ventricular failure. Very similar line shadows may represent the smaller peripheral vessels, particularly engorged and therefore conspicuous veins draining from the septa.

Very faint septal or vessel line shadows may be seen in the radiograph of a very thin normal person with well-inflated lungs.

Obvious septal line shadows may be seen in some pneumoconioses, particularly if the lymphatic or surrounding tissue contains a heavy metal, such as tin. The nodular and other shadows in the lung will generally suffice to suggest a non-cardiac cause for the lines. They are quite often seen in fibrosing alveolitis (see p. 100) but are uncommon in sarcoidosis, and if present are few in number.

Septal line shadows may also be seen in lymphangitis carcinomatosa. The very conspicuous sub-pleural lymphatics so often seen in this condition, and at operation in some cases of mitral stenosis, are in fact invisible in the radiograph, since there is no air round to give them contrast, so unless the septal or deep lymphatics are affected, no radiological evidence of lymphatic engorgement may be seen.

Hair-line shadows running towards the hila (Kerley "A" lines)

Hair-line shadows, usually in the upper half of the lungs, may be seen running towards the hila, often unconnected with the main vessel shadows (Kerley " A " lines) (Fig. 189). They represent thickened intercommunicating lymphatics (Trapnell, 1963), that is, lymphatics jumping from a course alongside an artery to one alongside a vein or vice versa, and in passing from one to the other they travel through the lung without much in the way of a surrounding connective tissue sheath. They are seen particularly in lymphangitis carcinomatosa, with or without the basal horizontal line shadows, or in mitral stenosis with basal line shadows and an abnormality of the heart contours. They are also seen in some cases of left ventricular failure with pulmonary oedema and thus in association with the blotchy shadows seen in this condition.

They may be seen in lymphatic obstruction from a hilar gland lesion, usually a secondary deposit, or in Hodgkin's disease.

A combination of long line shadows ("A" lines), broad septal line shadows and indistinct rather wide vessel shadows is seen in some cases of acute viral pneumonia, and may well represent a true inter-stitial inflammatory response.

Isolated line shadow in the upper half of the lung

Scar.—An isolated line shadow in the upper half of the lung may be caused by a fibrous scar, commonly the end result of a healed tuberculous lesion.

Bulla.—A vertical hair-line shadow running downwards from the apex to the shadow of the clavicle commonly represents the wall of a bulla. The apex is often relatively transradiant, and the small vessels normally seen in this region are no longer visible. In some cases the mechanism seems to be that of scar emphysema, the scar being that of an old tuberculous lesion, or an inflammatory episode in a chronic bronchitic. For the pathological basis of these line shadows outlining a bulla, *see* p. 128.

A much longer and rather wider line shadow may be seen running almost vertically downwards in the middle third of a lung with a lateral convex curve, and both the upper and lower end of the line terminating against the heart shadow (Fig. 190). This may also be caused by a large bulla. In the lateral view it will usually be seen to be lying retrosternally or against the posterior chest wall. Tomograms will show an absence of vessel shadows and increased transradiancy in the region surrounded by the line shadow. A roughly horizontal line shadow below a clavicle with an inferior convex curve and no vessels above it will also indicate a bulla (Fig. 191). Sometimes a similar line is seen on both sides.

Small peripheral bronchus.—A short line shadow or two short line shadows joining to form a Y-shaped shadow, usually in the upper half of the lung field, may be caused by a peripheral bronchus filled with caseous material, and is seen in a predominantly bronchial form of tuberculosis. This appearance has been observed particularly in the lung contralateral to a tuberculous dilated bronchus, which has presented either as a 1–2-cm circular shadow, or a ring shadow, or a ring shadow with a tubular shadow connecting it to the hilum (" tennis-racket " shadow) (Fig. 203), the endobronchial nature of the lesion having been proved after resection.

Artefacts.—An upper-zone line shadow may be produced by clothing. Its nature can be presumed if the line can be traced beyond the lung field, otherwise it may need confirmation with a further radio-graph of the patient uncovered in that region.

Line shadow radiating out from circular shadow

Progressive massive fibrosis in pneumoconiosis (P.M.F.).—A number of lines radiating out from a roughly circular or oval and rather poorly defined shadow some 2–5 cm in size, commonly in the mid zone or just below the clavicle (Fig. 192), is seen in progressive massive fibrosis (P.M.F.), a compli-cation of many forms of industrial pulmonary disease (particularly that of coal miners, boiler scalers and haematite miners). The massive fibrotic lesion is often bilateral and is associated with the

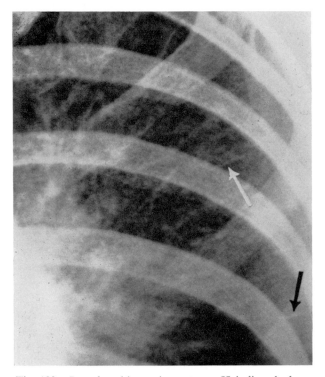

Fig. 189.—Lymphangitis carcinomatosa. Hair line shadows (opposite arrow). Dilated deep intercommunicating lymphatics choked with carcinoma cells. Also fine nodular shadows. Carcinoma breast.

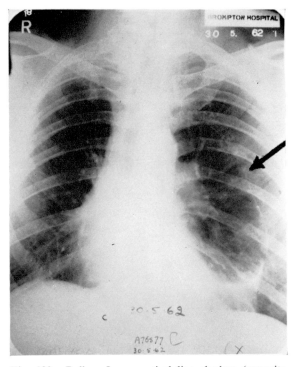

Fig. 190.—Bulla. Long vertical line shadow (opposite arrow) marks lateral wall of a large bulla. Fluid at bottom. Wall was essentially indented pleura. Surgical excision.

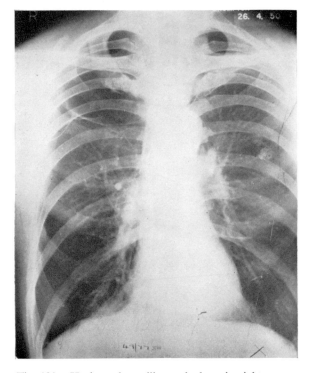

Fig. 191.—Horizontal curvilinear shadows in right upper zone with avascular area above mark the lower edge of bullae. Vessel narrowing lower zones (emphysema). Male aged 48 years. Cough, sputum and dyspnoea.

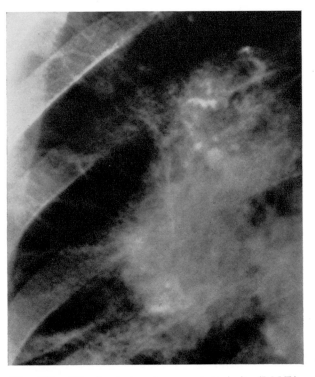

Fig. 192.—Fibrotic lesion in pneumoconiosis (P.M.F.). Circular 8 cm shadow with radiating line shadows. Male aged 68 years. Welsh coalfield-face worker for many years. Some dyspnoea. Only a few nodular shadows.

small circular shadows representing the basic nodule of the pneumoconiosis as described on p. 96. In some cases these basic nodules are inconspicuous and few in number, but can generally be detected with the aid of a magnifying glass in the periphery of the mid zone between the rib shadows. The exact aetiology of the fibrous mass is unknown, but infection, in some cases possibly tuberculous, acting on the already damaged lung may play a part in its growth. Avascular necrosis may also be a contributory factor. Sometimes a temporary central cavitation in the shadow may be seen in the plain film or on tomography, and may appear after the expectoration of a quantity of inky black sputum (*see* p. 131).

Tuberculous lesion.—A line shadow some 1–2 mm wide is quite frequently seen connecting a 1–3 cm circular shadow of a tuberculous focus to the hilum. The exact nature of this shadow is often difficult to determine. It is, in some cases at any rate, caused by a mixture of active tubercles and fibrous tissue situated along the course of the lymphatic channel connecting a primary tuberculous focus to the draining hilum gland, and is therefore situated in close proximity to the draining bronchus (which may be secondarily infected from this source) and the artery. Such a finding is common on histological examination of the specimen in cases of primary tuberculosis, but the lymphatic channel lesions are usually too small to be visible in a radiograph. Sometimes, however, fibrosis occurring months or years later will result in the lesions becoming denser, and therefore visible as a line shadow.

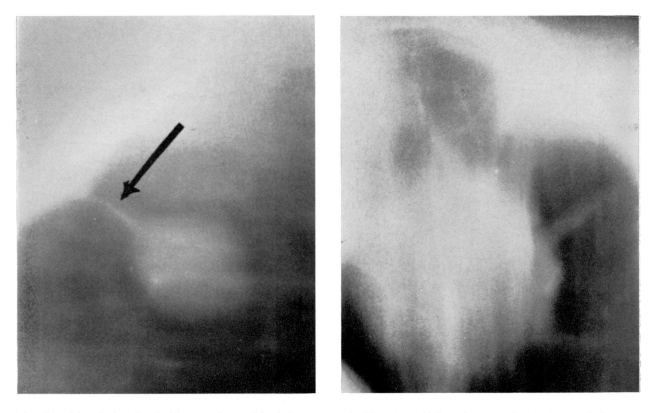

Fig. 193.—Line shadow (marked by arrow) caused by indrawn pleura and blocked bronchus. It lies distal to 2-cm circular tuberculous pneumonic focus, itself distal to a tuberculous bronchial occlusion. Male aged 45 years, mass x-ray finding.

Fig. 194.—Bronchial carcinoma. Line shadows radiating out from 4-cm circular shadow. One line represented airless alveoli around a blocked bronchus distal to the tumour. Male aged 67 years, with recent small haemoptyses.

More often when a line shadow is seen connecting a solid circular shadow or the ring shadow of a cavity with the hilum, it is obvious that the lesion is a post-primary tuberculous focus. Examination of the specimen in such a case may show tubercles and fibrous tissue along the line of the lymphatic channel somewhat similar to those seen in a primary focus. The bronchus draining the cavity or apparently solid focus is often thickened as well. The bronchial lesion, if it shows at all in the radiograph, is more likely to result in a tubular shadow than a single line shadow, so that occasionally three line shadows are seen running parallel to each other, two representing the bronchus, and the third the thickened lymphatic. In many of these examples showing thickening of the lymphatic channel the adjacent alveoli are either oedematous or collapsed, and this feature also contributes towards the formation of the line shadow.

Sometimes a short line shadow is seen extending from the circular tuberculous focus towards the peripheral pleura (Fig. 193). Such a line is sometimes caused by an indrawn tag of pleura adherent to the focus. An identical line shadow may be caused by a fibrous strand between the focus and the pleura, or by a zone of collapsed lung around the bronchus peripheral to the focus.

Neoplasm.—A line shadow or several short lines may also extend out in various directions from the circular shadow of a bronchial carcinoma (Fig. 194), as described on p. 86. These may represent vessels or lymphatics directly permeated by a mass of cells from the neoplasm, or a fibrous strand associated with a dilated lymphatic blocked by the neoplasm, or a zone of airless alveoli around a small dilated and secretion-filled bronchus obstructed by the tumour.

BAND-LIKE SHADOWS

Band-like shadows 2 mm or more in width may have truly parallel walls (tooth paste shadow) (Fig. 195), or be rather elliptical in shape, or have an enlarged peripheral end—the " gloved-finger shadow" (Fig. 196).

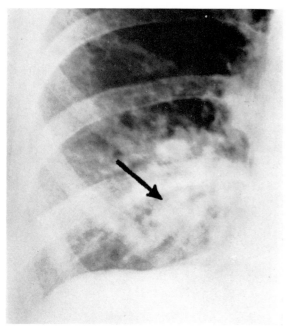

Fig. 195.—Bronchiectasis. Band-like (tooth paste) shadow (opposite arrow). This disappeared, leaving a parallel line shadow in its place. Asthma and allergic bronchopulmonary aspergillosis with eosinophilia.

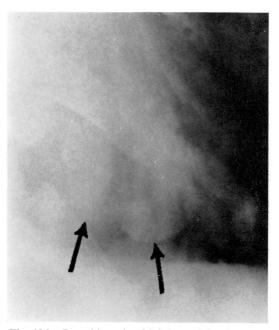

Fig. 196.—Bronchiectasis of left lower lobe (bronchographic proof). Gloved-finger shadows opposite arrows due to secretions in the dilated bronchi which are occluded distally. Diaphragm shadow below.

PLEURAL SHADOW

A band-like shadow with parallel walls is often caused by a pleural lesion, and is a wide version of one of the pleural line shadows mentioned above. Wide band-like shadows are seen particularly with adhesions in a pneumothorax.

Atelectatic lung; strands across cavities

Long 5–8 mm wide band-like shadows are seen in consolidation or collapse of some of the segments of the lung, particularly the anterior and posterior segment of the upper lobe (Figs. 126 and 128), and middle lobe (Fig. 110) (*see* p. 65) An elliptical homogeneous shadow is seen in some cases of middle-lobe bronchostenosis (Figs. 108 and 112), and in an interlobar effusion (*see* p. 39 (Figs. 56 and 57)).

Band-like shadows are occasionally seen traversing a very large cavity. They represent trabeculae or remnants of a vessel passing through the air space.

Inhaled foreign body

A short band-like shadow close to the hilum may be caused by an inhaled foreign body (such as a piece of bone) lodged in one of the larger bronchi.

Bronchial shadows

A single band-like (tooth paste) shadow, about 5–8 mm wide and 2–4 cm long, may be due to a dilated bronchus filled with secretions (Fig. 195). A variant of this is two divisions of a bronchus also filled with secretions producing a V or Y-shaped shadow 5–8 mm wide in an upper lobe or an inverted V or Y in a lower lobe. In some cases previous or later radiographs may show a tubular shadow in the same site if the bronchus happens to empty. In a lower lobe a tooth paste shadow may terminate with a horizontal upper margin or fluid level, and with a continuation of a tubular shadow above it towards the hilum.

Very much more rarely, a band-like shadow, 3–8 mm wide, which tapers and bifurcates as it passes distally, may be caused by a group of mucus-filled bronchi associated with a developmental defect of that part of the lung. Gloved-finger shadows are often seen in bronchiectasis (Fig. 196), which is by far their commonest cause. Rarely a group of caseous tuberculous pneumonic foci may have an elongated shape, and thus give rise to a similar appearance. In bronchiectasis the gloved-finger shadows may be crowded together, suggesting some lobar shrinkage, which may be confirmed in a lateral view by visible displacement of an interlobar fissure. The presence of tubular shadows nearby will indicate both shadows are due to dilated bronchi, the one filled with secretions, the other containing air.

In children a low-grade left basal inflammatory lesion quite often results in shadows which are very similar to the gloved-finger shadows seen with bronchiectasis. Since cough and sputum may be present in a pneumonia, bronchiectasis may be mistakenly diagnosed. The partial consolidation of a pneumonia will generally resolve within weeks, and the disappearance of the shadows together with the improvement in the clinical picture will often suffice to dispel the fear of bronchiectasis.

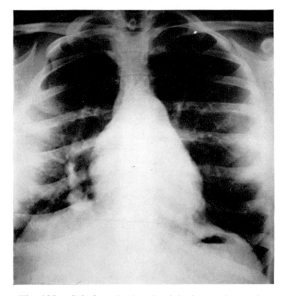

Fig. 197.—Scimitar shadow in right base. Anomalous pulmonary vein draining right lung into inferior vena cava. Female aged 17 years. Asymptomatic.

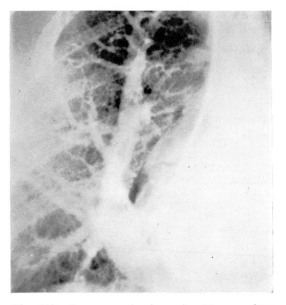

Fig. 198.—Same case (angiogram). Venous phase showing pulmonary veins draining into long trunk which joins inferior vena cava.

Vessel shadow

The dilated vessels leading to and from an arterio-venous aneurysm in the lung may be seen as band-like shadows, some 3–8 mm wide, and these may be an even more conspicuous feature than the shadow of the aneurysm where the anastomosis occurs (Fig. 146).

A large artery to a sequestrated segment may also cast a band-like shadow. This may be traced into one of the hilar vessels, or, if it originates from the thoracic or abdominal aorta, it may get lost when it reaches the central shadow or the diaphragm. The segment itself, if not aerated, will be seen as a circular or oval homogeneous shadow.

A long vertical band-like shadow, 0·5–1 cm wide, increasing in width as it passes downwards and with a lateral convex curve (like a scimitar in shape) (Fig. 197), is seen in one type of anomalous pulmonary venous drainage. The vascular nature of the shadow will be obvious in a tomogram, and it usually drains into the inferior vena cava, a feature which can be shown by catheter studies or angiography (Fig. 198). A rather narrower tortuous tooth paste shadow in a lower zone may be caused by a similar anomalous pulmonary venous drainage, but in this case it may enter the left atrium in a normal manner.

A rather rare anomaly is a pattern of branching vessels in an emphysematous area of lung.

A 2-cm wide band-like shadow, best seen in a lateral view extending forwards from the vertebrae at the level of D6 to reach the superior vena cava, is seen if the inferior vena cava enters the right atrium via the azygos vein and superior vena cava.

TUBULAR SHADOWS

In a normal person a rather faint tubular shadow consisting of a central transradiant band some 4–8 mm wide with a hair-line shadow on either side may be seen close to the hilum passing downwards and outwards in the line of the arteries. This represents a lobar or segmental bronchus, and the line shadows are in part bronchial wall and in part a composite shadow of bronchial wall and adjacent artery. There may be two or three such tubular shadows on either side.

A short tubular shadow may be caused by two normal vessels, perhaps situated on quite different planes, running parallel to each other for a short distance. Such normal vessel shadows, if traced farther, will be seen to taper, bifurcate and separate, and are thus easily distinguished from the shadow of a bronchus.

Tubular shadows with a hair-line wall and a lumen width appropriate for a bronchus at that level can be described as " tram line " shadows (Fig. 199). These are really extensions more distally of normal bronchial shadows described above. They are seen characteristically in a few children with asthma, in severely affected cases with cystic fibrosis (mucoviscidosis) and in some adult asthmatics with broncho-pulmonary aspergillosis with eosinophilia. In all these conditions the shadows tend to come and go and are rarely permanent. The pathological basis of the shadow is unknown. Since they are also seen in patients with pulmonary oedema from a raised pulmonary venous pressure, it is possible that oedema of the bronchial wall is a factor in many cases. Since the bronchial veins at this level drain into the pulmonary veins, bronchial wall oedema would be expected in some cardiac cases. In asthma, oedema may be part of the allergic response. Tram line shadows extend out for some two to three generations, which is often more than half the distance from the hilum to the periphery. They are often easier to see in the upper lobes than at the bases, but they occur in both situations.

More obvious tubular shadows are commonly multiple, and are usually caused by bronchiectases (Fig. 200). In some cases both the transradiant lumen and the white line of the wall are wider than in a normal bronchial shadow at that level. In others the transradiant centre only is relatively wide while the line shadows each side are only of hair-line width. Sometimes the transradiant zone shows a bulbous expansion just before it ends. Frequently such tubular shadows are crowded together, indicating some lobar shrinkage.

In an older child or young adult with fibrocystic disease (cystic fibrosis, mucoviscidosis), tubular shadows are often a very conspicuous feature extending upwards and outwards from the hilar regions. The transradiant lumen is not unduly wide, but the surrounding wall is often 1–2 mm wide. There may be no obvious increase in the width of the bronchial lumen between the " railway line " shadows in a bronchogram, but there may be moderate dilatation of the bronchi beyond this level, where no abnormal shadow is seen in the plain radiograph.

119

Tubular shadows due to dilated bronchi, especially if they lie behind the heart shadow, may be indistinct or even invisible in a routine anterior-view radiograph, but may nevertheless be clearly seen in an additional radiograph taken with greater exposure (Fig. 200). They may also be clearly seen in a lateral view or in well-exposed tomograms. Dilatation of the proximal branches is often associated with occlusion of the more distal ones, so that the abnormal tubular shadows do not extend as far distally as do the normal bronchi, and the shadows end some 2–3 cm above the diaphragm. In other cases the more peripheral branches are also dilated, in which case the abnormal shadows extend farther distally. In the case of bronchiectasis of the left lower lobe these dilated peripheral branches may be visible against the superimposed air transradiancy of the stomach, whereas in a lightly exposed routine anterior-view radiograph the more proximal dilatations cannot be seen through the general opacity of the heart behind which they lie.

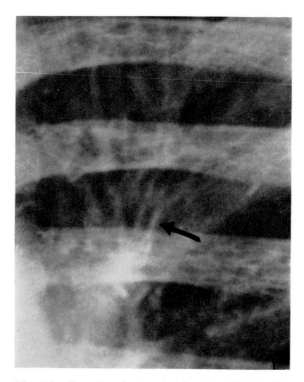

Fig. 199.—Tram line shadows in left upper lobe. Parallel line shadows (opposite arrow). Distance between lines (that is, lumen) is appropriate size for a normal bronchus at this level. Boy aged 9 years. Severe asthma since 2½ years old. Peak flow 44% of predicted normal. Lines disappeared at age 11 years.

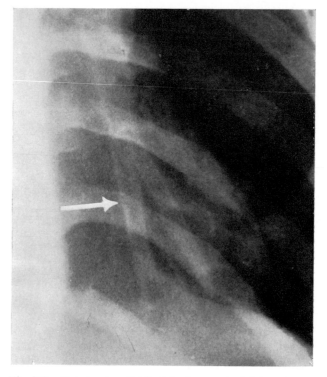

Fig. 200.—Tubular (parallel line) shadows at the left base due to bronchiectasis (one is marked by the arrow). Well-exposed radiograph. Child aged 10 years with cough and sputum. Bronchogram confirmed dilated bronchi in rather shrunken but aerated left lower lobe.

Tubular shadows are often associated with small areas of patchy clouding around them due to inflammatory changes in the nearby alveoli, or with areas of hypertransradiancy with vessel narrowing due to local emphysematous changes. The air presumably reaches these bullous areas by cross-aeration, since in a bronchiectasis the peripheral bronchi are usually occluded.

Obvious tubular shadows in the lower lobes may be seen in association with transposition of the heart (the left ventricle and aortic knuckle being on the right side), and small or absent frontal sinuses with evidence of infection of the antra (Kartagena's syndrome).

MODERATE-SIZED AND LARGE RING SHADOWS

A ring shadow is a roughly circular transradiant space surrounded by a relatively narrow zone of opacity. The size of the transradiant space varies greatly, and so does the width of the surrounding wall. Ring shadows may be single or multiple, isolated or in the midst of other kinds of shadow. A ring shadow should always be considered to represent an intrapulmonary cavity unless an extrapulmonary site is suggested either by some special appearance in the radiographs, supplemented when necessary by tomograms, or by some special feature in the history or clinical findings.

An intrapulmonary cavity is usually the result of destruction of lung tissue and its replacement by air: the air space, having been initiated in this way, may later be ballooned out by a check-valve action of the draining bronchus. Another type of cavity is formed by the dilatation of a bronchus or bronchiole as a result of bronchostenosis, or of an infection causing erosion and weakening of the bronchial wall. Yet another type of cavity is the result of necrosis deep in a neoplasm, and finally, a cavity may be part of a developmental abnormality.

ESTABLISHING THE PRESENCE OF A RING SHADOW

It is of course first necessary to establish with reasonable certainty that a ring shadow is in fact present in the radiograph. An intrapulmonary cavity may be very conspicuous or it may only be seen with difficulty; it is a useful procedure, therefore, whenever abnormal shadows are seen, to try to conjure up the image of a ring shadow amongst them. This may be partly obscured by superimposed or surrounding areas of pathological shadowing or by the superimposed shadows of normal structures such as the hilum, the heart, a rib, the clavicles, or the apex of the diaphragm. A cavity of this sort will be difficult to see in a single anterior-view radiograph, and may be more easily identified on fluoroscopy, since it may become more conspicuous on slight rotation of the patient. Alternatively, it may only be demonstrated in a lateral view or with greater certainty by tomography. The indications for tomography, and the features in a tomogram which will suggest the presence of a cavity, are discussed on pages 241 and 244.

RADIOGRAPHIC APPEARANCES OF THE LUMEN AND THE CAVITY WALL

Although a ring shadow is usually evenly circular or oval, the wall may have excrescencies into the interior so that the lumen is very irregular as in Fig. 201. Sometimes the lumen is even slit-like or crescentic in shape. It may be circular and centrally placed with a wall of even thickness; it may be eccentric in an otherwise circular shadow; or it may be placed almost anywhere within an irregularly shaped diffuse shadow, the size of which will indicate the amount of surrounding consolidation. This may occupy a whole lobe or only part of a segment, and there may or may not be evidence of shrinkage of the lobe due either to the cavity and surrounding lung lesions, or to an underlying bronchostenosis.

The word " ring shadow ", used in reference to the radiographic appearances of an air-containing cavity, is therefore given considerable latitude.

The thickness of the wall which forms the boundary of the cavity is also very variable, and is a feature which is sometimes of help in the diagnosis. A ring shadow with a wall of hair-line width is much more likely to be a bulla than a tuberculous cavity, whilst one with a very thick irregular wall will suggest a neoplasm. Such evidence is unfortunately not reliable, since a thick-walled cavity may be tuberculous (Fig. 201) and a thin-walled cavity may nevertheless be a neoplasm (Fig. 202). A thick-walled and eccentric cavity is more common in an acid-fast bacillus infection with " anonymous " bacteria (photochromagens, avian, Runyon) than with the ordinary tubercle bacillus, and the radiologist's report suggesting this may be the case will warn the bacteriologist to carry out the appropriate cultural tests.

The presence of other abnormal shadows in the surrounding lung, taken into consideration with the thickness of the cavity wall, is a further aid to diagnosis. For instance, a thick-walled peripheral cavity associated with a more proximal homogeneous shadow is likely to be a lung abscess distal to a neoplasm; a ring shadow with a thin hair-line wall, surrounded by a hypertransradiant zone, within which narrow widely spaced vessel shadows can be seen, is probably a bulla; or a ring shadow with a 2–3 mm wall, and a mixture of small circular and short line shadows in the lung around it, often with small calcifications in addition, will suggest a tuberculous lesion. In general, however, the diagnosis of the type of cavity is easier and more certain from the clinical and bacteriological or cytological findings than from the x-ray appearances.

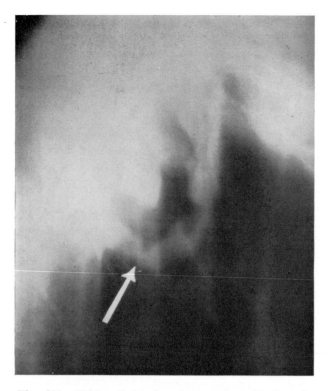

Fig. 201.—Thick-walled tuberculous cavity with irregular projections into the transradiant air space. Male aged 44 years. Recent onset of cough and sputum. Tubercle bacilli found. Specimen showed very irregular wall of cavity with liquefaction of a caseous pneumonia and some fibrosis.

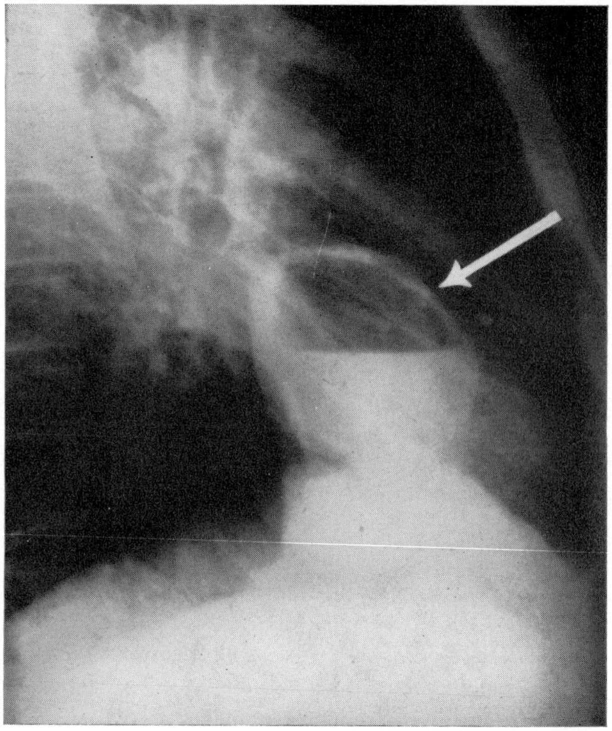

Fig. 202.—Thin-walled neoplastic cavity. Arrow points to thin wall. Fluid level in lower half. Male aged 40 years. Pains in joints. Dry cough and loss of weight. Right middle lobectomy revealed active and calcified tuberculous glands. Specimen showed wall of cavity consisted of squamous carcinoma cells.

THE CONTENTS OF THE CAVITY

There may be other contents in a cavity in addition to the air. The presence of fluid in it will be indicated by a horizontal upper limit to an opaque area occupying the lower part. If the contents are viscous or semi-fluid, the upper limit of the opaque area, that is, the fluid, may not be marked by a straight line, but may curve up at the ends where it meets the cavity wall, or may even bulge up in the centre.

If there is doubt concerning the presence of a fluid level, a radiograph should be taken with the patient lying down. If the appearances were in fact due to a fluid level, then the well-defined upper margin with the air transradiancy above it will vanish. If, on the other hand the shadow remains unchanged, it will suggest either an intrapulmonary solid lesion which happens to have a well-defined straight upper margin, or some artefact such as the straight horizontal upper border of a large transverse process simulating the fluid level, with some curvilinear vascular shadows superimposed on its upper part, simulating the wall of the cavity.

A fluid level is an important feature. In a case of doubt it may act as a pointer and lead to the demonstration of a cavity, the wall of which was perhaps indistinct or obscured by other shadows in the first plain radiographs. A fluid level may sometimes be a factor in the differentiation of a bullous cyst, in which it is rare, from other kinds of cyst in which it is not uncommon. During treatment, especially of a lung abscess, the height of the fluid level is an indication of how well drainage is proceeding through the bronchus.

A haemorrhage may occur into a cavity, and if the blood is retained and clots, and the clot subsequently shrinks, or if the cavity contains a fleshy mass of aspergilli mycelia (a mycetoma), a " halo " transradiancy may be seen. This is due to a small air space between the central blood clot, or mycetoma, and the cavity wall causing a 1–2 mm zone of transradiancy between the central homogeneous shadow and the ring shadow forming the wall of the cavity (Fig. 139) (*see also* p. 81).

In a hydatid cyst a small air leak may occur between the cyst and the adventitia surrounding it, which will also produce a " halo " transradiancy. Should some of the fluid contents of the hydatid cyst be coughed up, the cyst may shrink and the folded up membrane contrasted against the surrounding air which has replaced the fluid produces an appearance like a crumpled handkerchief or water-lily which is surrounded by the ring shadow of the outer covering of the adventitia.

A ring shadow may also contain small shadows of high radio-opacity due to calcifications in material which has sloughed off the wall, and is lying loose in the lumen. The presence of such cavernoliths (or broncholiths) may influence the decision as to the line of treatment—resection perhaps being preferable to a thoracoplasty, if haemoptyses occur despite successful chemotherapy (*see* p. 136).

TUBERCULOUS CAVITIES

A ring shadow (Fig. 203) with a diameter anything from 1 to 7 cm is a common finding in pulmonary tuberculosis. It may be the only shadow, or the only shadow in that area, but more often there are adjacent nodular shadows or areas of patchy clouding. There may be calcifications nearby or elsewhere, though these will not be present in an acute cavity. The ring shadow may be obvious, or will only be seen on careful inspection and when a ring shadow is specifically sought. It may only be seen in a tomogram (*see* p. 243).

In pulmonary tuberculosis it has been observed that cavities giving a similar radiographic picture may have several quite different histologies.

The wall of an acute tuberculous cavity may consist of caseous material, and this may often have the ghosts of the lung structure still visible in it, the central air space having resulted from the expectoration of part of a liquefied caseous pneumonic focus.

In a more long-standing cavity, the wall is composed of tuberculous granulation tissue, consisting of small active tubercles, endothelial cells, lymphocytes and varying amounts of fibrous tissue. This is a common finding in cases treated by resection after the prolonged period of rest and chemotherapy. Sometimes the tubercles and cellular elements predominate, and sometimes the fibrous tissue forms most of the wall.

In a very long-standing case, the cavity may acquire a smooth epithelial lining and a fibrous tissue wall, and a few small tubercles remaining in the wall or adjacent lung are the only histological evidence of its tuberculous origin. After successful chemotherapy even the tubercles may disappear (p. 124).

When the tuberculous process is virtually confined to the bronchus, resulting in narrowing or occlusion with dilatation beyond, or in local wall destruction with weakening and dilatation, the ring shadow is in fact a dilated bronchus, and the wall of the " cavity " has the histological features of bronchial wall with or without tuberculous foci in it. The rest of the bronchus, extending proximally towards the hilum, is often dilated as well, and its wall thickened by tuberculous involvement, so that a so-called " tennis-racket " shadow is seen on the radiograph (Fig. 204). The dilated bronchus may wax and wane in size just like a more distal intrapulmonary tension cavity.

The term " tension cavity " is sometimes used when a ring shadow suddenly appears in a radiograph, or suddenly enlarges, without any x-ray evidence of tissue destruction, such as an area of clouding representing consolidation. These rather dramatic changes cannot help but suggest the theory that the cavity enlarges as a result of an increase in intracavitary pressure, but it must be admitted that the pressures actually found in so-called tension cavities are very variable and sometimes not raised at all. Traction from the surrounding lung may then be a factor.

The draining bronchus of most tuberculous cavities, whatever the type, is either concurrently or secondarily infected. This may be another reason for the periodic rapid changes in size which are observed in " tension " and other cavities; for the thickened oedematous bronchus acts as a valve, air being admitted as it widens during inspiration, but expelled with difficulty as it narrows towards the end of expiration. Alternatively complete obstruction, or renewed free patency, of the draining bronchus may be a factor in the rapid closure of the cavity, and consequent disappearance of the ring shadow.

The cavity wall is usually much less well-defined histologically than it appears in the radiograph. A zone of oedematous alveoli, or compressed (condensed) airless alveoli, is often found around the wall, and variations in the width of this zone may account in part for the changes in the apparent thickness of the wall sometimes noted in serial radiographs.

After successful chemotherapy most tuberculous cavities disappear even if initially they were very large. Some persist, but the wall gets thinner and may end up as a ring with a wall only 2 mm wide. Histologically such a cavity wall will consist of fibrous tissue with no evidence of any residual tuberculous foci, and the cavity thus represents a post-infective cyst with an open bronchial communication.

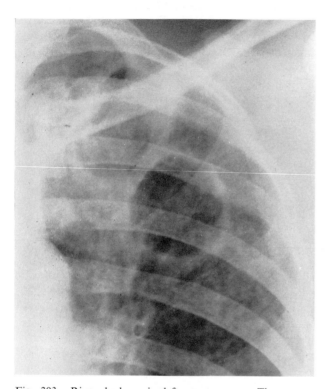

Fig. 203.—Ring shadows in left upper zone. These were tuberculous cavities. Female aged 32 years. Sputum: tubercle bacilli present. Haemoptyses. Some nodular and linear shadows nearby and below cavities.

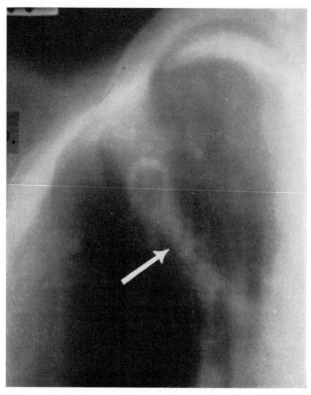

Fig. 204.—Tennis-racket shadow. The arrow marks the tubular shadowing extending from the hilum to an oval-shaped ring shadow. This " cavity " is a dilated bronchus, and " the handle of the racket " is the more proximal part of the same bronchus, which is dilated and thickened.

INFECTIVE CAVITIES

An infective cavity or lung abscess may be due to a specific non-tuberculous infection such as a staphylococcal pneumonia, or to mixed organisms as in suppurative pneumonia. In the acute stage with perhaps a gangrenous area of lung, the wall will consist of pneumonic consolidated or necrotic lung tissue. In the subacute or chronic stage the wall will be formed for the most part by granulation tissue with some surrounding consolidated or oedematous alveolar spaces. If it becomes chronic, fibrotic tissue will be present in increasing amounts.

The x-ray appearances of an infective cavity, whether due to a specific coccal infection or to a mixed infection, are very variable, depending to some extent on the stage of the abscess and on the degree of surrounding consolidation. In the early acute stage of a lung abscess, the only evidence of cavitation may be a small transradiant zone with or without a fluid level, lying in a well-defined 2–3-cm circular shadow (which may have quite a well-defined margin), or in an area of opacity indicating consolidation of the greater part of a lobe or segment. Rather later, the central air transradiancy enlarges and becomes more obvious as some of the fluid is coughed up through the draining bronchus. The size of the fluid level depends on how well the cavity is draining. The anatomical site of the lesion can also be determined from the radiographs.

Resolution may proceed quite rapidly, the fluid level vanishing, and the ring shadow getting smaller and in its turn becoming invisible on the plain radiographs, though persistence of a ring shadow for some time longer may be shown on tomograms. If the abscess becomes chronic, the wall becomes thinner and better defined, so that a typical ring shadow with a wall some 5 mm wide will be clearly seen. As healing proceeds, the wall becomes thinner, and if the cavity persists it will become virtually a post-infective cyst with a well-defined wall no thicker than 1–2 mm consisting almost entirely of fibrous tissue (Fig. 205).

In a staphylococcal pneumonia, particularly in a child, quite a large air space may appear in the opaque consolidated area in a matter of hours, often in the absence of much sputum, so that there is no evidence of expectoration of either necrotic lung tissue or of the pus from an abscess. The exact mechanism of production of these acute cavities is unknown, but it is always assumed they are tension cavities arising as a result of the acute inflammation producing a check-valve action of the bronchus.

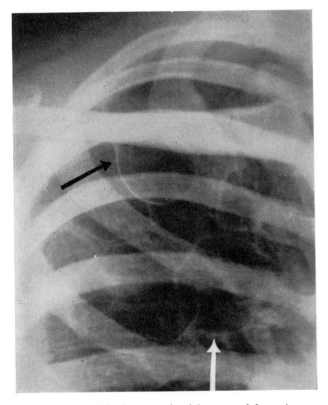

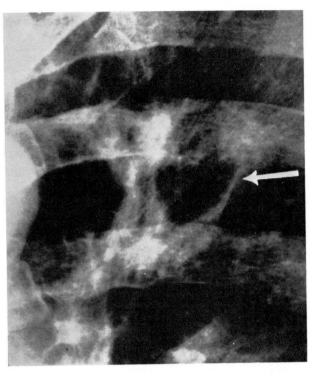

Fig. 205.—Post-infective cysts in right upper lobe. Arrows point to the hair-line wall of some of the cysts. Female aged 22 years. Boil on temple, followed by acute staphylococcal pneumonia. Penicillin; recovery. Now asymptomatic.

Fig. 206.—Bronchial carcinoma. Thin-walled cavity. Similar shadow on the other side. Both resected and both showed a wall of squamous carcinoma. Male aged 50 years. Many years cough and sputum. Malignant cells in sputum.

They are quite common in a staphylococcal infection, and uncommon in infection due to other organisms. They may be single and the consolidation confined to a lobe or part of a lobe; or they may be multiple either in close proximity to each other or scattered as small foci in several lobes, a distribution seen with embolic abscesses in staphylococcal septicaemia. In the early stages a fluid level is quite common, whilst if they do not resolve as the infection subsides, the cavity will usually fill on bronchography if this test is carried out.

After the pneumonia has subsided, which may be within a few days, the cavity may also shrink and finally disappear. Quite frequently, however, a ring shadow or several ring shadows with a hair-line thick wall remain indefinitely, and are often symptom free for long periods thereafter (Fig. 205).

A single large residual ring shadow some 2–5 cm in diameter with a wall only 1–2 mm wide will suggest that the abscess has become a post-infective cyst, the wall of which may consist mainly of fibrous tissue. The exact anatomical site (bronchiole or alveolar) is generally unknown.

Infantile tension cyst

A large relatively transradiant circular or oval avascular area in a lung may be caused by an infantile tension cyst complicating a staphyloccocal pneumonia (Fig. 207). The shadow of some normal lung at the apex separated by the white line shadow of the wall of the air space will distinguish the condition from a pneumothorax which might also complicate a staphyloccocal pneumonia. In infantile lobar emphysema (*see* p. 147) such an apical shadow of normal or compressed lung would not be seen and the clinical picture would be different, though either may cause respiratory distress and in either case surgical intervention with resection of the lobe or cyst may be a life-saving measure.

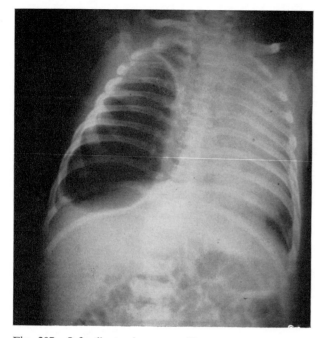

Fig. 207.—Infantile tension cyst. Note some aerated lung over the transradiant zone in the medial part of the apex. Heart and trachea to the left. Male aged 4 years. Six weeks previously a staphylococcal pneumonia. Very breathless when feeding. Lower lobectomy. Cyst had complete epithelial lining.

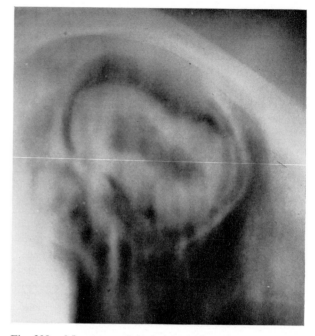

Fig. 208.—Mycetoma. Large ring shadow in left apex with central shadow. This shows a central oval transradiant zone, and a peripheral transradiant zone (halo transradiancy). Elderly female. *Aspergillus fumigatus* in sputum. Skin tests and serum precipitins + ve.

FUNGUS INFECTION WITH A CAVITY

In aspergillosis a well-defined ring shadow may be seen with the fungus mass occupying most of the lumen but, since the central fungus mass does not completely fill the cavity, a small crescentic transradiant zone of air can be seen between it and the cavity wall, producing the so-called " halo shadow " (Fig. 139) (*see also* pp. 81 and 122). In some cases the fungus mass is smaller in relation to the size of the cavity and a wider transradiant zone is seen. Rarely a transradiant zone or cavity occurs within the central fungus mass, producing a double cavity (Fig. 208). In other cases a 2–5 cm transradiancy is seen in an ill-defined area of clouding, the appearances simulating a chronic lung abscess. The finding of *Aspergillus fumigatus* in the sputum will suggest this diagnosis of the ring shadow, but the relation of the cavity to the fungus must be assessed with caution. The serology is often helpful in that in all cases the serum will show positive precipitins to the *Aspergillus fumigatus*. As regards the skin tests for sensitivity to this fungus, the cases can be divided into three groups. The first two are those patients without asthma, half of whom will show no reaction while the other half will show a positive reaction. These two groups will include patients with a pre-existing tuberculous cavity or pre-existing bronchiectasis. The third group consists of those patients with asthma and bronchopulmonary aspergillosis with eosinophilia, all of whom will show a positive skin reaction as well as a positive serum precipitin reaction. In a recent series of mycetomata studied by Dr. D. MaCarthy (personal communication), about one-third of the patients with a mycetoma came from each group. Histological study of the wall of the cavity after resection may indicate that it is a distended bronchus, a cyst, or an infarct breaking down, so that the aspergilli seem to have been a secondary invader. On the other hand, if the fungus is found to have invaded the wall and nearby lung, it will appear to have been the primary cause of the cavity. Sometimes the history and previous radiographs indicate that the fungus is a secondary invader of a pre-existing tuberculous cavity.

The advent of the fungus infection superimposed on a chronic tuberculous cavity (possibly sterilized by a long course of chemotherapy) is sometimes shown in the radiograph by a sudden increase in the thickness of the wall from a few millimetres to well over 1 cm.

In coccidioidomycosis a fine 1–2 cm ring shadow is often seen, particularly in the mid zone. It usually has a thin well-defined wall, and a fluid level may be present. The wall consists of granulation tissue with giant cells and fungi in it. At a later stage it may become fibrotic. The condition is found in the United States of America. The radiographic appearances simulate those of tuberculosis, but the bacteriological and serological findings will generally indicate the diagnosis.

In histoplasmosis a thin-walled 1–2 cm cavity is also sometimes seen. This form of the disease has not yet been reported in persons who have not at one time or another been in an area where the disease is endemic. Distinction from a tuberculous cavity can only be made on the clinical findings.

PARASITIC INFECTION WITH A CAVITY

The cavity seen after a hydatid has been coughed up (or removed) will appear the same as a lung abscess. The wall may be quite well defined, but often the margins are indistinct, so that it suggests an abscess with much surrounding consolidation. Histological examination may reveal the special features found in this condition. If no clinical clues are present, and the cavity boundaries poorly defined, then the diagnosis may be difficult unless previous radiographs before rupture are available, showing a well-demarcated circular shadow, or tomograms show a small well-defined homogeneous circular shadow from another previously unsuspected cyst.

DILATED BRONCHUS

A ring shadow due to a single dilated bronchus may be seen in one form of non-tuberculous bronchiectasis. The wall will have the structure of a bronchus, and the appearances in the radiograph will be the same as those of a post-infective cyst or other cause of a well-defined thin-walled ring shadow. It may attain a size of several centimetres.

Much more commonly several bronchi are dilated, the resulting ring shadows being about 0·5–2 cm in diameter (Fig. 209). They may be situated in one lobe, or the distribution may be quite widespread. The ring shadows are usually quite conspicuous, but if they lie medially so that the hilar shadows are partly superimposed on them, they may be obscured in an anterior view, though clear enough in a lateral view, or in tomograms. This form of bronchiectasis with localized ring shadows is sometimes seen in elderly patients with symptoms suggesting chronic bronchitis.

In a third form of cystic bronchiectasis, there are widely diffused ring shadows the walls of which are of hair-line thickness. This appearance is sometimes referred to as " cystic lung ". There may be few or no symptoms and no other changes in the plain radiographs. If fluid levels are present in these cystic bronchiectases, a half-moon shadow may be seen occupying the lower part of each ring shadow, which may be a more conspicuous feature than the ring shadow itself.

The presence of ring shadows should lead to a consideration of bronchography, but in the absence of specific indications for this (see p. 231) the diagnosis can often be made from the plain radiographs or from tomograms, even though these will not show the extent and character of the dilatations as clearly as the bronchograms.

NEOPLASTIC CAVITIES

In a bronchial carcinoma a lung abscess distal to the growth is not uncommon, and will have the same pathological features as a lung abscess due to other causes. If the neoplasm is small and near the hilum it may be invisible in the plain radiographs, in which case the only visible abnormal shadow will be that of the distal abscess.

Sometimes the central part of a rather more peripheral growth becomes necrotic and is coughed up, and the thick wall, which is a common finding in such a neoplastic cavity, will consist of neoplastic cells. Usually a growth is several centimetres in diameter before such a cavity forms.

A well-defined 2–5-cm ring shadow with a thin wall 2–3 mm wide may also, in spite of its atypical appearance, represent a cavity lined with neoplastic cells (Fig. 202). Since, as in the case illustrated, there may be no history of cough or sputum, it is unlikely that the central air space has resulted from the coughing up of a central necrotic area of a neoplasm. A possible explanation is that the neoplasm in its early stages had obstructed a relatively small bronchus, causing it to become distended and cystic, and had subsequently grown into this cyst, and given it a secondary lining of neoplastic tissue. Sometimes the cavity is quite small (Fig. 206) and like a typical tuberculous cavity.

Secondary deposits may also cavitate and be seen as 2-cm ring shadows with a wall thickness of 3–5 mm. Rarely several similar cavitating secondary deposits may be seen, suggesting the propensity to cavitate is something to do with the type of neoplastic cell and its blood supply, rather than an incidental local mechanical event. Rarely, a rheumatoid nodule may cavitate.

Infarct cavities

A rather thin-walled cavity may develop as a result of a pulmonary infarct. This may represent an aseptic necrosis following a thrombo-embolic infarct, or necrosis secondary to a local vascular lesion (thrombotic or mural occlusive) such as may occur in diffuse lupus erythematosus or Wegner's granulomatosis. In the case of a septic infarct the cavity will result from a mixture of necrosis and infection. In both an infarct and a Wegener's granuloma the cavity wall may be thick and 1–2 cm.

BULLAE

A hair-line ring shadow with a central avascular transradiant zone may be due to a bulla.

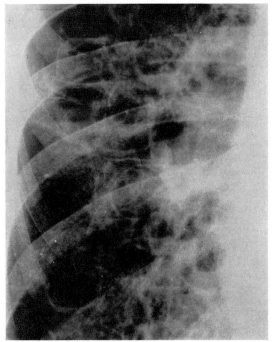

Fig. 209.—Cystic bronchiectasis; 2-cm hair-line ring shadows, some with small fluid levels. Male aged 40 years. Much cough and sputum.

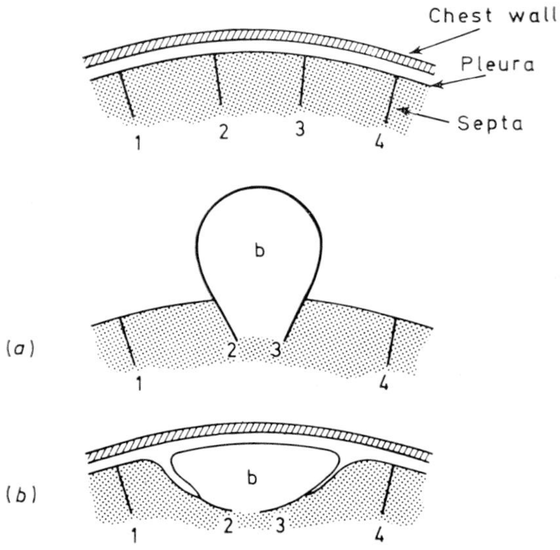

Fig. 210.—Diagram illustrating one way in which a bulla may be demarcated by a hair-line shadow: (a) out of the body, the bulla and its pleural covering project like a "mushroom"; (b) in the body it and the pleura over it are invaginated into the lung by the chest wall. (Reid, 1967.)

A bulla is a local distension with some destruction of the alveoli. The process may start with atrophy or some destruction of the alveoli and the distended air space thus formed is then ballooned out by a check-valve effect. In the resected specimen a bulla will cause a local elevation of the pleura, which is shown diagrammatically in Fig. 210. Since the chest wall will prevent any outward bulging of the lung and pleura, the bulla with its pleural covering will be indented into the lung adjacent to it, as shown in

Fig. 210, and the two layers of pleura together with the remains of connective tissue septa and perhaps a few compressed alveoli will be responsible for the line shadow seen in the radiograph (Figs. 211 and 214). In the apical region, particularly near stellate shadows of old scars, the line may form a ring; but with larger bullae part of the ring will be lost in the general opacity of the chest wall against which it lies, so that only a part of the wall will be seen represented by a curvilinear shadow (*see* below) (Fig. 214).

Bullae can be divided into three types, shown diagrammatically in Figs. 211–213. In type I the bulla has a narrow neck and in the specimen projects like a mushroom. When indented into the adjacent lung by the unyielding chest wall, the pleural covering will also be indented and will produce the well-demarcated curvilinear shadow shown in the radiograph (Fig. 211). This type of bulla represents only a small area of lung greatly over-distended. In a type II bulla the neck is wider and the line of indented pleura may be less easily seen, or may even be invisible in one view but can be seen in another projection.

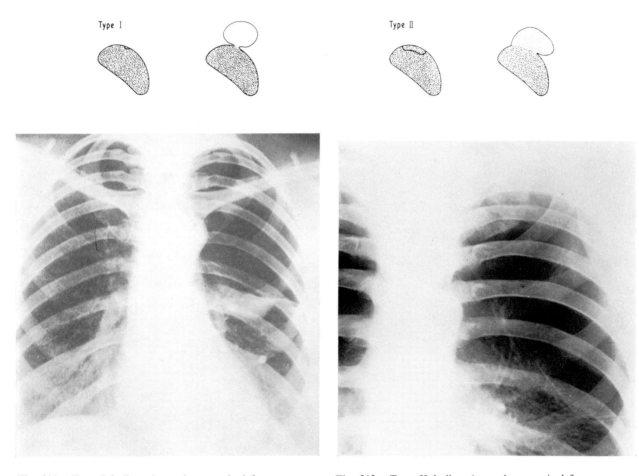

Fig. 211.—Type I bulla. Avascular area in left upper zone demarcated below by a line shadow. This represents a small amount of lung greatly over-inflated. Narrow neck (mushroom bulla). Contents: empty air space. Female aged 47 years. Asymptomatic.

Fig. 212.—Type II bulla. Avascular area in left upper zone poorly demarcated below by thin line shadows. Neck wider than in type I. Tendency to compress nearby lung. Contents: emphysematous lung with much-dilated air spaces.

It represents a larger volume of distended lung than a type I bulla and often causes displacement of the nearby fissure or crowding together and displacement of vessels in the adjacent lobe (Fig. 212). In spite of this the functional improvement following its removal is often slight. In type III there is slight dilatation of a larger volume of lung, and the architecture of the major vessels is more or less intact (Fig. 213). Because of the high intra-alveolar gas pressure, blood flow will be greatly diminished, so that in the plain radiograph the vessels may not be seen, and the apparently avascular area may be mistaken for an empty air space such as is seen in a type I bulla. The vessels may, however, be seen in a tomogram. Since the neck is very wide and the distension relatively slight, there is no indentation of the pleura and the avascular transradiant area is thus not demarcated by a white line (Fig. 213). It may then be described as a bullous area or area of emphysematous lung, in contradistinction from the well-demarcated empty air space of a type I bulla. The distinction is less obvious in a type II bulla since the line may be invisible in an anterior view but seen clearly in a lateral view.

Type III

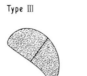

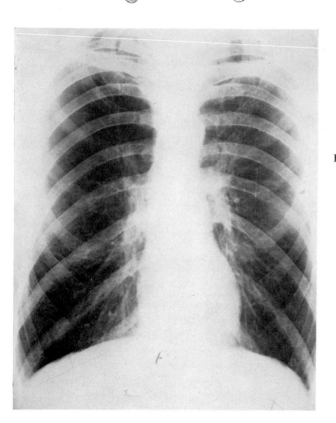

Fig. 213.—Type III bulla—or emphysematous lung. Avascular area in right upper zone. Horizontal fissure not displaced. Tomograms showed some vessels in the otherwise avascular area. On resection—contents: dilated alveoli with major vessels intact within the lobe. Low flat diaphragm and small vessels left base, so local accentuation of widespread emphysema. Male aged 46 years. Cough, sputum and dyspnoea. P.F. 100 l/min.

A bulla may be a purely local incident and then, even if it occupies the whole of one hemithorax (Fig. 215), it will not cause symptoms. It may also be seen as a local accentuation of a more widespread or general emphysema, and then will contribute to the dyspnoea by the amount of lung loss it represents. Only about a third of the cases of widespread emphysema do in fact show a bulla. In chronic bronchitis the symptoms will usually be caused by the bronchitis and not by the bulla. Compression of nearby lung is only of importance when it is gross, and symptoms may be relieved if the compressed lung is otherwise normal, and therefore when allowed to re-expand will contribute to respiration.

A type I bulla is so peripheral that a bronchogram may appear normal. In a type II or III bulla the more proximal bronchi may be seen filled with the contrast medium within the transradiant area, but peripheral filling will not occur.

A fluid level may occur in a bulla but is relatively uncommon. It may persist for months but will usually disappear in the course of time.

When a hair-line ring shadow is seen in close proximity to stellate or amorphous shadows from the scars of regressing tuberculous lesions, or a complicated pneumoconiosis, it may be difficult to decide whether the ring shadow represents a destructive lung cavity or a bulla. Tomograms may reveal features that favour one interpretation rather than another (*see* p. 245 and Fig. 345).

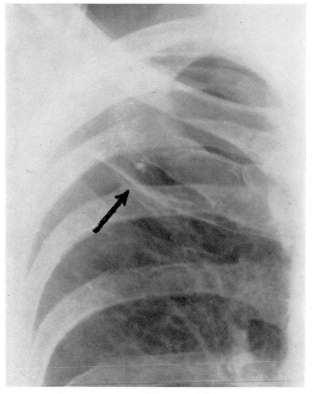

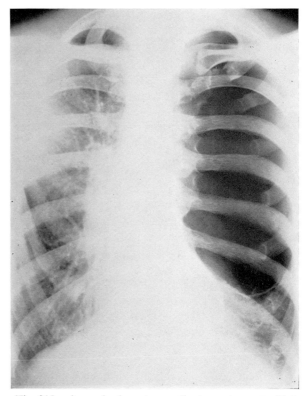

Fig. 214.—Bulla in right apex demarcated below by line shadow (above arrow). Type I in a chronic bronchitic. Male aged 53 years. Cough and sputum, some dyspnoea. No widespread emphysema.

Fig. 215.—Avascular hypertransradiant area in most of left lung, demarcated below by a line shadow. Large bulla in left upper lobe compressing lower lobe. Vessel shadows right lung normal. Male aged 42 years. Asymptomatic.

DEVELOPMENTAL AIR-CONTAINING CYSTS

A similar radiographic appearance to that of an isolated bulla may be caused by a cyst of developmental origin. Such a cyst may arise as a result of a local developmental bronchial defect causing a mechanical distension (by a check-valve effect) distal to it, or it may form inside a cellular growth, as in the case of a bronchogenic cyst or sequestrated segment with a bronchial connection. The latter type of cyst will be found to have elements of ciliated epithelium, mucous glands, cartilage, or muscle in its wall, and perhaps a blood supply from a systemic artery.

CAVITY IN PNEUMOCONIOSIS

Radiating lines spreading out from the poorly defined outer margins of a thick-walled ring shadow are typical of a pneumoconiosis, the cavity resulting from the expectoration of the central necrotic part of an area of massive fibrosis. The central transradiancy of the lumen of the cavity may be quite clear or may be made recognizable by the presence of a fluid level, or it may be indistinct until clearly demonstrated in tomograms. The very small circular shadows of the basic lesion will also be seen in both lungs, especially if they are sought. The wall of the cavity will consist of the surrounding fibrous tissue. The sputum may be inky black during the phase of expectoration of the necrotic central substance, and will usually not contain tubercle bacilli (*see* p. 116).

CAVITY IN SARCOIDOSIS

Occasionally in the late stage of sarcoidosis with massive residual ill-defined opacities and shrunken upper lobes, a 2–3-cm ring shadow with a central transradiancy is seen. The specimen in one such case showed a cavity with a wall of featureless collagen tissue. Such a cavity may therefore be equivalent to a large honeycomb space seen in fibrosing alveolitis, particularly if this is due to xanthomatous granulomata.

INTRAPULMONARY RING SHADOWS: SUMMARY

It is thus apparent that an intrapulmonary ring shadow may represent a great variety of lesions, ranging from an air space resulting from tissue destruction, often further ballooned out by a check-valve action of the draining bronchus, for example, a lung abscess or a tuberculous cavity, to a dilated bronchus, a breaking down infarct, whether thrombo-embolic, from a local arteritis in periarteritis, Wegener's granuloma or diffuse lupus erythematosus, an intrapulmonary neoplasm, a developmental cystic space, or an intrapulmonary distension space with or without tissue destruction, such as a bulla or area of emphysema.

As a general rule bullae, bullous areas, some post-infective cysts, and some cysts of developmental origin have a thin wall in relation to their size, and are thus fairly distinctive. When they are small they may more easily be confused with other forms of pulmonary cavitation.

PLEURAL AIR SPACE CAUSING RING SHADOW

An extrapulmonary ring shadow may be caused by an encysted pleural air space, and differentiation of such an air space from an intrapulmonary cavity may be particularly difficult. After an old abandoned pneumothorax for instance, or a recent lobectomy, it is sometimes impossible to tell immediately whether a localized transradiancy near an apex sharply demarcated by a ring-like shadow is a residual pleural air space, and therefore relatively harmless, or whether it is a recent intrapulmonary cavity, and therefore menacing. A diagnostic pneumothorax after a lobectomy would be impracticable, and careful clinical and radiological observation may be needed before a certain answer is possible.

An idiopathic spontaneous localized pleural air space can occur, but is uncommon, and most so-called " pleural rings " turn out to be intrapulmonary pathological air spaces of one kind or another.

An encysted hydropneumothorax or pyopneumothorax similar to that illustrated in Fig. 59 may be demarcated in part by a line or band, and may closely simulate a lung abscess, especially if a bronchial fistula is also present. Distinction between these two conditions is not always possible even during surgical drainage.

MEDIASTINAL AIR SPACE CAUSING A RING SHADOW

Mediastinal cyst

A mediastinal cyst such as a paratracheal or para-oesophageal cyst, or a sequestrated segment may become infected and develop a bronchial or oesophageal fistula as a result of this, so that some of the contents are replaced by air. If the shadow lies rather more laterally than usual, it will closely simulate an intrapulmonary cavity, but its position near or within the central shadow will suggest the diagnosis.

Diaphragmatic hernia

Another mediastinal air space may be the result of a diaphragmatic hernia containing stomach or intestine and will show in the radiographs as an intrathoracic air space, with a relatively thin wall and perhaps a fluid level. This shadow must therefore also be distinguished from an intrapulmonary cavity. Naturally if the condition is suspected, a barium meal will be given to confirm the diagnosis and determine the type of hernia (see p. 211). The thickness of the wall of the ring shadow, and the presence of band-like shadows projecting into the transradiant zone will not only suggest the diagnosis of a hernia, but will indicate which part of gut is herniated.

In the case of the stomach the width of the shadow of the wall will vary between 2 and 8 mm—the smaller figure only being seen if the stomach is much distended with air. Wavy band-like shadows about 3–5 mm wide are often seen running across the transradiant area, and are due to the gastric rugae. These rugal folds are much more conspicuous in some cases than others.

The wall of a loop of herniated colon may be almost as wide as the stomach shadow, but the band-like shadows passing from the wall across the transradiant zone are straighter, and often show short circular expansions in one or two places.

A loop of small intestine has a rather thinner wall, and the band-like shadows of the valvulae conniventes running across are finer, being only 1–2 mm wide, and are spaced more closely, being often about 1 cm apart.

A roughly oval or rather elongated ring shadow with a central transradiancy may be caused by a part of the stomach or upper small intestine lying in the thorax following an anastomosis after resection of the lower third of the oesophagus. The shadow tends to be more elongated than that of a more usual type of hernia, and generally lies centrally and to the left. It is only likely to be a cause of difficulty in diagnosis if interpretation of the radiographic appearances is attempted without knowing the clinical history.

SMALL MULTIPLE RING SHADOWS (HONEYCOMB SHADOWING)

A honeycomb shadow refers to a closely set group of small ring shadows, each with a wall about 1–2 mm wide surrounding a more or less circular central transradiant zone 3–8 mm in diameter. In some cases the walls are rather wider and less well defined although the central transradiancies are clearly seen; in others, the walls are of narrow hair-line width and well defined.

If the ring shadows are larger, for example over 1 cm, the appearance is sometimes described as "cystic lung" (*see* p. 127), although "large or coarse honeycomb shadowing" would be a better description. If the ring shadows are smaller and more numerous, the appearance superficially simulates a "reticular or net-like pattern", but by careful inspection the ring shadow can be identified.

Honeycomb lung

Small 3–8 mm clearly defined hair-line ring shadows occurring in a group close to each other are referred to as honeycomb shadows (Figs. 216 and 217). In fact, the ring shadows are usually separated from each other by nodular or short line shadows, and in serial radiographs nodular shadows usually precede the appearance of honeycomb shadows, which are often a late complication of lesions producing initially nodular shadows (*see* p. 97). They include such conditions as fibrosing alveolitis which may be cryptogenic or related to a known noxious agent such as asbestos, or to an agent producing an immunological reaction, or to allergic alveolitis as in farmers' lung (*Micropolyspora faenis, Actinomyces vulgaris*) bird fancier's lung (particularly budgerigars, pigeons and parrots), or to another disease of unknown aetiology such as rheumatoid arthritis, diffuse systemic sclerosis or xanthomatosis (Fig. 217).

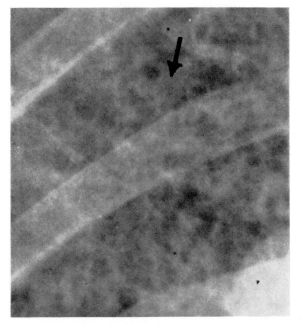

Fig. 216.—Honeycomb shadows. A group of hair-line ring shadows 8 mm in diameter (below arrow). Fibrosing alveolitis. Ring shadows smaller than in Fig. 217. Female aged 60 years. Severe dyspnoea. DLco 4·9; F.V.C. 1,600; F.E.V. 1,500. Died 6 years after onset. Fibrosing alveolitis.

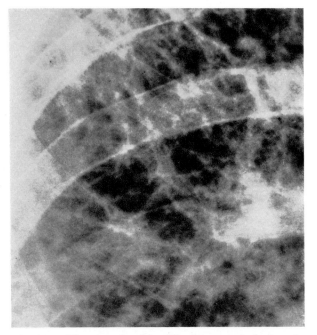

Fig. 217.—Fibrosing alveolitis. Fine honeycomb shadows in lower half of both lungs. Male aged 44 years. Dyspnoea and clubbing, and rheumatoid arthritis. Biopsy: alveolar wall thickening with macrophages, fibrosis, and in some areas clefts with fibrous walls, representing dilated alveoli and bronchioli.

Honeycomb shadows may also be seen in one manifestation of ordinary bronchiectasis, in which case they will be outlined in a bronchogram. This is in contrast to fibrosing alveolitis when the honeycomb spaces do not fill with the contrast medium. The only abnormality seen is that the terminal branches fail to decrease in calibre as in a normal bronchogram, and the millimetre pattern is not seen.

The honeycomb appearance may be widespread or only seen in one or two areas. If the honeycomb shadows are situated near the hilum they may pass undetected because of superimposed vessel shadows, but may nevertheless be clearly seen in a lateral view, particularly if they are in the anterior segment of the upper lobe. If they are situated in the left lower lobe they may be obscured by the heart shadow in a routine anterior view radiograph, but may be seen in a more exposed radiograph, or they may sometimes be seen contrasted against the superimposed transradiancy of the gastric air bubble lying in front of the posterior inferior part of the lung, or they may best be seen in a lateral view.

The honeycomb shadows often seen in a late stage of fibrosing alveolitis are easily identified pathologically as dilated air spaces. The wall of such an air space may show collagen and fibrous tissue with either remnants of alveoli or bronchioli. In fact the same air space may show elements of both these structures in different parts of the wall. In bronchiectasis remnants of bronchial wall will be seen. Occasionally only a single small ring shadow is seen, or there are several but they are not in close proximity. These more isolated air spaces may show a pathological structure of the wall similar to those described above.

Mesodermal dysplasia

Honeycomb shadows of a similar nature are sometimes seen in a mesodermal dysplasia (tuberose sclerosis) in a mentally deficient person. Frequently small ill-defined shadows can be seen in a lateral view of the skull indicating intracerebral calcifications. In some cases there is no mental deficiency but the diagnosis may be substantiated if a small skin nodule is found with the histological features of adenoma sebaceum. A lung biopsy will show much muscle tissue around the alveolar spaces which tend to be dilated.

Endocrine disorders

In a rare type of pituitary disorder there may be honeycomb shadowing in the lung. The clinical evidence of the endocrine disorder will indicate the diagnosis.

Pneumoconiosis

In some forms of pneumoconiosis the abnormal shadows are honeycomb or net-like rather than nodular. The industrial history will usually suffice for the diagnosis.

Pulmonary vascular plethora

Plethora of the pulmonary circulation in some cardiac conditions, especially if the engorgement is predominantly of the peripheral vessels, may give rise to a fine honeycomb or almost reticular pattern. When such changes are present, the cardiac condition will be quite obvious clinically.

Lymphangitis carcinomatosa

The dilated lymphatics in lymphangitis carcinomatosa may be so superimposed as to give a similar honeycomb shadow. If the patient is known to have a primary carcinoma elsewhere, the nature of the lung shadows will be apparent. Generally some long line shadows and nodular shadows will also be present, and there may be enlargement of the hilar glands.

Normal bronchus

An isolated ring shadow 2–5 mm in diameter is often seen near the upper and outer part of the hila in normal persons. Usually there is one each side and it is due to an anterior branch of the anterior bronchus seen end on. Sometimes there are two such ring shadows on each side; the lowermost on the left may be an anterior division of the superior division of the lingula bronchus. The wall of the ring shadow may show a transient increase in width from time to time in those conditions in which transient tram line shadows are seen (see p. 119), for instance in asthma, cystic fibrosis, and in asthmatics with bronchopulmonary aspergillosis and eosinophilia.

CHAPTER 4

HIGH-DENSITY SHADOWS AND HYPERTRANSRADIANCIES

SOME LESIONS are distinctive radiologically not by their size, shape, or position, but because of their relative radio-opacity or hypertransradiancy. Relatively high radio-opacity is due to the presence of atoms of high atomic number in the structure causing the shadow; whereas hypertransradiancy is generally caused by air occupying regions normally occupied by cellular tissues.

SHADOWS FROM ENDOGENOUS LESIONS OF HIGH RADIO-OPACITY

Relatively dense shadows are commonly due to calcifications in normal or in pathological tissue, and since these are often of little clinical significance, they are frequently given no more than a cursory glance. Nevertheless they are sometimes important, and their size, shape, position and relation to nearby shadows may assist the diagnosis.

Their most common cause is the deposition of endogenous calcium either in normal structures the blood supply to which is poor—such as the costal or tracheal cartilages—or in pathological tissue—such as a tuberculous focus—in which not only is the blood supply poor, but the infection is relatively quiescent or even obsolete. Calcification may also occur in cartilaginous nodules within tumours or whenever ectopic bone nodules are present in the lung. More rarely the relatively high density of the shadow is due to the deposition of endogenous iron molecules in pulmonary tissue.

INTRAPULMONARY RELATIVELY DENSE SHADOWS

Calcified small tuberculous foci

The most common intrapulmonary calcifications are those seen in small chronic regressing tuberculous foci. There may only be one such calcification, but more often there are several either in a localized group or scattered in other parts of the lung fields.

Considerable variations in the size and shape of the calcifications are seen. Some are smooth in outline and circular, others are oval, linear, Y-shaped, or with irregular margins and of no particular shape. They vary in size from a minute spot to several millimetres in width.

A calcification may be the only abnormal shadow or it may be surrounded by the low-density shadow of the unresolved and uncalcified part of the focus, appearing as a small dense spot in the middle of a less dense 1-cm shadow (Fig. 155), or lying eccentrically usually in relation to a rather smaller shadow. Several calcifications may be grouped together in one focus, giving it a mottled or woolly appearance.

In asymptomatic patients under 30 years of age, the finding of calcifications associated with small (minimal) lesions is of no clinical importance. Their presence does not affect the prognosis should separate shadows of low density be also present due to unresolved or more recent tuberculous foci, or should new shadows of fresh foci appear in subsequent radiographs. On the other hand, among asymptomatic patients over 30 years of age, these calcifications have a slightly beneficial effect on the prognosis, being associated with a lower rate of spread of the lesion over the next few years, and a smaller tendency for tubercle bacilli to be isolated on culture than is the case when no conspicuous calcification has been seen in the initial radiograph (Springett, 1956).

Since there are other causes of intrapulmonary calcifications than regressing tuberculous foci, the presence of these shadows does not always assist the diagnosis in a doubtful case. Even if the calcifications do represent tuberculous foci, their presence will not exclude the coexistence of another kind of lesion around or nearby such as a sarcoid, a neoplasm, or a suppurative pneumonia, any of which might be responsible for shadows of low density in their neighbourhood.

In rare cases the calcified tuberculous focus may be directly related to the symptoms. A recurrent haemoptysis may occur, for instance, because a calcified lesion is eroding a vessel or being extruded into a small bronchus. It is essential to exclude other causes of haemoptysis as far as possible before assuming the calcified focus to be the cause.

The combination of a solitary pulmonary calcified focus with calcification of the hilar gland in the region of its drainage is evidence of a tuberculous infection in the past (Gohn's focus), though an identical appearance may be seen in histoplasmosis. The shadows should not be dismissed without careful inspection, since a discrepancy between the position of the pulmonary focus in relation to that of the gland would indicate the possibility of some displacement of the focus, and in some cases this might be the most obvious evidence in the plain radiograph of a lobar displacement from an old bronchostenosis.

Calcifications in large circular shadows

Calcifications are sometimes seen in a large 2–4-cm low-density shadow. If the lesion is tuberculous, whether a healing primary focus or a massive post-primary focus, the calcifications are sometimes in the form of narrow concentric rings. In some cases only a small central spot of calcification can be seen in the large shadow, and in others, a fairly large central calcification, rather shapeless and either woolly or homogeneous in texture. These appearances may also be sometimes seen in a hamartoma or a dermoid.

Calcifications in cavernoliths and broncholiths

If a calcification is seen to be superimposed on a ring shadow in the anterior view, a lateral view and, if necessary, tomograms are indicated to see whether it represents a calcified body (cavernolith) in the cavity or another focus remote from the cavity. Anterior views taken with the patient first sitting and then lying on one side, and with the x-ray beam horizontal, will show whether the dense shadow moves in relation to the cavity wall, and is therefore lying loose in it, or whether it bears a constant relation to the wall and is therefore embedded in or adherent to it. The presence of a cavernolith will suggest that a thoracoplasty is not the most suitable method of encouraging cavity closure if some other equally safe method is available (see p. 123).

The relation of a calcification to any nearby major bronchus can be determined by tomography, and if it is found to be intraluminal it is a broncholith. Such a finding might explain an otherwise obscure haemoptysis or series of febrile respiratory episodes. A broncholith may be a cavernolith on its way out towards the trachea, or part of a calcified tuberculous gland which has ulcerated through the wall and has finally been extruded into the lumen of the bronchus; alternatively, it may have arisen in its present position as a result of a localized tuberculous bronchitis.

Hilar gland calcifications

Calcifications in the hilar glands may be obvious or may pass undetected in the plain radiograph. A large group of paratracheal calcified glands may be invisible in the routine anterior view though clearly seen in a radiograph taken with more exposure or in the lateral view. Slight degrees of calcification can often be seen only in tomograms, whether they are in the lungs, the hilar glands or the paratracheal glands. This fact must be remembered when only plain radiographs are being used for epidemiological studies, or when bronchostenosis is suspected which may possibly be caused by a tuberculous and perhaps calcified gland.

Sometimes ring calcifications are seen around hilar glands, particularly in some of the pneumoconioses such as those of coal or china clay workers. In such cases widespread small nodular shadows will also be seen in the lungs. The ring of calcification is sometimes described as an egg-shell calcification.

WIDESPREAD SMALL DENSE (RADIO-OPAQUE) NODULAR SHADOWS

The calcifications in the lungs in histoplasmosis, and those in rheumatic fever, with or without evidence of cardiac involvement, in microlithiasis alveolaris, and the dense shadows produced by endogenous iron particles in haemosiderosis, have been described on pages 98 and 99.

Calcifications in small non-tuberculous foci

Calcification can occur in scars due to non-tuberculous inflammation, or around fibrotic nodules which have been caused by the inhalation of silica-containing dust. Some of the nodular calcifications often seen in the upper zones of the lungs may belong to this category, but proof that the originating lesion was non-tuberculous is often unobtainable. A very common cause of fibrotic nodules is chronic bronchitis with emphysema, but these scars do not usually calcify. A healed infarct may eventually calcify, but no proved example of this has come to the author's notice.

Calcifications in the tracheal and bronchial cartilages and the pulmonary vessels

Calcifications in the tracheal rings or cartilages of the main bronchi are sometimes sufficiently marked in elderly people to cast shadows in the radiograph. The distribution of the calcium is patchy, but the general position of the shadows is such that their nature can be readily appreciated. A part of the left main bronchus may be seen as a dense tubular shadow, which may simulate a vessel calcification.

Radiographs of resection specimens of the lungs often show a few small spots of high-density shadowing, which are due to calcified deposits in the more peripheral bronchial cartilages, but these are rarely detected in the routine chest radiographs.

Calcifications in the pulmonary arteries within the lung fields are uncommon and rarely diagnosed.

PLEURAL CALCIFICATIONS

A pleural calcification may be small and quite localized resulting in a dense vertical linear or narrow band-like shadow usually just above a costophrenic recess. A more elliptical shadow may be seen if the calcification is in the residue of a fibrin body initiated during an artificial pneumothorax refill.

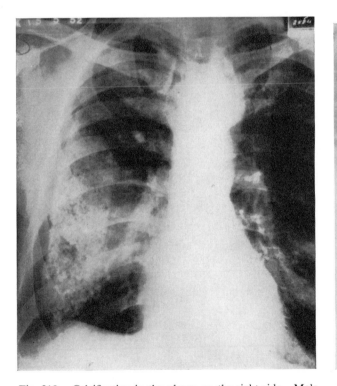

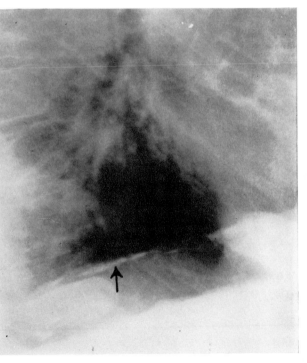

Fig. 218.—Calcification in the pleura on the right side. Male aged 50 years. Six weeks previously lump noticed in lower right chest wall. Abscess and rock-like mass excised. In spite of previous radiographs indicating the calcified pleura had been present for 20 years, active tuberculous lesions were present in the adjacent abscess.

Fig. 219.—Dense horizontal line shadow (of pleural calcification) running just above left dome of diaphragm (above arrow). Worked with asbestos. Asymptomatic.

A linear calcification in the axilla or parallel to the upper surface of the diaphragm is seen in asbestosis (Fig. 219). Such an x-ray finding may result in obtaining a more detailed occupational history than normal, and this may lead to the diagnosis. A similar linear calcification may be due to another cause such as an organizing pleural haematoma or old rheumatoid pleurisy, though actual proof of the initiating lesion cannot always be found.

A dense mottled shadow extending over a considerable area (Fig. 218) is a characteristic appearance of calcification in a sheet of thickened pleura. On fluoroscopy or in a lateral or oblique tangential view the position of the shadow just beneath the ribs is easily confirmed. Such a shadow is usually asymptomatic and found by accident, and generally indicates an old tuberculous pleurisy, which may not, however, be completely sterile. In one such case (Fig. 218) the shadow had been present for 20 years before the development of a small chest wall abscess made treatment necessary. Examination of the specimen after resection of the abscess and thickened pleura revealed several active caseous foci adjacent to the pleural calcifications. Similar calcification of a sheet of thickened pleura can result from a traumatic haemothorax or an old partly inspissated non-tuberculous empyema. A few rather more scattered 1–2 cm long irregular pleural calcifications may be seen in asbestosis.

CALCIFICATIONS IN MEDIASTINAL STRUCTURES

Extrapulmonary calcifications in mediastinal tumours are described on page 207; those in the pericardium, on page 179; and those in the heart and great vessels, on page 180.

EXTRATHORACIC CALCIFICATIONS

Extrathoracic calcifications can usually be distinguished from intrathoracic ones if care is taken to locate the position of the shadow accurately from the anterior and lateral views, supplemented when necessary by an anterior view taken on expiration, by fluoroscopy with careful rotation of the patient, or by tomography. A tangential view may be useful to confirm some point seen during fluoroscopy.

Unusual calcifications in a rib or costal cartilage are possible sources of confusion, but these will be seen to bear a constant relation to the rib during respiratory movements. Their relation to the rib can, if necessary, be clearly demonstrated by tomography.

A calcification in an intercostal space, even if it is in contact with the pleura, can often be localized by the same means. The calcification may be in a lymphatic gland in the lower neck or upper axillary region, or it may be in callus around a rib fracture whether spontaneous, traumatic, or from a cough.

Cysticerci may lodge in the intercostal muscles or in the muscles covering the thorax and, when calcified, produce a characteristic spindle-shaped shadow about 5–10 mm long.

In myositis ossificans of a chest wall muscle, the shadow in one view will be seen to extend beyond the lung margins.

DENSE SHADOWS FROM EXOGENOUS SUBSTANCES OF HIGH RADIO-OPACITY

INHALED FOREIGN BODY

An inhaled foreign body of high radio-opacity and characteristic shape such as a pin or small metal ball presents no particular difficulty in x-ray diagnosis and the foreign body can generally be localized to a particular lobar or segmental bronchus. If the foreign body is less radio-opaque and of ill-defined shape, such as a piece of tooth or a meat bone, it may be difficult to demonstrate, or it may be mistaken for a calcified gland. Similarly a calcified gland may be wrongly diagnosed as an inhaled foreign body. When such a suspicious but indeterminate shadow is seen, tomography should be undertaken to make sure it is in fact in a bronchus before bronchoscopy is undertaken to remove it.

If no foreign body can be demonstrated by radiology in spite of the history, an attempt should be made to determine whether it is likely to be sufficiently radio-opaque to be visible, in which case a failure to show it will exclude it, or whether like many artificial teeth, it is not sufficiently radio-opaque. If one of several teeth is missing from a denture, the opacity of the remaining ones can be rapidly checked. The denture should be placed on the patient's back over one lung, and an anterior view taken to see if it casts a shadow on the radiograph. If the test is negative and no shadow is seen, bronchoscopy may be indicated to exclude a non-opaque foreign body.

The presence of a foreign body may be suggested if a lung shadow is seen typical of an atelectasis, or of an area of consolidation, either of which might occur distal to a bronchostenosis from a non-opaque foreign body in one of the larger bronchi, or if the lung or a lobe fails to deflate like that on the other side in a radiograph taken in expiration (*see* p. 145).

If no abnormal shadows can be seen in the lungs, and the patient is not even sure whether he inhaled or swallowed the foreign body, or if there is a suspicion that he has a wrong impression of which way it went down, it will be necessary to search for it radiologically in the pharynx, oesophagus, or even the abdomen.

INHALED RADIO-OPAQUE DUSTS

Small widely disseminated very dense shadows varying from pinpoint size to about 5 mm may be due to the inhalation of particles of substances containing atoms of high atomic weight such as iron, barium, tin, and calcium (talc) as described on page 98.

IODIZED OIL SHADOWS

The characteristic dense shadows due to iodized oil residues after bronchography are described on page 98.

If some iodized oil is inadvertently injected into the neck tissues instead of the trachea during an attempted cricothyroid injection for bronchography, the opaque medium will tend to disperse in a thin layer in the paratracheal or retrosternal tissues, where it will remain indefinitely. It may also remain in a sinus or other walled-off space if it cannot drain away after injection. It will sometimes collect in small 5–10-mm globules in the pus in an empyema cavity or a bronchiectasis.

TRAUMATIC FOREIGN BODY

A metallic foreign body in the thorax resulting from trauma may require identification and localization. Sometimes the foreign body is very obvious, and its position easily determined in relation to the chest wall, the heart, or the lung. If it is in the lung it may be possible to see either from anterior and lateral views or from tomograms in which segment it lies. Sometimes accurate segmental localization is very difficult, either because the patient is too ill for elaborate radiography, or because associated lung or pleural damage have resulted in an effusion or pneumothorax, and have thus made recognition of the normal landmarks difficult or impossible.

Given reasonable co-operation with the surgeon, the radiological problem often resolves itself into a decision whether the limited radiography available gives sufficient information, or whether delay is justified in the hope that the patient may soon be fit enough for more elaborate radiography, including perhaps fluoroscopy or tomography, or even a parallax method of depth localization.

HYPERTRANSRADIANCIES

A slight generalized hypertransradiancy of both lungs is difficult to detect because there is as yet no measure of normal lung transradiancy, and excessive blackening of the lung fields in the radiograph may be the result of technical factors and thus of no clinical significance. The hypertransradiancy may, however, be detected if the blackening of the lungs is assessed in relation to the body build of the patient and the density of the rib and thoracic coverings. Its significance should be judged in conjunction with the cardiovascular pattern.

A local hypertransradiancy, on the other hand, can be detected by comparing it with the blackening of the other presumably normal parts of the lung fields.

EXTRATHORACIC CAUSES OF LOCAL HYPERTRANSRADIANCY

Extrathoracic causes of hypertransradiancy are generally unilateral and often local. An exception to this will be a patient with gross wasting or poor development, a condition which will be obvious on clinical examination, or from observation of the thinness of the shadow of the extrathoracic soft tissue layer in the lower axilla.

Scoliosis, or faulty development, atrophy or removal of a muscle overlying the lung fields or of a breast, will give rise to a localized area of hypertransradiancy in which there will be a normal vessel pattern. The cause will be obvious on examination of the patient, or may even be obvious on the radiograph.

Localized extrapleural air pocket

A pocket of air in an abnormal site overlying a lung field may give rise to a localized area of transradiancy in the anterior-view radiograph. Such an air pocket may remain for several days in a fascial space after a radical mastectomy, and the appearances, sometimes even including a fluid level, may simulate an intrapulmonary cavity. A localized transradiancy due to air in the extrapleural space is seen after a thoracoplasty or a ball or pack " plomb ", and since it is inevitable in the first few days, it is of no importance provided it tends to shrink rapidly. It will become significant if the amount of fluid or air increases rapidly, suggesting the possibility of haemorrhage, infection, or a fistula into the space.

Generalized subcutaneous and extrapleural emphysema

Air transradiancies are sometimes seen over a wide area around muscle bundles and in fascial spaces, producing a series of spindle-shaped and linear transradiancies (Fig. 223). These usually extend into the axillary or lower neck regions so that their extrathoracic position is obvious even from the anterior-view radiograph. There may be a history of trauma, thoracoscopy, or a pneumothorax refill, or it may be an idiopathic condition particularly in asthmatics or associated with a spontaneous pneumothorax from a ruptured bulla. Rarely, but more ominously, it may be an upward extension of a mediastinal emphysema from a ruptured oesophagus, and the air transradiancies in the lower neck region may be seen in the radiograph before the air can be detected clinically (see p. 141).

INTRATHORACIC BUT EXTRAPULMONARY LOCAL HYPERTRANSRADIANCIES

Pneumothorax and extrapleural pneumothorax

Air in the pleural cavity, whether the result of a therapeutic induction or refill, or whether spontaneous, will result in a transradiancy which may be very obvious, especially if there is a lot of air present. If in addition the lung edge is clearly visible, the diagnosis of a pneumothorax will usually present no difficulties.

On the other hand, if there is only a small quantity of air present, so that the pneumothorax is shallow, the hypertransradiancy may be very inconspicuous and the lung edge invisible or only seen with difficulty. If there is a history of recent chest pain on one side, this condition should be suspected and the white hair line of the lung edge carefully sought. If necessary an additional film should be taken during deep suspended expiration, since the white hair line of the lung edge and the transradiancy of the pleural air space may then be more conspicuous. The transradiancy of the pleural air space is free from any vessel shadows unless, as a result of a broad band of adhesions, some lung tissue lies in front or behind it, the vessels in which will then be superimposed on the transradiant zone.

A small localized pneumothorax may easily be confused with a bulla, a bullous area (Fig. 220), or a small thin-walled intrapulmonary cavity, and distinction between these conditions may not always be possible on the initial radiograph (see p. 245). The line demarcating a bulla is usually more horizontal than the line of visceral pleura over a localized pneumothorax. If there is doubt whether a localized transradiant avascular area represents a bulla or a localized pneumothorax, it will almost certainly be due to a bulla, and a needle should not be introduced with a view to expanding the lung since, if the lesion is a bulla, it may result in a disastrous pneumothorax as well. A pneumothorax of such a small size will not cause symptoms, and does not need aspiration of the air.

Difficulties of diagnosis may also arise with a very large spontaneous pneumothorax with almost total relaxation of the lung. The large hypertransradiancy occupying most of one side of the chest, possibly with displacement of the heart and trachea to the opposite side, and some depression of the dome of the diaphragm on the same side, may look very like a large bullous or other kind of air-containing cyst. In the pneumothorax the relaxed or positively compressed lung can be seen close to the hilum, whilst in a large air-containing cyst the shadow of some still aerated or partly compressed lung can be seen at one point around the cyst, either in the region of the cardiophrenic or costophrenic angles, or medially near the apex. In the same way an " infantile tension cyst " (Fig. 207) must be distinguished from a spontaneous pneumothorax, since resection of the cyst may be a life-saving measure.

Diaphragmatic hernia

A diaphragmatic hernia with much air in the stomach or intestine is another cause of an extrapulmonary hypertransradiancy. Usually the diagnosis is fairly obvious, but if the stomach or a short length of colon lying in the thorax becomes obstructed, it may become so distended that it occupies the whole of one side and will thus simulate a spontaneous pneumothorax or hydropneumothorax (Fig. 221). The absence of the typical shadow of the compressed lung near the hilum, and of the normal gastric air bubble below the left dome will suggest the possibility of this condition. Sometimes there is surprisingly little clinical evidence of the condition in spite of the gross distension.

Care must be taken not to confuse the large gastric air bubble seen below an elevated left dome with an intrathoracic transradiancy such as that seen with a diaphragmatic hernia or left basal air-containing cyst. The absence of the left dome shadow in its normal position (Fig. 2) will indicate the diagnosis.

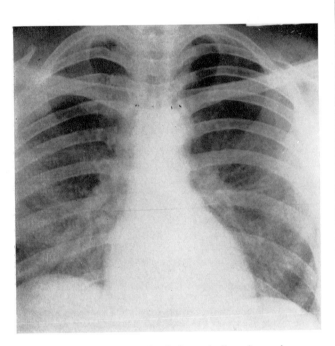 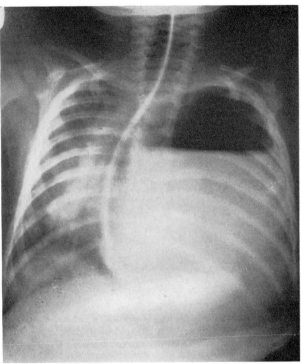

Fig. 220.—Pneumothorax simulating a bulla. Avascular area in left upper zone, edge of lung seen with difficulty.

Fig. 221.—Diaphragmatic hernia of stomach with obstruction causing distension. Female aged 41 years. Five days lower abdominal colicky pain settling in epigastrium. Vomiting of all food except some liquid. No shock, and no abdominal physical signs. Hernia through defect in anterior half of left dome. Reduction and recovery.

Mediastinal emphysema

Mediastinal emphysema will be suggested if a narrow 3–5 mm transradiant zone is seen surrounding a part of the heart shadow (Fig. 222). This may be the only radiographic abnormality. Sometimes the transradiant zone is separated from the lung by a hair-line white shadow running parallel to the heart border (Fig. 222). This represents the mediastinal pleura displaced away from the heart by the intervening gas. There may in addition be a similar narrow transradiant zone adjacent to the oesophagus and trachea, which is best seen in a lateral view.

In many cases the gas spreads along the tissue planes into the neck and thoracic wall, resulting in the characteristic transradiant areas of surgical emphysema with gas outlining the muscle bundles (Fig. 223).

Mediastinal emphysema may result from a spontaneous tear of the oesophagus, which will be suggested by a characteristic history. The patient, usually an elderly man, experiences a sudden severe retrosternal pain after vomiting or straining during defaecation, and enters a state of collapse. The tell-tale gas transradiancies in the mediastinum will be valuable radiological collaborative evidence, but the tear itself will not be demonstrable.

Mediastinal emphysema with less immediate clinical manifestations may follow perforation of the oesophagus during oesophagoscopy or gastroscopy or, very rarely, of the trachea or main bronchus during bronchoscopy. It may be seen with a small bronchial tear or complete rupture following external trauma, and is occasionally seen spontaneously after a severe attack of asthma. Except for cases of spontaneous rupture of the oesophagus, absorption of the air is the rule without surgical intervention. In some cases there is an associated pneumothorax or pyopneumothorax.

Primary emphysema

An extensive avascular area with relative hypertransradiancy in the upper or lower half of both lungs (Figs. 228 and 229) will suggest primary emphysema, especially if the patient has dyspnoea without cough or sputum. The site of the vessel narrowing is as commonly in the upper as the lower half of the lungs. Some cases may develop cough and sputum after the onset of the dyspnoea. If the

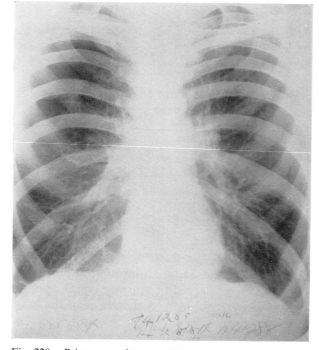

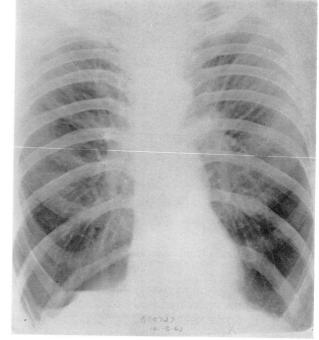

Fig. 228.—Primary emphysema. Vessel narrowing and loss in upper half. Long vertical hair-line on right demarcates bulla. None on left. Diaphragm normal. Male aged 38 years, with increasing dyspnoea for 6 years. F.E.V.$_1$ 375; DLco 9·7. P.M.: panacinar emphysema grade III upper half, II lower.

Fig. 229.—Primary emphysema. Vessel narrowing and loss in lower half and low flat diaphragm. Male aged 47 years, with 5 years' increasing dyspnoea. F.E.V.$_1$ 600 (40%); DLco 6; O_2 sat. 95%; Pco_2 42 mm Hg. Panacinar grade I–II upper, III–IV lower half.

lower half is affected, the diaphragm will be low and flat and the heart narrow and vertical. The x-ray appearances are very similar to those of widespread emphysema in chronic bronchitis, except that the distribution is rather more symmetrical and regional. In a late stage the two conditions will have the same x-ray appearances, and, as a part of one lobe will be less affected than the rest, marker vessels will be seen here (Figs. 242 and 243) (*see* p. 153).

In primary emphysema the lesion is panacinar grade III–IV, fairly widespread, with dilated alveoli and some of the lung architecture still intact. There is no evidence of bronchial or bronchiolar disease, so that the air trapping appears to be at alveolar level, and the mechanism is predominantly atrophy. It would seem that the air trapping is at small airway level due to premature collapse of these airways on expiration resulting from an interference with the local lung elasticity secondary to the alveolar atrophy.

Infantile lobar emphysema

Acute respiratory distress in a baby or young child may be due to infantile lobar emphysema. In the radiograph there is a large upper zone or unilateral area of hypertransradiancy with no visible vessels and gross displacement of the heart and trachea to the opposite side (Fig. 230). There is usually depression of the diaphragm on the affected side with widening of the intercostal spaces. The compressed lower lobe may be visible behind the heart shadow. Resected specimens have shown panacinar emphysema grade III throughout the lobe with the general architecture intact. There is air trapping, and since no bronchiolar disease can be demonstrated, the mechanism of the check-valve effect is uncertain. A recent investigation of three resected lobes by Lynne Reid (personal communication) showed that there were too many alveoli in a part of the lobe rather than emphysema, suggesting the primary disorder in some cases is a growth acceleration. How this leads to air trapping is uncertain.

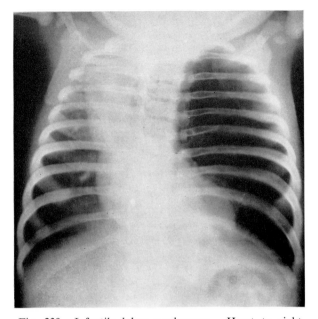

Fig. 230.—Infantile lobar emphysema. Heart to right. Avascular transradiant left upper lobe pushing lower lobe downwards and medially. Female aged 3 months. The dilated alveoli were panacinar. Acute respiratory distress, so lobectomy. Cause not elucidated from specimen. Bronchi normal.

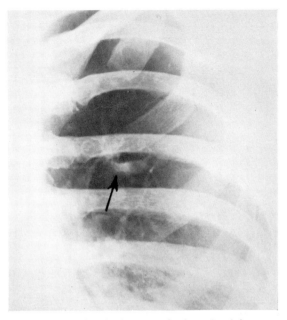

Fig. 231.—Atresia of apico-posterior bronchus left upper lobe. Avascular transradiant area left upper zone. Arrow to 2-cm ring shadow with fluid level. Female aged 27 years. Asymptomatic. Findings as Figs. 232 and 233. Missing bronchus confirmed in bronchogram. Lobectomy.

In some cases the degree of distension reaches a limit and becomes stabilized, and the condition becomes chronic; but many cases show progressive distension clinically with progressive respiratory distress, and the child's life can only be saved by lobectomy or decompression of the over-inflated lobe. The absence of fever, rapidity of deterioration and degree of over-inflation in the radiograph will distinguish the condition from an acute staphylococcal pneumatocoele or tension cyst (*see* p. 125).

EMPHYSEMA FROM IRREVERSIBLE BRONCHIAL OBSTRUCTION

Developmental–atresia of a segmental bronchus

A relatively hypertransradiant zone with too few vessels which are also small and narrow will suggest a local emphysema. This can be confirmed by showing air trapping in this area in a radiograph on expiration, when it will remain hypertransradiant, and the trachea may be deviated to the opposite side. A feature which will indicate the diagnosis in some cases will be the presence of a 1-cm hair-line ring shadow (Fig. 231) produced by the dilated proximal end of the atretic bronchus, as shown diagrammatically in Fig. 232. Sometimes the mucus secreted is not dispersed and a fluid level is seen in the ring shadow for a time, or if it fills up fully with secretions a 1-cm circular shadow is seen. In other cases only a part of the wall of the dilated bronchus is seen represented by a few hair-line linear shadows. If an angiogram is done it will show a poor flow to the affected segment and any vessels seen within it will be very small.

A bronchogram will show that the bronchus which should supply the area is not filled and that the absent one usually is either the apico-posterior or anterior bronchus. In addition, there may be minor variations in the pattern of branching, or nearby bronchi may be abnormally small to underline that the condition is a congenital defect and not acquired from disease. The transradiant area is usually in the left upper zone, but it may be in the right upper zone and very rarely in the right lower zone.

Examination of the specimen revealed a dilated bronchus at the hilum, the proximal end of which did not communicate with the trachea but sent out distally normal sized branches into the emphysematous segment of the lung (Fig. 233). The emphysema is panacinar and the mechanism of production seems to be hypoplasia. Because of the atresia the segment can only obtain air from nearby normally aerated segments by collateral air drift through the pores of Kohn and Lambert (*see* p. 71). This type of respiration is more efficient in inspiration when the channels of communication are widest, but as they narrow

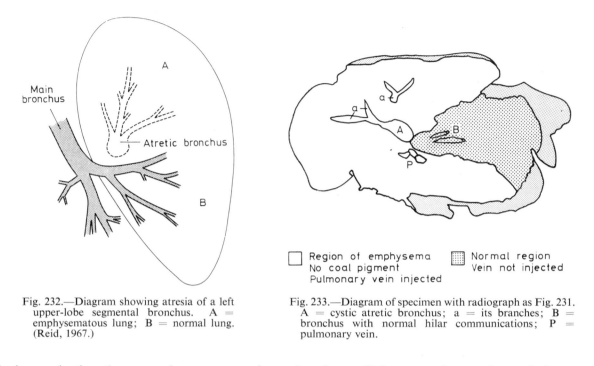

Region of emphysema
No coal pigment
Pulmonary vein injected

Normal region
Vein not injected

Fig. 232.—Diagram showing atresia of a left upper-lobe segmental bronchus. A = emphysematous lung; B = normal lung. (Reid, 1967.)

Fig. 233.—Diagram of specimen with radiograph as Fig. 231. A = cystic atretic bronchus; a = its branches; B = bronchus with normal hilar communications; P = pulmonary vein.

during expiration they may close prematurely so that there will be some air trapping and the segment will tend to remain suspended in inspiration. This will limit the ventilation and the blood flow of the segment, and, since the condition is present from birth, the normal increase in alveolar number between birth and the age of 8 years will therefore be less than normal. The volume of the segment will, however, be normal or greater than normal because of the air trapping. Thus there will be too few alveoli and, since they must occupy the relative large volume of lung, they will be larger than normal and emphysematous.

Emphysema with Bronchitis or Bronchiolitis Obliterans—Occurring in Childhood

Unilateral hypertransradiancy with a normal but very small lung vessel pattern (Fig. 234) will suggest Macleod's or Swyer and James syndrome. A radiograph in expiration (Fig. 235) will show that there is air trapping on the more transradiant side and therefore dilated alveoli (emphysema).

The heart on inspiration may be normal in position or displaced to the transradiant side indicating a small volume lung. On expiration it will be displaced to the opposite side (Fig. 235) and the normal side will deflate and become opaque, whereas the hypertransradiant side will remain hypertransradiant and unchanged. The diaphragm may show some restriction of movement but is usually at a normal level relative to the opposite side on inspiration.

The hilar vessels' anatomy will be normal with the basal artery and upper lobe vein clearly defined, but these vessels will be much smaller than on the opposite normal side, a feature which may be seen most clearly in a tomogram (Fig. 236). An angiogram will confirm these features and there will be poor flow into the transradiant lung, and any vessels which fill will be small. Bronchograms invariably show obliterative lesions. These may be quite proximal and in the first five generations (Fig. 237), or they may be in the middle regions (Figs. 238 and 239) or the terminal airways. There may or may not be dilatations (bronchiectasis) as well. In some cases the terminal airways may show circular dilatations (pools). The finding of normal airways here and there is also a common feature (Fig. 237). In most cases there are a few obliterative lesions on the other side, so that the lesions are often not quite as unilateral as would be suggested from the plain radiographs. In some cases earlier radiographs were normal. In one such case the child developed measles complicated by extensive consolidation of the left lung. This resolved, but a few weeks later the left lung showed hypertransradiancy with evidence of air trapping, and a bronchogram showed obliterative lesions on the left side.

Examination of the specimens has shown that there is panacinar emphysema, alveolar hypoplasia and patchy obliterative lesions with scars in the conducting air passages (Reid, 1967, p. 121).

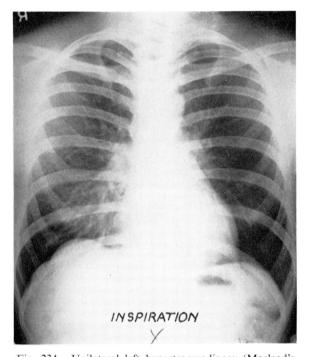

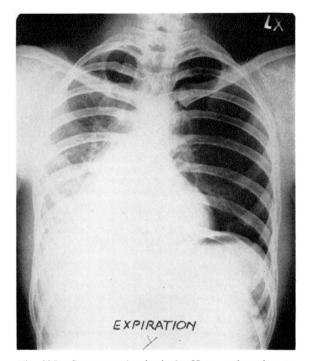

Fig. 234.—Unilateral left hypertransradiancy (Macleod's syndrome). Left hilar and lung vessels smaller than on right, but normal shape. Heart to left because lung small. Female aged 21 years. Asymptomatic.

Fig. 235.—Same case (expiration). Heart and trachea to right, normal clouding in right lung from deflation, but left lung remains hypertransradiant due to air trapping. Right dome 5 cm; left, 4 cm. Bronchoscopy normal. Bronchogram: peripheral occlusive lesions on left.

If the airway's obliterative lesions occur before the age of 8 years, that is, before the alveolar number has reached a maximum, the mechanism producing the emphysema will be the same as that in congenital atresia of a segmental bronchus (*see* p. 148). The occluded airway causes air trapping, and the lung can only be aerated by collateral air drift from regions which still have a patent airway. As a result of this the lung remains suspended in inspiration, and the restricted ventilation and blood flow will lead to restricted alveolar development. There will be too few alveoli, and since the lung volume is nearly normal they will be too large. There will thus be emphysema with hypoplasia. If the obliterative lesions of the airways only occur after the age of 8 years, hypoplasia will not be an important factor, while the air trapping itself will be the most important cause of the alveolar dilatations, and the lung volume will be normal or almost normal.

Respiratory function tests in these cases have confirmed the air trapping and have shown poor ventilation and perfusion of the hypertransradiant side. Although the condition is usually asymptomatic, some cases developed cough and sputum in the late forties probably from co-incidental chronic bronchitis, and a few, as they got older, complained of dyspnoea on exertion. In a few dyspnoea came on much earlier.

Sometimes the condition is confined to a single lobe which will then appear relatively hypertransradiant with small vessels, and will show some obliterative bronchial lesions in a bronchogram, usually with dilatations as well. In such cases examination of the specimen has shown the same lesions as in unilateral hypertransradiancy.

The diaphragm in by far the majority of cases of gross emphysema will move less than 3 cm between the inspiration and expiration pair of radiographs, which is less than in the majority of normal persons. In severe cases it remains flat on expiration, but in less severe cases of air trapping it may become normally curved in expiration, so that it is important to ensure the routine radiograph is taken in full inspiration. Sometimes the diaphragm is so flattened that the costophrenic recess is no longer seen or,

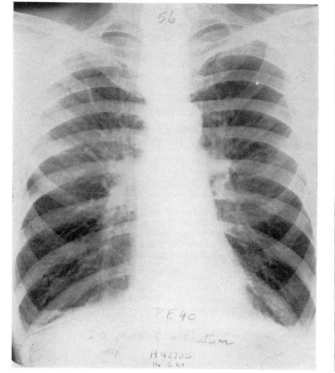 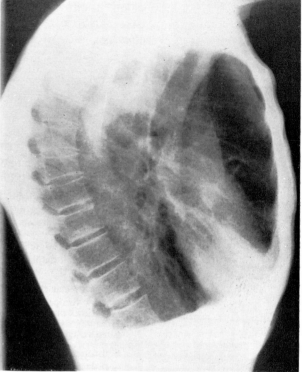

Fig. 240.—Widespread severe emphysema. Diaphragm rib level 7½, flat. Heart 11 cm; narrow vertical. Marker vessels left upper zone, rest small (more obvious on original because of small scale of reproduction). Male aged 43 years. Severe dyspnoea some years. Sputum: *H. influenzae*. F.E.V.$_1$ 500 (18% of F.V.C.); DLco 9; O_2 sat. 84%; Pco_2 51 mm Hg.

Fig. 241.—Widespread severe emphysema (lateral view) showing large retrosternal transradiant zone and flat diaphragm with superior concave curve. Retrosternal space 3 cm below sternal joint is 5 cm deep and lower limit 4 cm from diaphragm.

because of a high lateral attachment, the recess is occupied by a portion of diaphragm muscle simulating an effusion. In very severe cases the diaphragm may even show a superior concave curvature. The flattening is usually confirmed in the lateral view, but if the curve is normal in the anterior view flattening in the lateral view is a sign to be accepted with caution, since it seems to occur in some normal persons.

The size of the retrosternal relatively transradiant area

The area of relative blackening, caused by the two lungs in contact behind the sternum and in front of the aorta, is sometimes called the retrosternal space in the radiograph. Enlargement of this area of blackening is often an unsatisfactory sign of widespread emphysema. In most normal persons it is only 2–3 cm deep, measured from a point about 3 cm below the sternal joint, and does not extend very low so that its lower limit is 7 cm or more from the diaphragm (*see* p. 30). In widespread emphysema it is often 4–5 cm deep and may extend down to within 3–4 cm of the diaphragm (Fig. 241). Unfortunately the marker points are often ill defined and thus accurate measurements are not possible. Both by measurements and by visual inspection it is large in widespread emphysema, but it is also large in a few apparently normal persons, in some chronic bronchitics without emphysema, in some asthmatics in childhood (but rarely in asthma of late onset), in a few patients with cystic fibrosis, and last but not least in a bulla or area of local emphysema affecting one upper lobe only and without abnormal respiratory function tests or symptoms. This is often a non-progressive condition.

THE CARDIOVASCULAR CHANGES

The heart shadow

The heart tends to be of the narrow vertical type with a transverse diameter of 11·5 cm or less (Fig. 240). This is solely due to the low position of the diaphragm, and the heart may still be small even if there is right ventricular hypertrophy. However, it will not be small if the patient develops polycythaemia or cor pulmonale, or if there is independent heart disease such as ischaemic heart disease.

The main pulmonary artery

A slight lateral convexity of the left heart border just below the aortic knuckle due to the main pulmonary artery is seen in about half the cases of severe emphysema (Fig. 240), and is due either to rotation of the heart as it becomes narrow and vertical or, more commonly, to some real dilatation of the artery secondary either to peripheral vasoconstriction or to the loss of capillary bed which may not over all be sufficient to cause pulmonary hypertension. If there is pulmonary hypertension the dilatation of the pulmonary artery may become more marked.

The hilar vessels

The hilar vessels may be normal or they may be dilated. Measurements from tomograms (Table 5) show that there is on average dilatation of the right basal artery and left main pulmonary artery, but that there is considerable overlap between the emphysema cases and the normals.

TABLE 5
MEASUREMENTS IN TOMOGRAMS OF HILAR VESSELS IN EMPHYSEMA

	Normals		Emphysema		Other C.L.D.*	
	Average	Range	Average	Range	Average	Range
Right basal artery	13·8 mm	7–19 mm	21·5 mm	11–30 mm	15·5 mm	10–19 mm
Transhilar	11·9 mm	10–14·5 mm	14·7 mm	12·5–17 mm	13·4 mm	12·5–15 mm
Left "A"	24 mm	18–32 mm	36 mm	29–47 mm	32 mm	22–49 mm

* Chronic lung diseases

The lung vessels

Vessel narrowing or actual disappearance of vessel shadows in some areas is the most important sign of widespread emphysema. Three types of vessel change may be seen. Firstly, the vessels may be present but narrowed in most areas. Secondly, in some areas the axial pathway vessel may be normal or even large, but there will be fewer side branches, a condition described by Laws as vessel pruning. Finally there may be complete absence of vessel shadows in some areas, particularly if there is a large bulla with no contents other than air, as illustrated in Fig. 211. A similar appearance may be seen in an area of severe panacinar emphysema with the main vessels still intact when the specimen was examined, as was the case in the right upper lobe illustrated in Figure 212. Vessel narrowing or in some cases disappearance of vessel shadows is probably due to diminished flow through the affected area resulting from the high intra-alveolar gas pressure raising the resistance to flow, or to local vasoconstriction from local hypoxia because of poor air flow. If vessels are visible they will tend to be small for the same reason. In the past there has been some difficulty in recognizing that vessels were small, but an objective method is now available, namely the recognition of " marker vessels " and using these as a measure of vessel size.

Identification of "marker vessels"

It is known that the cardiac output is well maintained in emphysema in spite of the considerable loss of capillary bed. It is also known from morbid anatomical studies that the damage to the lung is uneven, some areas being spared or at any rate less affected than others, and, as might be expected, the blood tends to be diverted to these areas. Vessels of normal or even increased calibre will be apparent in these more normal areas, and these constitute the " marker vessels " which are then used for comparison with vessels in other parts of the lung at similar sub-segmental levels. In Fig. 242 the vessels to the left upper lobe are the marker vessels and are larger than the vessels elsewhere in the lungs. An angiogram (Fig. 243) confirms that this is so, and the total flow to this area is greater than elsewhere. In by far

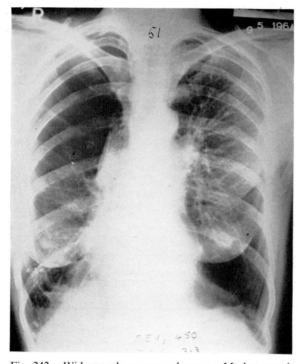

Fig. 242.—Widespread severe emphysema. Marker vessels in left upper zone. Female aged 51 years. Severe dyspnoea. F.E.V.) 450 (33% of F.V.C.). Low flat diaphragm. No chronic bronchitis (primary emphysema).

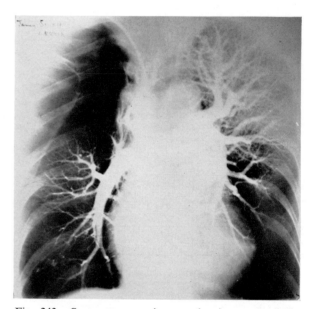

Fig. 243.—Same case; angiogram showing most of the contrast medium and thus blood flow is to the left upper zone (region of marker vessels). P.A. 35/8; O_2 sat. 85%; DLco 3.

the majority of cases of widespread emphysema such marker vessels can be identified without difficulty. Sometimes they are concentrated in one lobe, sometimes in two separate regions. To sum up, vessel narrowing, and for that matter vessel loss, can be proved by reference to the marker vessels, and such evidence is virtually necessary before a diagnosis of emphysema can be made. In addition, the zones in which such changes are present can be recorded.

It is known that if one lung is healthy, a patient can lead an almost normal life after the removal of the other lung by a pneumonectomy, or when one lung does not function because it is compressed by a very large bulla as in Fig. 215.

The elimination of normally functioning lung by emphysema in three out of the six zones (three each side) into which the lung can conveniently be divided by drawing lines across it at the level of the anterior ends of the fourth and sixth ribs respectively should therefore not cause dyspnoea. If between three and four zones are diseased, the patient may have some dyspnoea, while if more than four zones show areas of vessel narrowing or loss, the patient will almost certainly suffer from dyspnoea on moderate exercise.

Those patients showing involvement of less than four zones may be classified as having local emphysema, while those with four or more zones of involvement have widespread emphysema. The former may have no symptoms, the latter will either have dyspnoea or will develop dyspnoea in the near future. In Fig. 244 there is vessel narrowing throughout the left lung and in the right upper zone, that is, four zones. The patient could therefore be said to have extensive but still local emphysema, and at that time had cough and sputum but no serious dyspnoea. Six years later the radiograph was unchanged but the dyspnoea was severe, the combination of extensive though local emphysema and chronic bronchitis eventually leading to respiratory insufficiency.

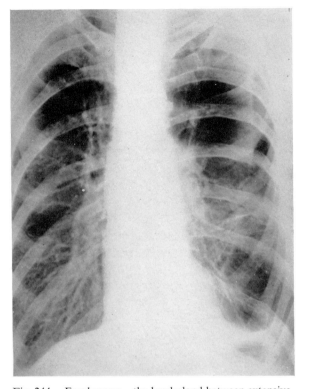

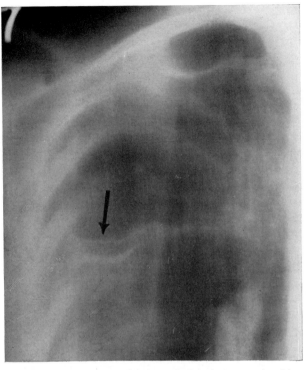

Fig. 244.—Emphysema—the borderland between extensive local and widespread emphysema. Avascular left lung, right upper zone and part of mid zone. Good vessel pattern 1½ zones right lower. For 4 years asymptomatic; last 3 years, increasing dyspnoea. Radiograph unchanged. Now aged 62 years. Right diaphragm normal.

Fig. 245.—Emphysema with large bullae (tomogram). Line shadow below the apex marks one bulla. Line shadow below the arrow marks another. Neither of the shadows was obvious in the plain radiograph. Small lung vessels in mid zone.

Bullae in widespread emphysema

Complete vessel loss and hypertransradiancy in a limited area, which may (Fig. 245) or may not be demarcated by a white line shadow, will suggest a bulla (*see* p. 128). Bullae or bullous areas are only seen in one-third of cases with radiographic evidence of widespread emphysema. The bulla must be included in the zonal assessment but, since it represents a local emphysema, it is not in itself a fundamental factor in the diagnosis of *widespread* emphysema.

Changes in the thoracic cage

Changes in the thoracic cage such as high rib angles, wide intercostal spaces or a large antero-posterior diameter are not of value in the diagnosis of widespread emphysema. They may be seen in some normal persons, in chronic bronchitics, asthmatics and so on. Kyphosis does not in itself cause a large retrosternal transradiant area but a curved sternum, which may be unrelated, may do so.

ALTERATIONS IN THE WIDESPREAD " EMPHYSEMA PATTERN "

It is relatively uncommon to find the transition from a normal x-ray appearance to the emphysema pattern as illustrated in Figs. 246 and 247, presumably because there are no symptoms until the condition is well established, and therefore no indications for a chest radiograph. In two cases observed by the author the interval since the normal radiograph was 7 and 12 years, and there are thus no clues as to whether the transition was rapid or gradual, and what factors, for example an infection, preceded it.

There is usually no change in the emphysema pattern once it is present, although the patient gets more short of breath. This may be because the lung reserve is used up and the loss of some more alveoli,

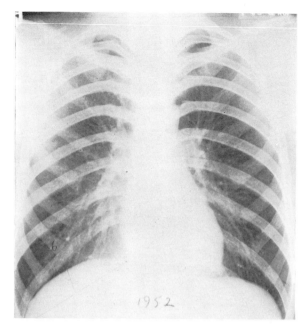

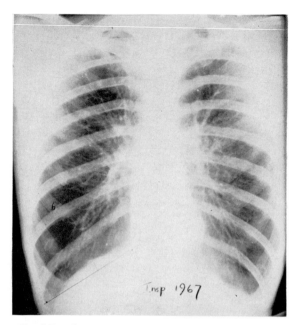

Fig. 246.—Normal chest (1952). Male aged 20 years. Asymptomatic; routine employment radiograph. Vertical from costophrenic to cardiophrenic line to well-curved diaphragm is 3 cm. In Fig. 247 reduced to 12 mm.

Fig. 247.—Same person 15 years later with severe widespread emphysema. Diaphragm lower and flatter; narrow heart. Marker vessels left upper zone. Now severe dyspnoea. P.F. 160; O_2 sat. 95%; PCO_2 50 mm Hg.

which may be too slight to be detected in the radiograph, will cause a disproportionate increase in the dyspnoea. Occasionally a bulla enlarges, or the diaphragm becomes lower and flatter, but such radiological evidence of deterioration is uncommon, and the radiograph is of little value in recording progress.

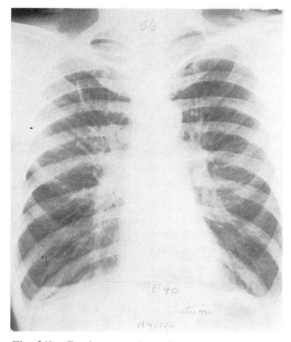

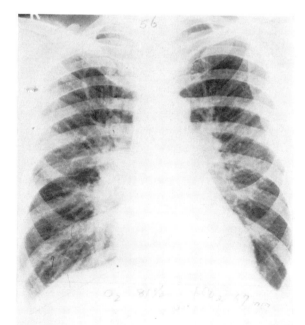

Fig. 248.—Emphysema. Low flat diaphragm. Heart 11 cm. Marker vessels right lower zone, rest narrow. Many years cough, sputum and dyspnoea. P.F. 90 l/min; Hb 106% (15·7 g). Male aged 56 years.

Fig. 249.—Same patient. Emphysema pattern lost during incident of cor pulmonale in failure. Diaphragm higher and curved. Heart larger; 15 cm. Lung vessels dilated in all zones. O_2 sat. 81%; PCO_2 67 mm Hg. Cyanosis; J.V.P. ↑ 10 cm. Ankle oedema.

The emphysema pattern may disappear under two unfavourable circumstances. One is the onset of polycythaemia which, although more common in chronic bronchitis without emphysema, may also occur in the presence of widespread emphysema, and this will result in dilatation of the pulmonary vessels which previously appeared small, and the marker vessels may no longer stand out clearly. The other is left ventricular failure, whether part of the hypoxic failure in cor pulmonale or from independent coronary insufficiency.

If this occurs the diaphragm may become elevated and curved, the heart dilates and the previously narrowed lung vessels also dilate, so that the emphysema pattern is completely lost (Fig. 249) and the appearances are the same as in chronic bronchitis with cor pulmonale in failure. The correct diagnosis can only be made if a previous radiograph is available showing the emphysema pattern or, if following successful treatment, the emphysema pattern returns (Fig. 248). About 16 per cent of patients with the emphysema pattern develop right ventricular hypertrophy; only some of these will go into failure.

RELATION OF X-RAY APPEARANCES TO PROGNOSIS

If one studies a group of patients with chronic bronchitis who are sufficiently disabled to attend a doctor because of it, about 15 per cent will have the emphysema pattern. Once this is seen the prognosis is poor, 50 per cent being dead within 5 years and very few surviving after 12 years. These figures are not very different from those chronic bronchitics without gross emphysema but with severe airways obstruction (forced expiratory volume in 1 second of less than 1,200 ml, or expiratory peak flow rate of less than 150 litres/minute), of whom the same percentage will develop right ventricular hypertrophy and changes in the radiograph (*see* p. 157). On the other hand, the prognosis of those patients with chronic bronchitis with lesser degrees of airways obstruction is considerably better, as is that of patients showing only local emphysema.

In the group of chronic bronchitics with very severe airways obstruction as defined above, the radiograph may be entirely normal and there may be no emphysema or only trivial emphysema when they die. There will be gross hypertrophy of the mucous glands, but the thickening of the bronchial wall due

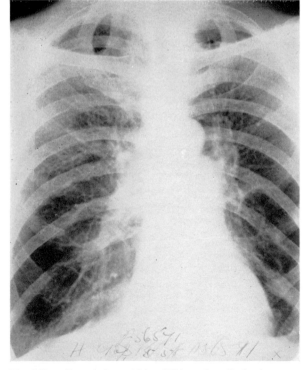

Fig. 250.—Chronic bronchitis. "Dirty chest." An impression of increased shadowing, but on closer inspection only normal vessels rather clearly seen. Died from his chest disorder but at P.M. no emphysema. Mucus gland hypertrophy. Male aged 66 years. F.E.V.$_1$ 1,000 (33%); P.F. 150 l/min; Hb 97%.

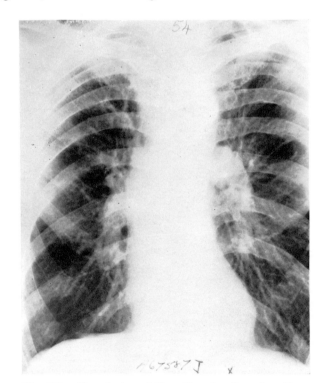

Fig. 251.—Chronic bronchitis with polycythaemia. Very large hilar vessels, normal lung vessels. Low but curved diaphragm. Male aged 54 years. Cough, sputum and dyspnoea many years. F.E.V.$_1$ 650; P.F. 60 l/min; O$_2$ sat. 87%, PCO$_2$ 50 mm Hg; P.C.V. 50%. E.C.G.: right ventricular hypertrophy.

to this is too slight for it to be detected in the radiograph, nor are there inflammatory changes of a degree which might cause bronchial walls of the larger bronchi to become visible in the radiograph. An appearance of lung vessel plethora, sometimes called " the dirty chest " (Fig. 250), has no basis in pathology, and in one such case the specimen showed singularly normal-looking bronchi and vessels and no emphysema, the only real change being the mucous gland hypertrophy.

There are two types of radiographic change which will indicate a poor prognosis. One is upper-lobe blood diversion (*see* p. 165 and Fig. 265), the other is a large heart with dilatation of the main pulmonary trunk and hilar vessels (Fig. 256), but normal lung vessels (Fig. 257). Such cases tend to have hypoxia, carbon dioxide retention and polycythaemia, pulmonary hypertension and cor pulmonale with episodes of failure.

INCREASED TRANSRADIANCY AND ALTERED VESSEL PATTERN IN ASTHMA

A patient may die of status asthmaticus and there may be no emphysema when the lungs are examined. On the other hand, if the lungs are of large volume, alveoli are perhaps dilated.

The majority of children with asthma will have a normal radiograph even when respiratory function tests just prior to the x-ray have shown severe airways obstruction.

Three abnormalities may, however, be seen. The first is tram line shadows (Fig. 199) (*see* p. 119) which are often transient. Secondly, the lungs may appear to be of large volume with a low but curved diaphragm, with the right dome below the anterior end of the sixth rib (Fig. 252). Because of the low

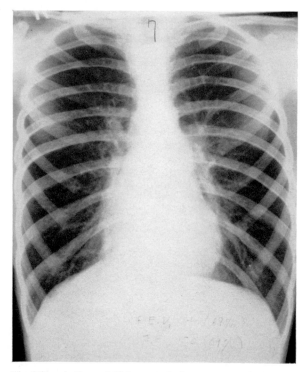

Fig. 252.—Asthma. Mild over-inflation pattern. Diaphragm low but curved, pulmonary vessels normal. Child aged 7 years. Asthma since age of 3. F.E.V.$_1$ 1·1 1 (67% predicted); P.F. 166 (69%).

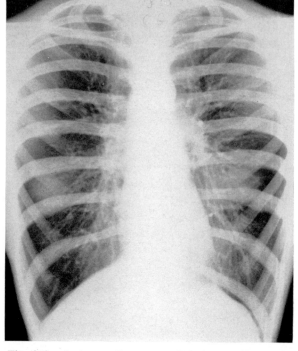

Fig. 253.—Asthma. Severe over-inflation pattern. Diaphragm low but curved. Hilar vessels large relative to pulmonary vessels. Child aged 14 years. Asthma since 10 years. F.E.V.$_1$ 0·9 1.

diaphragm the heart is narrow and vertical. The contrast between the lung vessels and the surrounding air is high so that the lungs give the impression of being hypertransradiant, although this may be because the patient is very thin, Finally, in some cases not only are the lungs of large volume, and the heart narrow and vertical, but the hilar vessels appear large relative to rather small lung vessels and stand out very clearly against the alveolar air background (Fig. 253). Occasionally the diaphragm is flat as well as low. The retrosternal transradiant zone is often large, and the sternum may be bowed forwards.

The radiographic appearances in a series of 85 children with asthma of varying degrees of severity are shown in Table 6. In those with a normal radiograph the severity of the airways obstruction, found by tests just before the radiographs were taken, varied from the trivial to the gross. Many cases showing radiographic abnormalities were treated with steroids or Intal, and became clinically normal with normal function tests and a normal radiograph.

TABLE 6

INCIDENCE OF ABNORMAL RADIOGRAPHIC PATTERN IN AN UNSELECTED GROUP OF CHILDREN WITH ASTHMA

Normal radiograph	66 (21 F.E.V.$_1$ less than 55% of predicted)
Tram lines or mild over-inflation pattern	5 (5 ,, ,, ,, ,, ,, ,,
Gross over-inflation pattern with large hila	14 (6 ,, ,, ,, ,, ,, ,,

In adults with asthma of late onset, the majority showed a normal radiograph however severe the airways obstruction, and only a few showed the simple over-inflation pattern while none showed the over-inflation appearance together with the large hilar vessels. Abnormal shadows were seen in those complicated by allergic aspergillosis with consolidations and eosinophilia (*see* pp. 49, 87, 102, 119).

Differential diagnosis

There are various x-ray appearances which must be differentiated from that of emphysema. A hyper-transradiant lung with conspicuous vessels is seen in otherwise normal people in whom the contrast between the air spaces and vessels is higher than average. The vessels are not narrow or widely spaced, and the balance between the size of the hilar vessels and those farther within the lungs is within

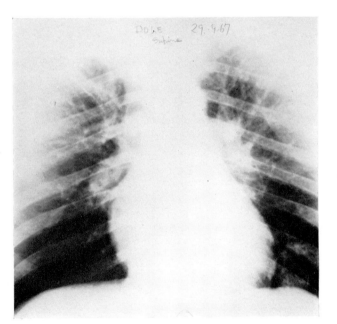

Fig. 254.—Acute massive pulmonary embolus; 3 hours after collapse (posterior view supine). Hyperaemia upper half, oligaemia lower half and plump hilar vessels (normal radiograph day before). Female aged 27 years.

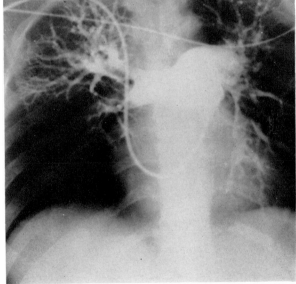

Fig. 255.—Same patient, same time (angiogram). Concave defect bifurcation right main, defect left basal artery. Flow mainly to upper half. Emboli removed from main vessels. Recovery.

normal limits. The range of diaphragmatic movement is good. An over-exposed radiograph may give an impression of vessel narrowing and vessel loss. However, if the radiograph is viewed in a stronger light, or another one taken with less exposure, the vessel pattern will appear normal, and there will be no local accentuation of vessel narrowing and no marker vessels.

An occlusive or spasmodic narrowing of the vessels may occur distal to a neoplasm. In one such case, although apparent narrowing of the vessels was seen lateral to a 2-cm circular bronchial carcinoma, no area of collapse suggesting that the narrowing was a compensatory emphysema was found on resection, nor was there any evidence of emphysema on histological examination. The appearances were therefore probably due to vascular spasm. Occlusive vascular lesions from acute large emboli will show areas of vessel narrowing, and may even show local dilatation as well (Figs. 254 and 255), that is, marker vessels; but the diaphragm will be normal in shape and there will be no clinical evidence of airways obstruction to account for the dyspnoea. In chronic pulmonary embolism with pulmonary hypertension the lung vessels may be small, but the large heart shadow, large pulmonary trunk and normal diaphragm are often characteristic (Figs. 258–260).

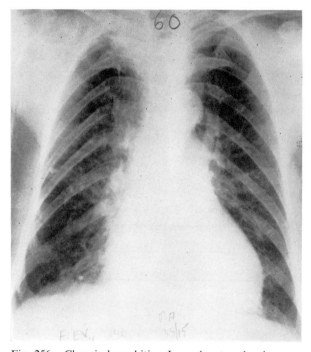

Fig. 256.—Chronic bronchitis. Large heart and pulmonary artery, even-sized lung vessels (normal). Normal diaphragm. F.E.V.$_1$ 1,000, P.F. 180; DLco 11; O$_2$ sat. 70%; Pco$_2$ 74 mm Hg. Male aged 60 years. Cough, sputum and dyspnoea many years.

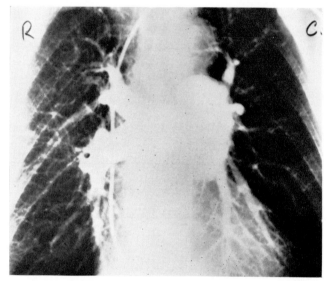

Fig. 257.—Same case (angiogram). Dilated pulmonary artery and hilar vessels. Slow flow into lung vessels which are of even calibre. P.A. 35/15; on exercise 55/25. Ankle oedema and large liver. Hb 14 g.

In pulmonary ischaemia, particularly when it is due to a congenital heart lesion, such as pulmonary stenosis, the x-ray appearances of the lung fields, in which the vessels are all small and the background hypertransradiant, may superficially resemble emphysema, except that the hilar vessels will be small, and the diaphragm normal. The clinical findings will clearly indicate a cardiac condition, so that confusion between the two will not arise.

CHAPTER 5

THE PULMONARY VESSELS IN LUNG DISEASE

A careful study of the pulmonary vessels should always be made since any alteration in their course or size may be the only abnormality in the radiograph, or such alterations may give important evidence of the nature of the lesion, even if other abnormalities are seen. The vessel patterns in normal persons are described on p. 22. In certain lung diseases the vessel pattern may be altered, and such changes may be local or generalized.

INCREASE IN SIZE

INCREASE IN SIZE OF THE MAIN PULMONARY ARTERY

A prominence of the left heart border below the aortic knuckle will suggest an increase in size of the main trunk of the pulmonary artery. This appearance may be due to rotation of the patient or to scoliosis (*see* p. 15) or to dilatation of the artery. It is seen in some cases of emphysema without pulmonary hypertension (Fig. 264); in pulmonary hypertension whatever the cause—whether secondary to chronic bronchitis with hypoxia and polycythaemia (Fig. 257), emphysema with or without chronic bronchitis (Fig. 242), cor pulmonale from gross diffuse lung disease such as fibrosing alveolitis, gross bronchiectasis or the late stage of sarcoidosis, or to occlusive disease of the pulmonary arteries from emboli, intimal thickening, periarteritis or from more distal obstruction from perivenitis, or idiopathic with presumably arteriolar muscular constriction (primary pulmonary hypertension; Figs. 258–260).

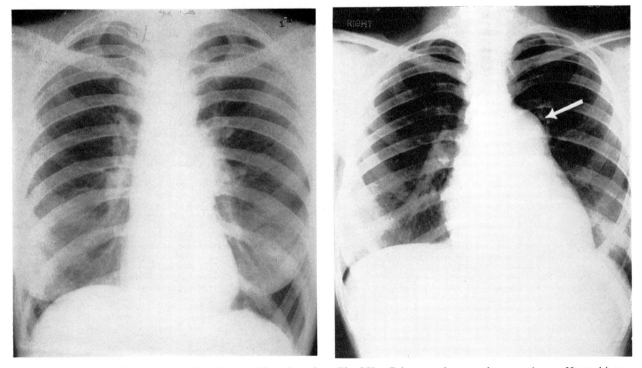

Fig. 258.—Pulmonary hypertension. Small heart, dilatation of pulmonary artery and, to less extent, the hilar vessels. Lung vessels normal. Female aged 42 years. P.A. 55/20 (ex 88/43). E.C.G.: right ventricular hypertrophy. Some dyspnoea. Diaphragm normal.

Fig. 259.—Primary pulmonary hypertension. Heart 14 cm. Thorax 28 cm. Large pulmonary trunk (opposite arrow), small hilar and lung vessels. Female aged 15 years. Increasing dyspnoea, worse at periods. P.A. 57/30 mm Hg. P.V.R. 8 units; O₂ sat. 94 %. Diaphragm high.

Dilatation of the main pulmonary artery may be developmental and of no significance, and of course is seen in many cardiac lesions with either increased pulmonary artery flow or pressure, or both, and usually there is a murmur (*see* p. 175). In emphysema or chronic bronchitis the dilatation of the main pulmonary artery is usually relatively slight (Figs. 229 and 256); in pulmonary hypertension from other causes it is more variable and is often gross (Figs. 258–260).

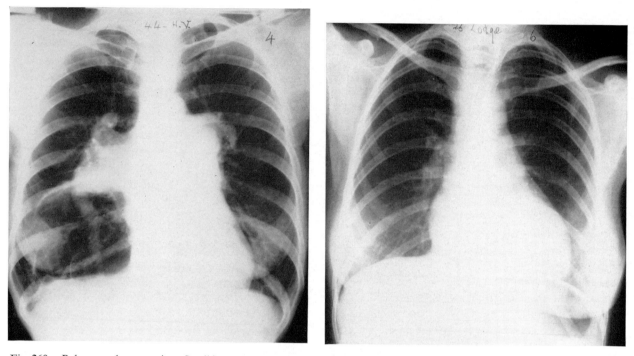

Fig. 260.—Pulmonary hypertension. Small heart, greatly dilated pulmonary artery and hilar vessels, small lung vessels. Female aged 44 years. P.A. 65/35; P.V.R. 8·5 units; O₂ sat. 90%.

Fig. 261.—Primary pulmonary hypertension. Large heart. No dilatation of pulmonary artery. Normal hilar and lung vessels. Female aged 26 years. R.V. 80/17; P.V.R. 23 units. P.M. arteriolar muscle hypertrophy. No emboli or intimal disease.

INCREASE IN SIZE OF THE HILAR VESSELS

Bilateral hilar vessel dilatation without visible dilatation of the main pulmonary artery is seen in some cases of widespread emphysema (Fig. 248), in some cases with severe chronic bronchitis before persistent pulmonary hypertension has developed (Fig. 251) and very occasionally in pulmonary hypertension whatever the cause.

Unilateral dilatation of the hilar vessels may be secondary to blood diversion from disease of the contralateral lung as in Macleod's syndrome (*see* p. 148). At first the dilatation may only be relative to the small size of the vessels on the side of the disease (Fig. 234) but may become absolute 20 years or more later, particularly if in middle age the patient develops chronic bronchitis as well. Occasionally unilateral dilatation of one pulmonary artery is a developmental defect.

In some cases with severe chronic bronchitis there may be a thrombus in the dilated basal artery on one side which will then appear dilated and often have a very well-defined margin (Fig. 251).

INCREASE IN THE SIZE OF THE MAIN PULMONARY ARTERY AND HILAR VESSELS

An increase in size of the main pulmonary artery and hilar vessels is characteristic of pulmonary hypertension (Figs. 258 and 260), whether from multiple minor emboli, chronic large artery emboli, peripheral arteriolar lesions or apparently from peripheral vasoconstriction. There is often enlargement of the heart shadow as well. The range of x-ray changes is very great, sometimes the main artery dilatation being most obvious, sometimes the heart or hilar vessel enlargement, and sometimes combinations of these changes. They are indicated in Figs. 258–262 where a series of patients with primary or embolic hypertension are grouped empirically by the x-ray appearances.

An increase in the heart size, main pulmonary artery and hilar vessels, is seen in some patients with severe chronic bronchitis (Figs. 256), the lung vessels being within normal limits, and appearing equal in size in the upper and lower zones. These appearances can be confirmed in angiograms (Fig. 257) which show a slow rate of flow of the contrast medium beyond the hilar vessels, though eventually peripheral filling may appear almost normal. These appearances may precede the onset of gross polycythaemia or pulmonary hypertension (at rest).

INCREASE IN SIZE OF THE HILAR AND THE PROXIMAL LUNG VESSELS

A generalized increase in the size of the hilar and proximal lung vessels may occur in polycythaemia. This may be due to a non-pulmonary cause, or more commonly is secondary to the chronic hypoxia of severe chronic bronchitis (Fig. 251). More rarely hypoxia and secondary polycythaemia may complicate a case of chronic bronchitis and emphysema, when enlargement of the heart and lung vessels will abolish the classical emphysema pattern of a small heart and narrow vessels (Fig. 248). A similar situation may arise if a patient with emphysema develops cor pulmonale with failure (see p. 157), when large hilar and large lung vessels may be seen together with a large heart shadow (Fig. 249).

INCREASE IN SIZE OF THE SMALL PERIPHERAL VESSELS

Dilatation of the small peripheral lung vessels may be seen in some cases of polycythaemia vera. In addition, there may be some small nodular shadows and a faint ground-glass haze in the lower half of the lungs. The changes are not always easy to detect, but may be seen more easily if earlier radiographs, taken before the onset of the polycythaemia, are available.

Dilatation of the peripheral vessels may occur in infants who develop respiratory distress and cyanosis. The pathology of the condition is still uncertain.

LOCAL INCREASE IN LUNG VESSEL SIZE

In emphysema

The marker vessels (see p. 154) in widespread severe panacinar emphysema may be normal but will appear large in contrast to the narrow vessels elsewhere, or they may in fact be dilated (Fig. 243).

After pneumonectomy

After pneumonectomy there is as a rule no convincing x-ray evidence of an increase in the size of the vessels in the remaining normal lung in spite of the diversion of all the blood to this side. Comparison of the normal side before and after the pneumonectomy is difficult because the displacement of the heart bares the hilar vessels on the normal side, and makes identification of vessels at similar levels in the pre- and post-operative radiographs rather unsatisfactory. In rare cases where the remaining lung is abnormal so that most of the ventilation and perfusion are through a single lobe, a great increase in the size of the arteries and veins may be seen in that lobe (Fig. 263).

In upper-lobe blood diversion

Dilatation of the upper lobe vessels so that they appear larger than the lower lobe vessels, instead of being the same size or smaller, will indicate diversion of blood from the lower to the upper half of the lungs. This type of blood diversion is commonly seen if there is a rise in pulmonary venous pressure as in mitral stenosis or left ventricular failure. The possible mechanisms in these conditions are discussed on page 184.

Blood diversion from the lower to the upper half of the lungs will also be seen if the lower half is diseased, as in lower zone emphysema (Fig. 264) or gross lower-lobe bronchiectasis.

Blood diversion to the upper half is seen in some patients with severe chronic bronchitis (Fig. 265). Examination of the lungs in one such case showed no appreciable amount of emphysema and no occluded arteries. Radioactive gas studies in other cases have shown a low dynamic distribution index

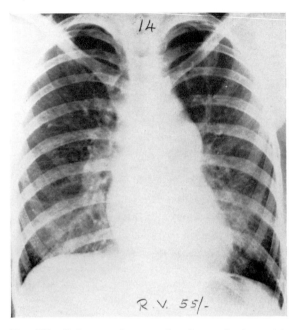

Fig. 262.—Pulmonary hypertension from mixed arterial and venous sclerosis. Large pulmonary artery, hilar and lung vessels, and basal septal line shadows. Female aged 14 years. Increasing dyspnoea for 2 years, no murmurs. P.A. 55/35 (ex 135/65); P.V.R. 6 units. Pathology: venous sclerosis small veins.

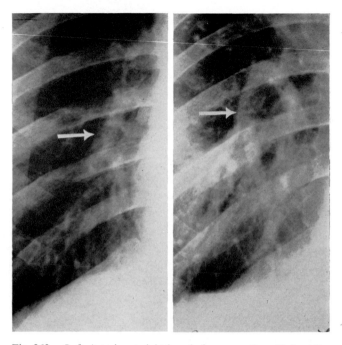

Fig. 263.—*Left.* Arteries at right base before operation. *Right.* After operation of left pneumonectomy, and loss of function in upper lobe from a tuberculous lesion with scarring (arrows point to the main descending artery). The enlargement after the pneumonectomy is obvious, and was confirmed in tomograms.

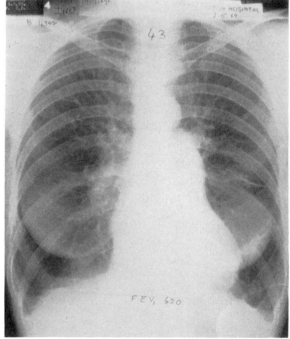

Fig. 264.—Upper-lobe blood diversion due to lower zone emphysema. Low flat diaphragm and narrow vessels in lower half. Female aged 43 years. Sputum and dyspnoea 4 years. F.E.V.$_1$ 620 (27%); DLco 5·3; O_2 sat. 86%. Xenon studies confirmed poor flow and poor mixing bases.

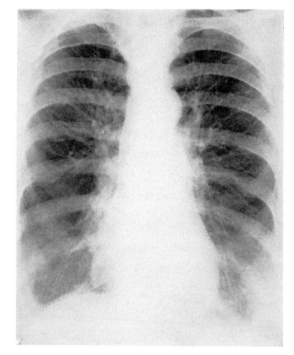

Fig. 265.—Upper-lobe blood diversion in a chronic bronchitic. Female aged 55 years. Cough, sputum and increasing dyspnoea 5 years. F.E.V.$_1$ 35% of F.V.C.; DLco 7. P.M. a few small thrombi, a little emphysema, dilated mucous glands. Right ventricular hypertrophy.

(D.D.I.), indicating poor blood–gas mixing in the lower zones, possibly the result of the uneven distribution of plugs of mucus allowing ventilation in some alveoli but not in others nearby, and yet poorly and well-ventilated alveoli are close enough for perfusion to each area to be the same. This will lead to local hypoxia and a local vasoconstrictive response. Upper-lobe blood diversion is also common in chronic bronchitis with cor pulmonale. Sometimes the diversion precedes the incident of failure; sometimes it is first seen during the incident. It may disappear on recovery but often persists after recovery, indicating it was not the result of simultaneous left ventricular failure with a rise in pulmonary venous pressure.

Finally, upper-lobe blood diversion will be seen with lower zone pulmonary artery occlusions from emboli. If the right and left lower-lobe arteries and some of the left upper lobe arteries are occluded, diversion may be limited to the right upper lobe, the appearances simulating the marker vessels in emphysema (Fig. 254). The normal diaphragm and clinical absence of airway obstruction will indicate the diagnosis.

The causes of upper-lobe blood diversion are summarized in Table 7.

TABLE 7

CAUSES OF UPPER-LOBE BLOOD DIVERSION

A rise in pulmonary venous pressure
Mitral valve disease
High end left ventricular diastolic pressure (left ventricular failure, decreased compliance)

Lower zone disease
Local basal emphysema
Severe lower-lobe bronchiectasis

Severe chronic bronchitis
Severe airways obstruction with $F.E.V._1 < 1,200$
Peak flow < 150. Often hypoxia and CO_2 retention

Lower-zone artery occlusions from emboli

Dilated vessel shadow between a circular shadow and the hilum

Sometimes a localized circular shadow may be associated with evidence of an increased blood supply, as in an arterio-venous aneurysm in the lung when the aberrant and enlarged vessels may be clearly seen in the plain radiograph or in tomograms (Fig. 136) (*see also* p. 78). Occasionally the shadow of a dilated aberrant (intercostal) artery can be seen extending from the descending aorta to supply an opaque area of lung representing a sequestrated segment in a tomogram or more clearly in an aortogram.

It is improbable that there is an increased blood supply from the pulmonary artery in other types of lung lesion. An appearance of a dilated vessel leading to the opacity of a tuberculous focus is usually due not to a dilated vessel but to tubercles and fibrous tissue seeded along the lymphatics adjacent to the bronchus and its accompanying artery.

DECREASE IN SIZE

LOCAL DECREASE IN VESSEL SIZE

A local decrease in vessel size is one of the main diagnostic features of localized severe panacinar emphysema grade III–IV (*see* p. 153). The hilar and lung vessels will be smaller on one side if the ventilation and perfusion to one lung is diminished because of many bronchial or bronchiolar occlusions leading to air trapping and producing a unilateral hypertransradiancy (*see* p. 149) or if there is diminished ventilation and perfusion due to pleural fixation following a long-sustained pneumothorax or pleural effusion.

Local vessel narrowing is a common finding in cases of acute or subacute major artery pulmonary emboli, and such oligaemic areas will be confirmed in angiograms (Figs. 254 and 255). They may be confined to one lobe, one lung or all zones except for one small area where the vessels may actually be dilated. It may be the only finding in the plain radiograph, although sometimes there may be small shadows of associated areas of infarction, or the hilar vessels may be dilated or rounded and pear shaped, or one dome of the diaphragm may be elevated.

In the majority of cases the plain radiograph will confirm the clinical suspicion and give a fairly good prediction of the sites not being perfused because of the arterial occlusions. Sometimes the plain radiograph to demonstrate the oligaemic areas fails because there is some flow past the embolus or, because of severe scoliosis or old lung disease, the assessment of the vessel pattern is unsatisfactory.

An absent main left pulmonary artery may be associated with a slight decrease in the size of the lung vessels on that side, depending on how efficient alternative sources of blood supply happen to be. There is therefore no evidence of relative hypertransradiancy in most cases, and no evidence of air trapping in a radiograph taken in expiration. The actual hilum shadow may be small. Similar findings are seen with acquired occlusion of a right or left pulmonary artery. An angiogram may show no evidence of the artery on one side, and it is only the evidence of a previous radiograph with normal hilar and lung vessels which will indicate not an absence but an acquired occlusion of the artery to that lung. True hypoplasia of one lung may occur (mechanism unknown) so that one lung is too small with small hilar and lung vessels, but no evidence of air trapping and a normal bronchogram except for a slight reduction in the calibre of the bronchi.

Small hilar and lung vessels with some vessels taking an unusual course may be seen on one side in partial pulmonary agenesis (Fig. 343). The heart and trachea will be displaced to the affected side which is usually somewhat opaque. In total agenesis of the right lung any vessels seen will in fact be in the left lung which has herniated across to occupy a part of the right hemithorax. The true situation may be confirmed in a posterior-view tomogram which will show only a left bronchus and left hilar vessels, a finding which may make bronchograms or angiograms unnecessary in an asymptomatic patient.

In agenesis of one lobe, usually a right upper lobe, a somewhat similar appearance may be seen in the plain radiograph, but a tomogram or bronchogram will show the presence of a right main bronchus and hilar vessels although they may be small. The one lobe present may be larger than normal, though smaller than the whole lung of one side. The vessels in it will appear rather small, and often take an abnormal course. Since the bronchi run with the arteries, the abnormal course may be confirmed in a bronchogram (Fig. 344).

General Decrease in Lung Vessel Size

A general decrease in the size of the lung vessels will be seen in those rare cases of emphysema with an excess of air in the lungs but in whom no marker vessels can be identified. It is only possible to be certain that the lung vessels are small if the hilar vessels are large, or in the unlikely event of a previous radiograph being available for comparison.

A decrease in the size of the lung vessels is seen in some cases of acute massive pulmonary embolism with virtually complete occlusion of the main trunk and main arteries on each side. The hilar vessels may appear normal in size or the basal artery may be dilated and appear rather rounded and pear shaped because of the abrupt decrease in the size of the vessels leading out from it. The small size of the lung vessels may be obvious or may be detected by comparison with a previous radiograph should one be available.

Another cause of small lung vessels is primary pulmonary hypertension. The large heart and hilar vessels with a normal diaphragm will suggest the diagnosis (Fig. 259). However, in many cases of primary pulmonary hypertension the lung vessels are not small but appear so in relation to the large hilar vessels. A decrease in the size of the hilar and lung vessels is usually seen in patients with severe scoliosis. This hypoplastic type of pulmonary circulation is almost invariably present in severe idiopathic scoliosis starting in infancy, and is commonly seen even if the spinal deformity only starts in adolescence, whether due to poliomyelitis or whether it is idiopathic. Nor is it related to the amount of exercise which the young person takes, being seen even in energetic patients whose limb musculature is normal (Fig. 358).

LOCAL VESSEL DISPLACEMENTS

Displacement of a vessel or group of vessels by a localized lung lesion is common. They may be spread out around a cyst or neoplasm or crowded together in lobar shrinkage. With a shrunken but still aerated lower lobe the basal vessels in an anterior view will show a slight lateral concave inclination instead of passing downwards and outwards almost in a straight line, while in the lateral view they will have an anterior concave inclination. If the line of the displaced interlobar pleura can be seen this will confirm the lobar shrinkage, but if not the altered vessel pattern may be the only evidence of an underlying bronchitis obliterans with or without bronchial dilatation.

CHAPTER 6

CARDIOVASCULAR ABNORMALITIES

THE PLACE OF THE PLAIN RADIOGRAPH IN CARDIAC DISEASE

The first duty of the radiologist in a case of suspected lesion of the heart or great vessels is to report, from the chest radiograph, the size, shape and position of the heart, changes in the size or position of the great vessels and whether the lung vessels are normal, dilated or small and any abnormal lung shadows.

These observations together with the initial radiograph will act as a base line from which the progress of the condition can be observed, and any improvement or deterioration detected, often before it is apparent clinically.

When drawing conclusions from these observations it is important to concentrate on those features which will be of most help to the clinician. Often the diagnosis is already known (as in cases of systemic hypertension, mitral stenosis and so on), and the radiograph is not needed for diagnosis but may nevertheless be useful for other reasons. Abnormalities in the heart size or shape reflect the adverse effects of the lesion, while changes in the lung vessels may give some indication of the haemodynamic consequences of the lesion and thus aid in the selection of cases for catheter studies or angiography with a view to possible surgical treatment. Only occasionally is the plain radiograph a pointer to the diagnosis when this is not obvious clinically, or a corrective to an initial clinical diagnosis later proved faulty. A study of the changes in the lungs or lung vessels is often more informative than a study of the heart shadow, even when this is abnormal.

When necessary, the plain anterior-view radiograph will be supplemented at least by a lateral view and in some cases by fluoroscopy, though there seems to be no indication for this as a routine procedure in many cases. Other procedures such as oblique views or a barium swallow are also only needed when there is an indication for them. Finally, the limitations of all these procedures are well known, and many cases will require catheter studies and angiograms; however, these are usually only undertaken in special units and, since the personnel in such units will not read this book, detailed consideration of these procedures has been purposely omitted.

THE CARDIAC SHADOW

The Size of the Heart Shadow

The size of the heart shadow can be measured from the cardiac volume or a rough estimate can be made from the transverse diameter (T.D.). The difficulties and limitations of both these methods in detecting early or slight heart enlargement have been referred to on page 16, where it is suggested that the criteria for early heart enlargement in an adult should be an increase of more than 1·5 cm since an earlier radiograph, or a T.D. of more than 15·5 cm, the reliability factor for these figures being over 95 per cent.

Thus in some conditions such as valvular disease or some cases of hypertension, in which early detection of heart enlargement might be important in the future, the initial radiograph for measuring the heart size should be taken as soon as convenient after the diagnosis has been made. The importance of comparison with an earlier radiograph is thus stressed.

In babies heart enlargement can only be detected when it is very gross, since it is often difficult to obtain a radiograph with the baby straight and in reasonably full inspiration. In children with heart disease, increases in size in serial radiographs must take into account the natural increase in size as the child grows. A chart showing the mean increase and percentile variations in the T.D. of normal children is shown in Fig. 266. However, it must be remembered that these are average figures, and the graph may wander somewhat within the range of the percentile lines in individual cases, as illustrated in Fig. 267.

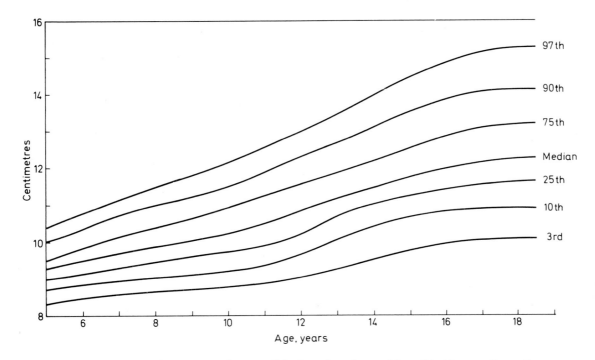

Fig. 266.—Increase in transverse diameter of the heart in males aged from 5 to 18 years. Percentiles.

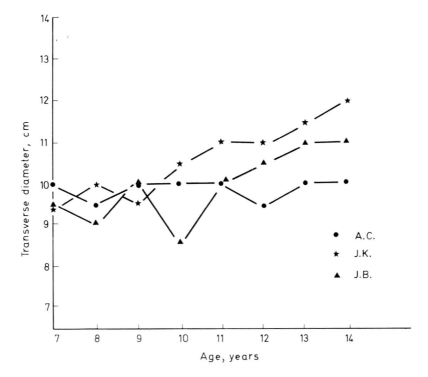

Fig. 267.—Increase of transverse diameter with age in 3 females.

Enlargement of the T.D. may be found with a heart of normal shape, but it is more often associated with a general alteration of shape, as in a large pericardial effusion (Fig. 270), or with a local prominence of one border caused by dilatation of one chamber, as for instance the left atrium in mitral stenosis (Fig. 283). Thus in assessing heart size the shape should also be taken into consideration. In some cases of aortic stenosis the work load is increased but the T.D. is normal, the hypertrophied muscle causing a filling out of the left border above the apex (Fig. 272). A similar appearance may be seen if the volume load is increased in aortic incompetence.

Marked hypertrophy of the muscle round a chamber will not necessarily cause any enlargement of the heart shadow, though gross hypertrophy of the muscle round the left ventricle may cause a local prominence above the apex. On the other hand, enlargement is always seen when there is dilatation of a chamber with an increase in the amount of blood in it.

In assessing either the size or shape of the heart, it is of course important to make sure that the lower part of the central shadow is in fact caused by the heart, and that the whole or one border of the heart is not obscured by an abnormal mediastinal, pleural, or pulmonary shadow. This is not always easy and a barium swallow may be needed to exclude an oesophageal mass such as a leiomyoma. In other cases catheterization and angiography may be required, but sometimes even these will fail to distinguish between a pericardial shadow and a shadow caused by an adjacent mediastinal, pleural or pulmonary lesion.

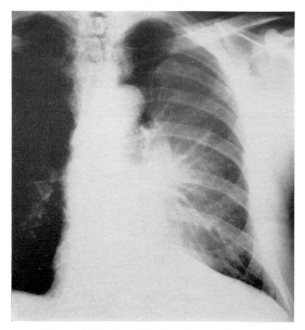

Fig. 268.—Vanishing heart shadow due to atelectasis of the left upper lobe including the lingula.

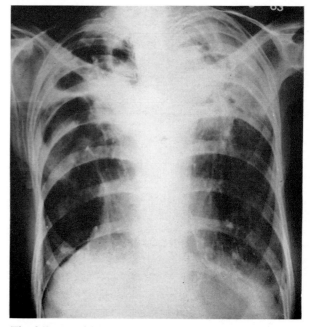

Fig. 269.—Vanishing heart shadow due to shrinkage of both upper lobes and pleural retraction retrosternally.

Sometimes the heart shadow may be invisible in the anterior view, an appearance referred to as the vanishing heart (Figs. 268 and 269). This occurs when there is no aerated relatively transradiant lung around it, but atelectatic or consolidated lung or a pleural effusion, which will be of the same density as the heart and thus only a diffuse ill-defined shadow is seen. Under these circumstances measurement of the heart size may not be possible. In a lateral view the shadow of the atelectatic or consolidated lobe or anterior pleural effusion may be clearly seen superimposed on the heart shadow.

THE LARGE HEART SHADOW

THE LARGE HEART SHADOW—WHICH CHAMBER IS DILATED?

There is a tendency to take oblique views and give a barium swallow as a routine in heart disease (the cardiac work-up), to tell in particular which chamber is dilated. In the majority of patients with heart disease such procedures are not indicated and, resources in money and manpower being limited, these additional investigations should be reserved for cases with special problems.

In most cases if a chamber is dilated, it will be obvious clinically which one it is. In systemic hypertension it will be the left ventricle, in pulmonary stenosis the right; alternatively, the electrocardiograph will give certain evidence. The information obtained from the radiograph is not always of value. For instance, in mitral stenosis the finding of some dilatation of the left atrium is of little importance since the diagnosis is made on clinical and not radiological grounds, nor is slight left atrial dilatation a factor in assessing severity. When the left atrial dilatation is moderate or gross it can be assessed from the well-exposed anterior view. In this view the left atrium can be assumed to be dilated if there is a prominence of the left border well below the aortic knuckle due to the left atrial appendage, or if there is a double outline of the right border (Fig. 283), the upper and medial edge being caused by the confluence of the dilated veins as they enter the dilated left atrium, the right border by the right atrium. The medial shadow must not be mistaken for a similar shadow sometimes caused by a dilated ascending aorta. In case of doubt the lateral view will indicate the true state of affairs, where either the heart shadow will bulge posteriorly because of the dilated left atrium, or the dilated ascending aorta will be visible. (A lateral rather than oblique view is perhaps indicated as a routine.) In very gross left atrial dilatation this chamber may form the right heart border. Nor is it always possible to tell from the plain radiograph whether only the left atrium is dilated or whether both atria are dilated. In a well-exposed anterior view moderate or gross dilatation of the left atrium will be seen to displace the left main bronchus upwards and the subcarinal angle will be increased so that it is more than 90 degrees. The bronchus may also be narrowed, but atelectasis of the left lung from compression by the left atrium is uncommon.

In cases where it is uncertain which ventricle is dilated, the radiograph is often of little value. An example is assessment of the severity of the mitral incompetence in a case of mixed mitral valve disease, when radiological assessment from the plain radiographs as to which ventricle is dilated is too uncertain in this condition. The mitral incompetence should cause hypertrophy and then dilatation of the left ventricle, but in this case a left ventricular angiogram is needed to indicate, by the way the left atrium fills and the valve moves, the site, type and severity of the mitral incompetence. In complicated congenital heart lesions the appearances may suggest dilatation of a particular ventricle when in fact there may only be one. Finally, when the heart shadow is much enlarged and those cases are excluded in which the dilated ventricle can be diagnosed clinically, then the accuracy of x-ray assessment is not high. Any large heart will project posteriorly, and may show a large distance between the inferior vena cava and the posterior border even when the dilatation is predominantly right sided. Nor is encroachment of the heart shadow on the retrosternal transradiant zone reliable evidence of right ventricular dilatation, partly because the size of this zone is very variable in normal persons, and partly because any large heart tends to bulge forwards.

The accuracy of angiocardiography is so much greater than the plain radiographs in assessing the chamber volume, the presence of muscle hypertrophy or the dilatation of the individual chambers, it should be used when such information is needed to help the patient.

Large heart shadow from a pericardial effusion

In a large pericardial effusion there is enlargement of the T.D. and the central shadow assumes a rounded contour (Fig. 270). The angle between the superior vena cava and the right atrium is filled out giving an even convex curve to the right border, and the angle between the aorta and the left ventricle is filled out giving a similar convex curve to the left border. The cardiophrenic angles usually remain acute (Fig. 270), and there is diminished or absent movement of the heart margins on fluoroscopy.

If the clinical diagnosis is certain, the radiological findings can only be of value for confirmation, whilst if the diagnosis is in doubt, the radiological findings will often fail to narrow down the differential diagnosis. The difficulties of diagnosis in pericardial effusion and myocardial failure may be considerable, and are discussed in an Annotation (1955). Similar appearances to those of a large pericardial effusion may be seen with dilatation of the heart arising from myocardial failure from almost any cause. In acute rheumatic fever, especially, it may be difficult to tell whether the enlargement is due to a pericardial effusion or to acute rheumatic myocarditis.

A similar abnormal shape of the heart may be seen with certain uncommon congenital heart lesions such as transposition of the great vessels, idiopathic cardiomegaly, or Ebstein's anomaly (*see* p. 175).

Sudden enlargement of the heart shadow in serial radiographs will also suggest a pericardial effusion, especially if there is no clinical evidence of myocardial disease, or if earlier radiographs indicate a possible cause for the effusion, such as the shadow of a tuberculous lesion or neoplasm in the lung, or a pleural effusion.

A small pericardial effusion may cause no alteration in the heart contour, nor obvious restriction of movement. A moderate effusion will cause rather less alteration in size and shape than a large effusion, but distinction from moderate or gross heart enlargement from a myocardial disorder will still be difficult.

The ultrasonic echo scan is the simplest method of confirming a diagnosis of a pericardial effusion, but three radiological techniques are also available.

The first method is to pass a cardiac catheter into the right atrium and direct its tip to the right. In a normal heart or in myocarditis with a large heart the tip will be only 2–3 mm from the right border, while in a pericardial effusion it will be 1–2 cm from the border. This method is not entirely reliable, for the right border may be formed by the left atrium, or the pericardial effusion may be loculated and not on the right side.

The second method is therefore to inject a contrast medium down the catheter not only to outline the right atrium and thus show its relation to the right heart border, but also to outline the other chambers, and note their relationship to the other heart borders.

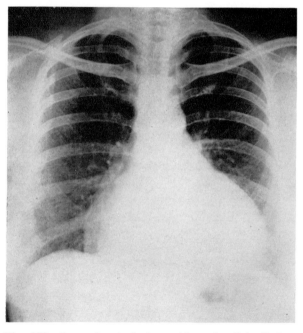

Fig. 270.—Large heart shadow with pericardial effusion. Female aged 25 years. Pain in chest and dyspnoea. Sterile pericardial fluid, resolved on anti-tuberculous therapy.

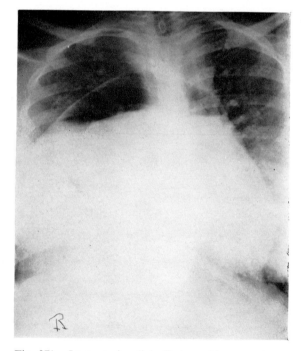

Fig. 271.—Large pericardial effusion with gas replacement after aspiration. No pericardial thickening.

A third method is to define the right border of the right atrium by injecting a bubble of carbon dioxide gas into it through a cardiac catheter, turning the patient onto his left side so that the right side is uppermost, and taking an anterior view with the x-ray beam horizontal. The relation of the right atrial cavity to the right border of the heart shadow will thus be shown.

Once the diagnosis is established by radiology or by aspirating some pericardial fluid, it may be of value to inject some carbon dioxide gas into the pericardial sac, and then radiograph the patient in various positions standing up, lying on the right and left side with the x-ray beam horizontal, so that the gas is uppermost (Fig. 271). These radiographs will show the thickness of the pericardium, and may outline a projection suggesting a tumour is causing the condition.

THE LARGE HEART SHADOW

Small heart shadow from pericardial constriction

Pericardial constriction may follow a tuberculous pericardial effusion after an interval of several months, or it may supervene while the effusion is still present; more often it arises, however, without a previous history of pericardial disease. In some cases the constriction follows an acute viral influenza-like illness; in others it may be the result of rheumatoid disease. The heart shadow is often small and rounded, and the angle between the superior vena cava and the right atrium is lost or even filled out, so that the right border forms one continuous convex curve from the top to the diaphragm. Diminution or complete absence of movement may be seen on fluoroscopy. The constriction may be generalized, or may be confined to one border. Constriction or rather restriction of diastolic expansion from pericardial disease can also be present with a large heart shadow. As a rule the hilar and lung vessels are small as the cardiac output is low. Occasionally restriction causes a rise in pulmonary venous pressure, when dilated upper-lobe vessels may be detected.

Large heart shadow associated with valvular disease

A large heart shadow in a patient with a murmur indicating stenosis or incompetence of one of the heart valves, will suggest that the obstruction or regurgitation is severe whether the patient complains of great disability or is without symptoms, and may thus indicate the time is appropriate for fuller haemodynamic investigations.

In aortic stenosis dilatation of the heart only occurs if failure is present. If there is doubt about the severity of the obstruction, and it is decided to observe the patient for a time with serial radiographs included, then any increase in heart size in these of more than 1·5 cm will be an indication for a detailed assessment of the case, and perhaps catheter studies to determine the gradient across the valve. Moderate enlargement of the heart shadow will indicate left ventricular failure and will suggest that the stenosis is severe, even if some of the dilatation is due to an associated myocardial factor.

Dilatation of the aorta due to a turbulence effect of the deformed valve, and upper-lobe blood diversion due to a rise in pulmonary venous pressure matching a rise in left ventricular end-diastolic pressure, will confirm that urgent relief of the stenosis is necessary. Calcification should be present if the patient is more than 20 years of age, and if none is seen it will suggest the stenosis is sub-valvular rather than valvular.

In aortic regurgitation the heart shadow tends to be much larger than in aortic stenosis for a given degree of disability, and there is often no valve calcium. The enlargement is to the left and downwards (Fig. 273), and obviously left ventricular. The type of pulse will be an indication of the stroke volume, so that vigorous pulsations of the ascending aorta, which may be seen on fluoroscopy, do not add any significant information.

In combined aortic stenosis and incompetence, or combined mitral and aortic valve disease, the size and shape of the heart will give an uncertain indication of the predominant lesion, so that an aortogram may be needed at some stage to assess the severity of the aortic regurgitation.

In mitral valve disease a large heart shadow may be due to a variety of causes. It may be due to aneurysmal dilatation of the left atrium, but if this chamber is not particularly large, the cause of the large heart should be considered with care. In mitral stenosis it often turns out to be due to previously unsuspected aortic regurgitation, mitral incompetence or tricuspid incompetence. In many other cases the dilatation is the result of a poor myocardium (Fig. 274). This may be inferred if atrial fibrillation is present, or if the cardiac contractions are poor either on fluoroscopy or when seen during surgical procedures. The slow rate of contraction and poor stroke volume are often aptly described as a lazy heart.

A rare cause of the large heart shadow in mitral stenosis is an unsuspected pericardial effusion. This has been confirmed at operation when it was large enough to add 1 cm to either side of the heart contour.

In pulmonary stenosis any enlargement of the heart shadow will indicate that the stenosis is severe, but unfortunately, severe pulmonary stenosis may be present with a heart of normal size (*see also* p. 191).

173

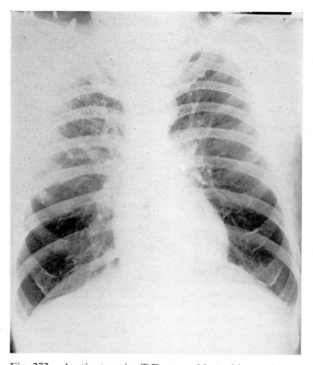

Fig. 272.—Aortic stenosis. T.D. normal but with prominence of left border just above apex. Upper-lobe blood diversion from raised end-diastolic pressure in left ventricle. Gradient across aortic valve 130 mm Hg. Male aged 21 years. Aortic systolic ejection murmur. Slow rising pulse. Valve replacement; improved.

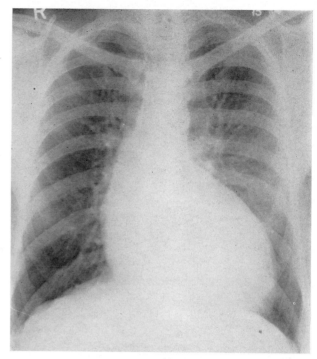

Fig. 273.—Aortic incompetence (regurgitation). Heart dilated and enlarged to left and downwards. Dilated upper lobe vessels. L.V. 135/20; L.A. 12/15. Male aged 27 years. Angina and dyspnoea. Aortic diastolic murmur. Valve replacement. Symptoms went.

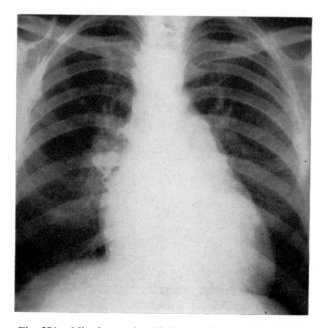

Fig. 274.—Mitral stenosis with large indistinct hilar shadows. The mid-lung field vessels are inconspicuous. Male aged 34 years. Ten years progressive dyspnoea on moderate exertion; fibrillating. Successful valvotomy. Dilated upper-lobe arteries and veins.

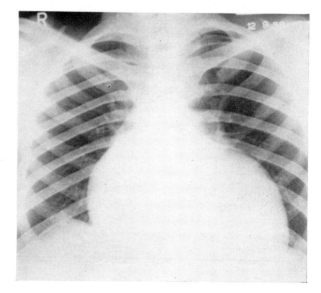

Fig. 275.—Pulmonary stenosis and tricuspid incompetence. Large rather rounded heart shadow. Hilar and lung vessels small. Male aged 22 years. Systolic ejection murmur. R.V. 125/25; P.A. 25/20. Diaphragm normal.

In tricuspid valve disease there are often other lesions, and these will contribute to the large heart shadow. In pulmonary stenosis or mitral stenosis the hypertrophied and later dilated right ventricle may lead to functional tricuspid incompetence. This will lead to dilatation of the right atrium which will cause a convex prominence of the right border, so that the enlarged heart becomes rather rounded in shape (Fig. 275). A similar appearance may be seen with organic disease of the tricuspid valve causing either stenosis or incompetence (Fig. 276). Pure right atrial dilatation is difficult to diagnose from the plain radiograph since in some normal persons the heart shadow shows a prominent and very convex right border.

A large rounded heart shadow which is rather inert on fluoroscopy may be due to Ebstein's anomaly, a condition in which there is a developmental defect with the tricuspid valve displaced as it were into the right ventricle, so that the right atrium is much enlarged; in addition, part of the ventricle has a thin wall like an atrium, and therefore has poor contractility. There is usually a murmur though this may not be very loud.

Large heart shadow from a shunt in congenital heart disease

The three common simple defects resulting in shunting of blood from the left to the right side are an atrial septal defect, a ventricular septal defect and a patent ductus arteriosus. For brevity, these will be referred to as an A.S.D., a V.S.D. and a ductus, respectively. They are usually associated with a systolic or, in the case of a ductus, a continuous murmur, and may give somewhat similar x-ray appearances.

In infancy they all show a rather non-specific enlargement of the heart shadow if the shunt is large.

In children the heart enlargement is relatively less than in infants or adolescents, even when the defect is quite large. After about the age of 15 years, if the shunt is still large, the heart will be enlarged and may increase further until old age. In an A.S.D. the heart enlarges almost entirely to the left (Fig. 294) in spite of the dilatation being predominantly of the right atrium and right ventricle, while in a V.S.D. or ductus there is better development of the left ventricle which will prevent the dilated right ventricle from moving so far across to the left. In some 20 per cent of cases with a V.S.D. there will be a double outline on the right border, indicating some dilatation of the left atrium.

In general, the larger the shunt the larger the heart shadow, or conversely a trivial shunt will show no heart enlargement. The heart size should be related to the vessel size as described on page 181.

Should the lung vessels be subjected to a high flow with a high pressure, or simply a high pressure, they are apt to develop organic wall thickening and the pulmonary vascular resistance may then rise, so that the shunt will be balanced or even reversed and blood will then pass from the right to the left side (the Eisenmenger situation). This will be indicated clinically by the onset of cyanosis, and, because of the reduced volume of blood shunted, the heart shadow may become smaller, which is an ominous sign.

Large heart shadow with no murmur or a trivial murmur

A large heart shadow is often seen in conditions which are obvious clinically; for example, systemic hypertension, coronary artery insufficiency producing ischaemic heart disease with or without evidence of myocardial infarction, primary pulmonary hypertension, hypoxic cor pulmonale, hyperthyroidism with auricular fibrillation, myxoedema and so on.

Systemic hypertension

In systemic hypertension the hypertrophied left ventricle may at first cause no enlargement of the heart shadow. At a later stage the heart may dilate because the coronary artery supply fails to keep pace with the needs of the hypertrophied muscle, so that a state of relative ischaemia is present. This or the consequences of renal damage (water overload; unidentified metabolic effects, other than the high blood urea) may result in heart failure. The heart shadow may then enlarge, or changes may be seen in the vessels and so on due to left ventricular failure (*see* p. 194).

Hyperthyroidism

In hyperthyroidism any dilatation of the heart is often part of the myocardial damage which has produced auricular fibrillation.

Myxoedema

In myxoedema the condition will be obvious clinically. A large heart shadow may be due to myxoedematous tissue amongst the muscle interfering with function, or to a pericardial effusion with myxoedematous tissue. The chief value of the radiograph is to trace improvement under therapy by the decreasing heart size.

Heart block

Heart block, which will be obvious clinically from the slow pulse rate and E.C.G. appearances, may result in a large heart shadow if the radiograph happens to be taken towards the end of a long diastolic pause.

Cardiomyopathies

In a group of conditions included under the term "cardiomyopathy" a large heart shadow is often seen but the cause may not be obvious either from the radiograph or from the initial clinical examination. The E.C.G. will usually indicate whether the enlargement is predominantly of the left or right side of the heart, or whether it is due to unsuspected ischaemic heart disease, but in some cases is unhelpful. In many cases there is no murmur but in others there is a non-specific systolic murmur often from secondary mitral incompetence, the great dilatation or elongation of the left ventricular cavity either stretching the ring, or lengthening the chordae so that mitral valve closure is inefficient.

The cause of the myopathy may eventually be deduced from the clinical or laboratory findings. A history of a severe influenza-like illness some 3 months previously from which recovery has been incomplete would suggest a Coxsackie viral myocarditis.

A history of a large intake of alcohol over a long period will suggest a myopathy partly due to alcohol and partly due to the associated inadequate diet with perhaps vitamin B_{12} deficiency.

Other rather rare causes of a myopathy are biochemical abnormalities leading to the deposition of amyloid in or around the heart muscle, haemochromatosis, sarcoidosis, periarteritis, or diffuse systemic sclerosis. In the last-named instance, if neither skin changes nor Raynaud's phenomenon are present, radiology may help in the diagnosis by showing calcifications in the finger tips or oesophageal inertia on a barium swallow (see p. 94). Finally, sub-endocardial elastosis may not only restrict diastolic filling and raise the pulmonary venous pressure, but may also cause the heart to dilate.

Another condition now perhaps being recognized more frequently is a lesion of unknown cause known as hypertrophic cardiomyopathy (Fig. 277). This in its turn may cause obstruction to left ventricular emptying, or it may result in congestive heart failure, the two types with their different haemodynamic disasters being known as obstructive or congestive hypertrophic cardiomyopathy, respectively. Other cases with an apparently similar pathology may have no symptoms, at least for a number of years. All degrees of cardiac enlargement are found from the trivial to the gross (Fig. 277). In those with trivial heart enlargement the T.D. may be within the normal range but there may be a prominence of the left heart border just above the apex, similar to that seen in aortic stenosis (Fig. 272), which may suggest the diagnosis. It is due to the hypertrophied muscle in this region. Owing to the huge bulk of muscle, left ventricular compliance may be diminished, and this may result in a rise in left atrial and thus pulmonary venous pressure. This may be diagnosed from the radiograph if there is evidence of upper-lobe blood diversion (see pp. 163 and 165).

In the cardiomyopathies not only is there difficulty in many cases of finding the cause of the myopathy, but there may also be difficulty in excluding a pericardial effusion (see p. 171) or Ebstein's anomaly (see p. 175). Therefore catheter studies are sometimes needed for diagnosis. Obstructive cardiomyopathy is characterized by a very high pressure reading near the apex of the left ventricle, with a lower pressure in the aorta, while the angiogram will show indentation into the undersurface of the lumen of the ventricle by the hypertrophied muscle (Fig. 278) and a very elongated but narrow chamber in systole (Fig. 279).

The shape of the heart shadow

In normal persons the heart shadow may be narrow and vertical or more horizontal with a large prominent convex left border. The shape depends to some extent on the level of the diaphragm, being more vertical when this is low, and more horizontal when it is high.

Alterations in shape are seen in disease, but are not always decisive in indicating either the diagnosis or which chamber is dilated. A large left ventricle will increase the bulge of the left border, but so may a large right ventricle. Prominence of the left border just above the apex is seen in some cases of right

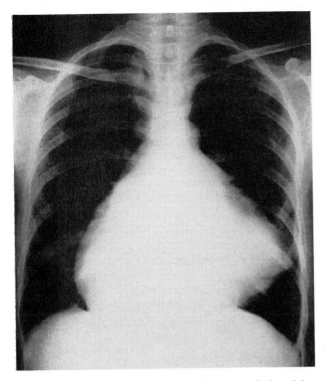

Fig. 276.—Tricuspid stenosis with dilatation of the right atrium (operative confirmation). J.V.P. much raised. Right atrial pressure 33/26 mm Hg. Hilar and lung vessels inconspicuous.

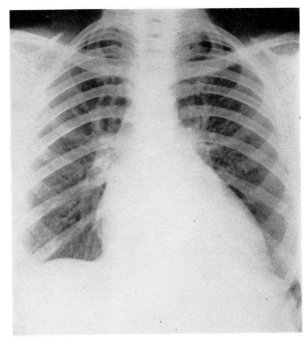

Fig. 277.—Hypertrophic cardiomyopathy. Heart 16 cm. Slight upper-lobe blood diversion, either from the mitral incompetence, or poor compliance of the huge left ventricular muscle mass. Female aged 35 years. Syncopal attacks and some dyspnoea.

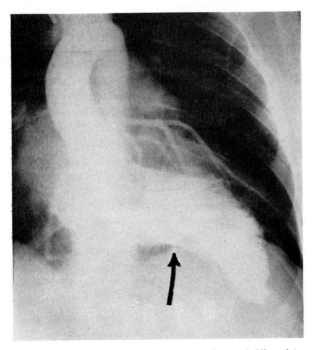

Fig. 278.—Same case (left ventricular angiogram) (diastole). Left ventricular wall thickness 2 cm. Indentation of undersurface (opposite arrow) from hypertrophied muscle. Filling of left atrium from mitral incompetence (possibly stretched chordae from long ventricular cavity).

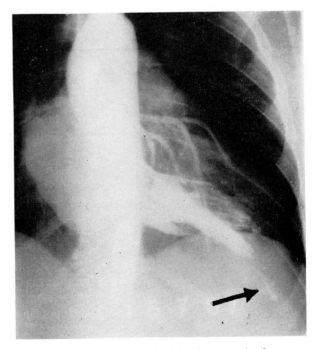

Fig. 279.—Same case (systole). Note long streak of contrast medium towards apex (opposite arrow). Large coronary arteries. L.V. 255/0. Aorta 75/50; L.A. 25/19; E.C.G. left ventricular hypertrophy. At operation: normal aortic valve, gross muscle hypertrophy.

ventricular dilatation, but is an inconstant finding, and a similar appearance may be seen from the hypertrophied muscle of the septum just above the chamber of the left ventricle in hypertrophic obstructive myopathy, or in some cases of aortic stenosis before dilatation occurs (Fig. 272).

A small pulmonary trunk with a very prominent left border, giving the heart the shape of the toe of a well-worn boot, is seen in children with pulmonary atresia (Fig. 280) and is uncommon in a true Fallot situation. In an elderly man a similar appearance (Fig. 281) would suggest a left ventricular aneurysm. This usually follows a myocardial infarct. The protuberance is commonly situated where the more horizontal part of the left border turns downwards, and the aneurysm tends to protrude upwards as well as laterally so that the shape again is that of the toe of a well-worn boot. In a right anterior oblique view the upper margin of the local bulge runs almost horizontally and then curves downwards to meet the sternal shadow, thus producing a step-like appearance of the anterior part of the heart shadow. In a left lateral view the protuberance is often seen end-on as a denser area superimposed on the anterior third of the heart shadow.

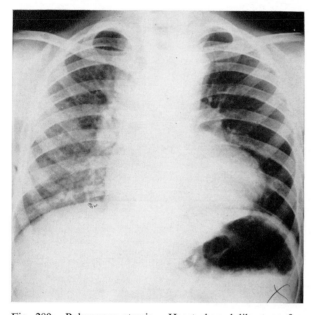

Fig. 280.—Pulmonary atresia. Heart shaped like toe of a well-worn boot. Cyanosed since birth, murmurs. Male aged 8 years. Left lung vessels small, right large as right pulmonary artery has been anastomosed to ascending aorta.

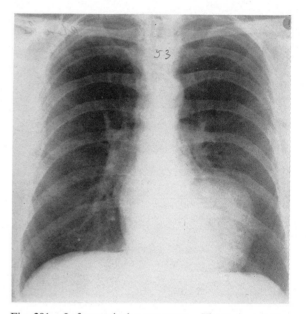

Fig. 281.—Left ventricular aneurysm. Heart shaped like toe of a well-worn boot. Male aged 53 years. Angina. Two episodes of heart failure. E.C.G. indicates myocardial infarct. Aneurysm excised, improved.

The clinical picture and evidence of a previous myocardial infarct in the electrocardiogram will often indicate the diagnosis, but the radiograph is of help in showing the extent of the lesion; if the patient remains much incapacitated as a result of the aneurysm and surgery is contemplated, then a left ventricular angiogram is indicated. This will show the size and site of the aneurysm and will give some indication of how much blood flows into it instead of into the aorta in systole, and how much good muscle remains in the rest of the left ventricle.

A large rounded heart is seen most frequently when there is aneurysmal dilatation of the left atrium in mitral incompetence (Fig. 282), but a similar appearance may be seen in mitral stenosis, or with great dilatation of the right atrium in Ebstein's anomaly. A large rounded heart may be seen in some cases of cardiomyopathy, and finally with a large pericardial effusion.

A local prominence half way down the left border due to a large left atrial appendage is in many cases a characteristic appearance of mitral stenosis (Fig. 283), but since the diagnosis will be obvious clinically, and the haemodynamic effects will be shown by alterations in the vessel pattern and so on, it is a sign of little value.

A rare cause of a small local prominence of either border is an anomalous, dilated, tortuous, coronary artery. The murmur associated with this condition may be continuous or suggest aortic incompetence, but without the other features. Such a clinical finding should lead to a careful scrutiny of the plain radiograph for a local though inconspicuous prominence. A coronary angiogram may be needed to confirm the diagnosis.

Another rare cause of an obvious prominence of the left border, usually high up in the region of the pulmonary trunk, is a developmental deficiency of a part of the pericardium which allows the heart muscle to bulge out laterally. A protuberance of the lower half of the left border is sometimes seen after surgical procedures, due also to a gap left in the pericardial covering.

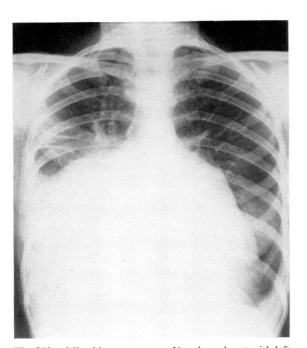

Fig. 282.—Mitral incompetence. Very large heart with left atrium reaching to *right* axilla. Female aged 33 years. Severe dyspnoea. Pansystolic murmur. L.A. 25/16. At operation: huge L.A., right atrium small. Upper-lobe vessels probably dilated. Line shadow (of fluid) in the horizontal fissure.

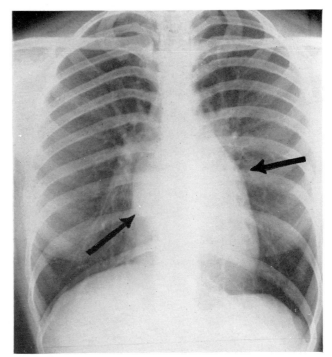

Fig. 283.—Mitral stenosis (classical appearances). Heart 12 cm. Right arrow points to the right margin of the left atrium medial to the right heart border. Left arrow to prominence caused by dilated left atrial appendage. Dilated upper lobe veins. Female aged 32 years. P.A. 27/23; L.A. 20/15. Valvotomy with improvement.

A localized convex prominence of one heart border may be due to encysted pericardial effusion. A similar x-ray appearance may be seen with fluid encysted in the mediastinal pleura adjacent to the heart, a mediastinal tumour or tumour of the heart muscle, or a hydatid cyst in the wall of the heart. Such a local prominence of the right heart border is often clinically silent and first discovered on a routine chest radiograph. It may be necessary in some cases to show the relationship of the right atrium to the shadow by cardiac catheterization and angiography, the latter being particularly helpful since it will indicate whether the shadow encroaches on the lumen of any of the heart chambers or whether these are unaffected by the lesion.

LOCALIZED HIGH-DENSITY SHADOWS WITHIN THE HEART SHADOW

Pericardial calcification

Pericardial calcification may occur without constriction. It may pass undetected in a routine anterior view, but be clearly seen in a more exposed radiograph, and is often most clearly seen in a lateral view (Fig. 284) or left anterior oblique view. It may stand out most clearly when the radiograph is taken with a Potter–Bucky diaphragm.

The shadow is often a 2–5-mm line or band which curves in an almost circular or semicircular manner round the heart, usually lying 1–2 mm deep to the actual border, and often thickest and most conspicuous along the lower border just above the diaphragm. Sometimes a shorter and wider band-like shadow is seen, and if it is of limited extent and lying posteriorly its position near the edge of the heart may only be appreciated in a tangential view.

Sub-endocardial and thrombal calcification

A pericardial calcification must be distinguished from a dense circular line shadow which is sometimes seen when there is sub-endocardial calcification in the wall round an enlarged left atrium in mitral stenosis. The clinical picture and the position of the shadow, lying as it does high up posteriorly, will generally serve to differentiate the two conditions.

A sub-endocardial calcification is indistinguishable from a calcification round the edges of an intra-atrial thrombus, or within a thin thrombus stuck to the endocardium of the atrial wall.

Myocardial calcification

A band-like calcification can occur deeply within the heart muscle, usually in the region of the inter-ventricular septum. It may be the result of an old infarct or haemorrhage, and may be seen in a patient without symptoms.

Coronary artery calcifications

Two high-density parallel line shadows 3–4 mm apart and 1–2 cm long may be seen superimposed on the heart shadow near the aortic valve and will represent atheroma with calcification in the wall of a coronary artery. In old persons such a change may be of little significance, and can occur without narrowing of the lumen. In a person under 50 years of age such a change may be more ominous, and coronary insufficiency may occur.

Valvular calcification

A local increase in the radio-opacity of the heart shadow may be caused by extensive valvular calcification, a complication quite common in severe mitral or aortic stenosis. This high-density shadow is generally rather mottled and rarely more than 1–2 cm long and 2–5 mm wide. It may be band-like, elliptical or in the form of a ring or a group of small spots. In an anterior view, calcification in the mitral valve will lie 2–3 cm to the left of the spine, and calcification in the aortic valve is usually super-imposed on the shadow of the vertebrae or may lie just to the left of the spine. In a right anterior oblique view with limited rotation of about 25 degrees, calcification in the mitral valve will lie more or less in the middle of the heart shadow and may show a rotary or almost horizontal type of movement. In a left anterior oblique view well round at about 60 degrees, aortic valve calcifications will lie centrally and mitral valve calcification more posteriorly. Aortic valve calcifications usually move horizontally at an angle inclined anteriorly and upwards, though sometimes the movement is more or less rotary.

In a lateral view the aortic calcifications lie just anterior to the middle of the heart shadow (Fig. 285), mitral valve calcifications more posteriorly.

Fluoroscopy will usually indicate which shadows lie in the region of which valve and sometimes whether the calcium is in the valve cusp or valve ring.

These calcifications are most convincingly demonstrated by fluoroscopy, when the small spot or mottled shadow shows a characteristic rotary or to and fro movement in phase with the heart beats. In addition, its position will show little change with respiration, whereas a calcification in a hilum gland or the lung would be seen to move downwards on deep inspiration, together with the adjacent vessels. Small calcifications are difficult to see by conventional fluoroscopy, but will be clearly visible if screen image intensification is used. For increased clarity the x-ray beam should be reduced to a field about 5 cm square.

LOCALIZED HYPERTRANSRADIANCY WITHIN THE HEART SHADOW

Pneumopericardium

A pneumopericardium may result from trauma or from rupture of an air-containing space adjacent to it, such as a pneumothorax or pneumomediastinum, or a gas may be introduced deliberately after aspiration of some pericardial fluid (Fig. 271).

If the amount of air is small, the resulting transradiant zone round the borders of the heart will be only 1–2 mm wide, and may be very inconspicuous, but can often be detected if the possibility of this condition is borne in mind. If the amount of air is larger, the transradiant zone may be as much as 2 cm wide, and may be made even more obvious by the presence of a fluid level. The transradiant zone is sharply demarcated by the 1-mm line shadow of the parietal pericardium which runs parallel to the heart shadow with a lateral convex curve and which is superimposed on either lung field. If, as a result of inflammatory changes or the deposit of fibrin from a haemopneumopericardium, the pericardium is much thickened, then the transradiant zone will be demarcated by a band-like shadow several millimetres wide.

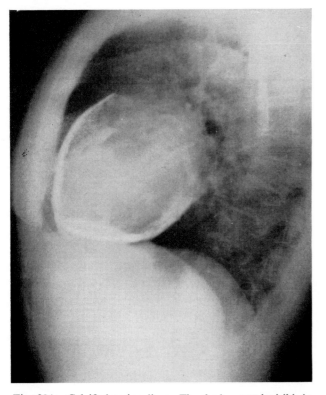

Fig. 284.—Calcified pericardium. The shadow was invisible in the routine anterior-view radiograph. It could be seen in a more exposed anterior view, and was most conspicuous in the lateral view. The white band-like shadow of the calcium forms most of the margin of the heart.

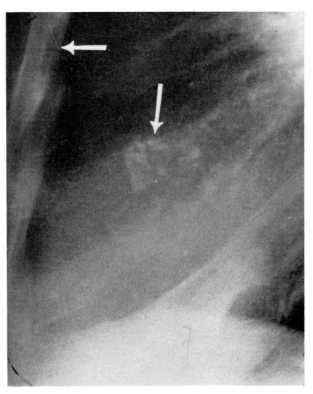

Fig. 285.—Aortic ring and valve calcification (below vertical arrow, horizontal arrow to sternum). Male aged 66 years with aortic stenosis and incompetence. Rotary movement on fluoroscopy (lateral view). The calcification is spotty and was partly in the cusps and partly in the valve ring.

THE PULMONARY VESSELS IN CARDIAC DISEASE

Considerable changes of pressure and flow may be present in the pulmonary circulation as a result of cardiac disease, and although these can be measured with greater accuracy by cardiac catheterization, some of the more severe changes may be reflected in the plain radiograph. The plain radiograph carefully studied may sometimes make cardiac catheterization unnecessary, or at least be a partial substitute should catheterization be contra-indicated at the time. When studying the plain radiograph the pulmonary vessel pattern should be studied as a whole, starting with the heart contour—particularly that part of the left border below the aortic knuckle which is formed by the outflow tract of the right ventricle and the pulmonary artery—then proceeding to the hilar vessels outwards into the larger intrapulmonary vessels, and ending with the smaller peripheral vessels. The larger pulmonary veins may also be separately identified.

DILATATION OF THE MAIN TRUNK OF THE PULMONARY ARTERY

Dilatation of the main trunk of the pulmonary artery may be diagnosed if there is some convexity of the left border of the central shadow just below the aortic knuckle. It can be graded by drawing a line from where the bulge meets the aortic knuckle to the point where it meets the left heart border and then drawing a perpendicular to this line to the left edge of the bulge (Fig. 294).

Grade 1: up to 4 mm
Grade 2: 4–9 mm
Grade 3: 9 mm or more

A shadow in this region may suggest dilatation of the artery when in fact none is present and the appearances are due to slight rotation of the patient or a scoliosis (*see* p. 15). Occasionally the appearances suggest dilatation of the artery but an angiogram shows the shadow has no connection with the artery at all. Sometimes grade 1–2 dilatation is present and is due to a developmental variation with no underlying haemodynamic abnormality.

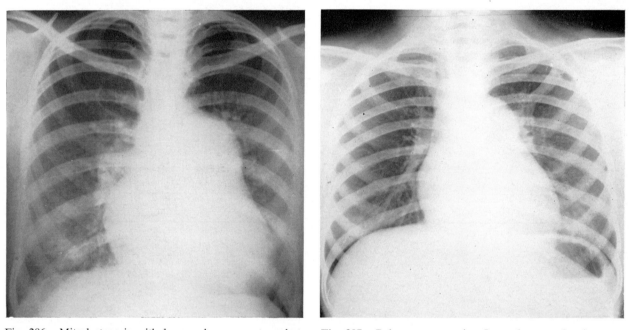

Fig. 286.—Mitral stenosis with large pulmonary artery, but small lung vessels. Horizontal line shadows above the costo-phrenic recesses. Female aged 23 years. Many years breathless on exertion, becoming more severe. P.A. pressure 100/45. Valvotomy. Very great improvement.

Fig. 287.—Pulmonary stenosis. Large heart and pulmonary artery. Small (normal) hilar and lung vessels. Female aged 12 years. Asymptomatic. R.V. 125/0; P.A. 15/5. Pulmonary ejection systolic murmur. E.C.G.: right ventricular hypertrophy. Angiogram: valve stenosis.

Dilatation of the pulmonary artery usually indicates one of four states. First is a high pressure and high flow situation seen in a large V.S.D., ductus, or a late stage of an A.S.D. (for symbols, see p. 175) Second is a high pressure but relatively small flow seen particularly in any of these conditions when the pulmonary vascular resistance is high (the Eisenmenger situation). The high pressure and low flow situation may also be seen in severe mitral stenosis with pulmonary artery hypertension and a high pulmonary vascular resistance (Fig. 286), and in primary or embolic pulmonary hypertensions (Figs. 257–259). The third situation is that of a high flow but at normal pressure, a situation found in many cases of A.S.D. (Figs. 294–296). Finally, dilatation of the main pulmonary artery may be seen in a situation where there is a low pulmonary artery pressure and normal flow, as in pulmonary stenosis (Fig. 287).

DILATATION OF THE HILAR VESSELS

Strictly speaking the hilar arteries and veins are those vessels in the hilar regions but outside the lung substance. For convenience when describing the size of the pulmonary vessels in heart or lung disease, the vessels may be divided up as follows.

Hilar vessels   Right and left main artery
Lobar arteries or veins
Proximal segmental upper lobe vessels

Mid-lung vessels   Branches beyond hilar vessels up to within 2 cm of the pleura
Peripheral vessels   Within 2 cm of the pleura

When hilar vessel dilatation is gross it will be obvious on inspection of the plain radiograph, but in case of doubt measurements can be made of the basal arteries and compared with the range of size found in normal persons (already referred to in Table 1, p. 21).

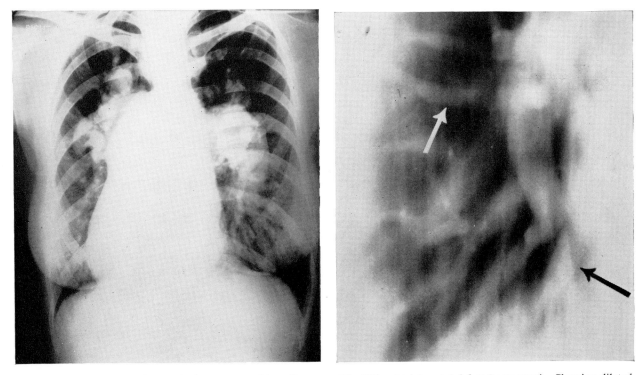

Fig. 288.—Atrial septal defect and mirror transposition. Large pulmonary trunk on the right and enormous dilatation of the hilar arteries. The intrapulmonary arteries are inconspicuous, but the lower veins dilated (confirmed in tomograms). Female aged 42 years with only slight disability.

Fig. 289.—Atrial septal defect (tomogram). Showing dilated upper lobe vein (white arrow) and lower lobe vein (black arrow). Basal artery dilated. Male aged 27 years, moderate disability. Pulmonary blood flow twice systemic, and normal pulmonary artery pressure.

Considerable dilatation of all the hilar vessels (arteries and veins) is seen when there is a left-to-right shunt with a high flow and normal pressure as in an A.S.D. (Figs. 288 and 289) and will indicate that the shunt either is or at one time was 2/1 or more. The dilatation tends to be rather less in cases with a high pressure but only moderate flow, a situation seen in many cases of V.S.D. or ductus. Very gross dilatation may be seen when the flow at one time was very large, but later the pulmonary vascular resistance rose because of the high flow damaging the small peripheral pulmonary vessels. The high resistance may diminish the flow in spite of a rise in pulmonary artery pressure. This course of events in an A.S.D. leads to the Eisenmenger situation (Fig. 299). The shunt then becomes balanced, or reversed so that blood is shunted from right to left, which will be indicated clinically by the onset of cyanosis.

Dilatation of the left main and left basal artery only is seen in some cases with pulmonary stenosis, the post-stenotic dilatation of the main trunk being continued into these vessels (Fig. 305).

Dilatation of the right pulmonary artery is an uncommon developmental defect seen in a Fallot situation, but with an absent pulmonary valve with pulmonary incompetence. The shadow may simulate a large hilar gland.

Dilatation of the upper-lobe hilar vessels

Dilatation of the upper-lobe hilar vessels (upper-lobe blood diversion) is seen particularly when there is a rise in pulmonary venous pressure and is perhaps the most important evidence of this in the plain radiograph. It is seen in the majority of cases of critical mitral stenosis (critical being defined as needing surgical relief of the stenosis), and an example is shown in Figs. 290 and 291. It really represents blood diversion from the lower to the upper half of the lungs. The exact mechanism inducing this is still debated. It seems that in the upright position the pulmonary venous pressure will rise more in the lower than the upper half of the lungs, and this may result in pulmonary oedema in the lower half of the lungs before the upper half. Alveolar wall oedema in the lower half may lead to relative local hypoxia and a local vasoconstrictive response. Alternatively, vessel sheath oedema may cause a local increase in resistance to blood flow, and hence blood diversion to the upper part where the resistance to flow may then be less.

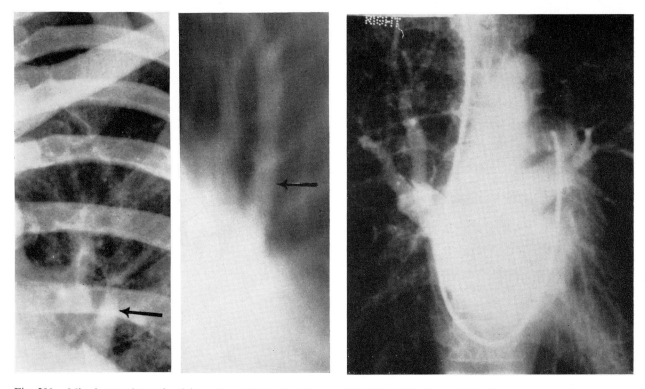

Fig. 290.—Mitral stenosis. *Left*. Plain radiograph showing large upper lobe vein. *Right*. Tomogram showing dilated vein opposite arrow.

Fig. 291.—Mitral stenosis (angiogram, venous phase). Showing large upper lobe but small lower lobe veins draining into the left atrium.

Another cardiac cause other than mitral stenosis for upper-lobe blood diversion is a high end-diastolic pressure in a failing left ventricle with a consequent rise in left atrial pressure which must overcome the residual ventricular pressure before atrial emptying can start. An example of this is acute or chronic left ventricular failure resulting from ischaemic heart disease secondary to coronary artery stenosis or occlusions. In other cases there may be no disease of the coronary arteries but they may fail to increase in size when there is a demand for an increased coronary flow from grossly hypertrophied muscle resulting from an increased work load, as in hypertension or aortic stenosis.

Another mechanism which may cause a rise in pulmonary venous pressure is poor compliance of the left ventricle. This may result from an excessively large muscle mass, as in hypertrophic cardiomyopathy, or from fibrosis beneath the endocardium which will impede diastolic expansion.

Sometimes patients with upper-lobe blood diversion show clinical evidence of left ventricular failure; sometimes the failure is not evident clinically and can only be proved by catheter demonstration of a raised left ventricular end-diastolic pressure.

Finally, there are other causes of upper-lobe blood diversion besides a rise in pulmonary venous pressure and these are listed in Table 7 (page 165).

In the radiograph the main upper-lobe vein to the apex lies lateral to the artery (Fig. 290), and in a high penetration radiograph or a posterior-view tomogram the shadow of the vein can be traced passing downwards and medially to the basal artery to meet the heart shadow before entering the left atrium (shown diagrammatically in Fig. 25). This feature is shown clearly in an angiogram (Fig. 291). In most cases of upper-lobe blood diversion the upper-lobe arteries are also dilated but this may not be noticed because the veins cast a more obvious shadow. The upper-lobe artery dilatation will be more obvious in some cases where there is also pulmonary artery hypertension, and this may be deduced from the radiograph if the lower zone vessels are obviously smaller than the upper-lobe vessels, and perhaps smaller than normal due to vasoconstriction and a reduced flow through them. The small size may be detected in some cases if there is a change in size since a previous radiograph. In many cases of upper-lobe blood diversion the dilatation of the hilar vessels will extend out to the mid-lung vessels.

Dilatation of the mid-lung vessels

Defining the mid-lung vessels as suggested above, any vessel beyond a segmental vessel and more than 2 cm from the pleura can be considered a mid-lung vessel.

Dilatation of mid-lung vessels is not usually great enough to be obvious in the radiograph, although it may be in a high flow, high pressure situation as in a large V.S.D., or in a high pulmonary venous pressure and flow associated with total anomalous pulmonary venous drainage.

In border-line cases it may be possible to decide whether the mid-lung vessels are normal or dilated by matching them against radiographs of normal persons (*see* p. 22). In some cases a pre-existing radiograph of the same patient may be available and can at least be used to see if the mid-lung vessels have become larger. This is apt to happen in acute left ventricular failure or cor pulmonale in failure.

Peripheral vessel dilatation

If peripheral vessels are defined as vessels within 2 cm of the pleura, or as vessels normally too small to be seen in the radiograph, then peripheral vessel dilatation can sometimes be diagnosed with certainty. The dilatation may be the predominant change at this level, or it may be associated with basal horizontal septal line shadows. Since the vein leads off from the medial end of an interlobular septum, the two shadows may form a continuous line. Peripheral vessel dilatation is seen occasionally in mitral stenosis when it may be so marked that it will suggest an almost reticular pattern in the lung. It is also seen in some cases with acute left ventricular failure. It is seen in some cases of V.S.D. with a high flow. In children the vessel dilatation may be uneven in different parts of the lung. For instance, gross mid-lung and peripheral vessel dilatation may be most marked in an upper lobe and, together with capillary flooding, may produce a general haze easily mistaken for an area of consolidation (Fig. 300).

Dilated vessels with indistinct outline

Normally the hilar and mid-lung vessels are fairly sharp in outline in the radiograph; however, with a rise in pulmonary venous pressure, especially if it is sudden as in acute left ventricular failure, the hilar and mid-lung vessel outlines become blurred due to oedema of the hilar structures including lymph glands, tissue spaces and the vessel sheaths (Fig. 274).

Mid-lung vessel tortuosity

Tortuosity of dilated segmental and sub-segmental arteries may be seen in some cases with a large V.S.D. and a high pulmonary vascular resistance (Fig. 293), that is, the Eisenmenger situation. This radiographic appearance reflects the haemodynamic abnormality and indicates the case is inoperable, since the high resistance will only arise with severe damage to the peripheral arterioles resulting from the continued high pulmonary artery pressure. Tortuosity is also seen in some cases of pulmonary artery embolism, and may be related to spasm of the longitudinal muscle. As the clot is absorbed, the tortuosity will disappear.

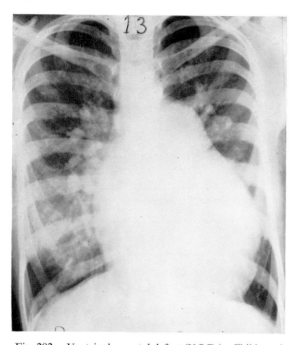

Fig. 292.—Ventricular septal defect (V.S.D.). Child aged 13 years. Large heart, pulmonary artery, hilar and lung vessels. Systolic murmur. O$_2$ sat. in R.A. 65, in R.V. 81; R.V. 120/0; flow 2·2/1; P.V.R. 4·5 units. Asymptomatic.

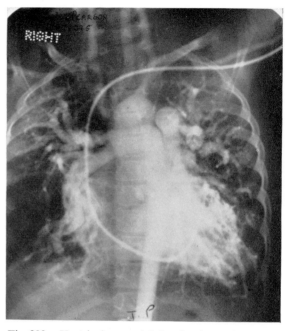

Fig. 293.—Ventricular septal defect (angiogram). Dilated lung vessels, capillary flush right upper zone, tortuosity of large vessels right lower zone. Female aged 5 years. Same case as Fig. 300.

Hilar and Mid-lung Vessel Narrowing

Small or narrow hilar and mid-lung vessels may be associated, or the hilar vessels may be normal while the mid-lung vessels are small. Either occurrence may be seen in severe pulmonary stenosis or atresia, provided that in the latter there is no large compensatory systemic supply. Vessel narrowing may be obvious with the lungs appearing empty, or it may only be detected by a matching technique (*see* p. 22).

Narrowing in lung disease is referred to on page 153, and in pulmonary embolism on page 166.

Pulmonary Plethora (Hyperaemia) and Ischaemia (Oligaemia)

Pulmonary plethora and ischaemia are expressions used rather loosely to suggest either an excessive amount of blood in dilated pulmonary vessels or too little in narrow vessels. For instance, one would expect more dilated vessels in a left-to-right shunt of 5/1 in an A.S.D. than in a patient with severe pulmonary stenosis. In addition, careful observation is needed to appreciate which vessels are dilated or narrow.

In an A.S.D. in an adult with a shunt of at least 2/1 there is often a large heart, pulmonary trunk and hilar vessels, but normal mid-lung vessels and peripheral vessels (Fig. 294). In severe pulmonary stenosis there is often dilatation of the pulmonary artery (Fig. 287), but when the radiograph is compared with those of selected normal persons of the same age, the hilar and mid-lung vessels are found no smaller than those in the normal control group. In a difficult case one often ends up by saying there is plethora or no plethora, and being more cautious in deciding whether or not ischaemia is present. In assessing vessel size, it is of great help to make observations on the radiographic appearances before knowing the clinical diagnosis, or if this is already known, to ignore its possible implications for the moment, and assess the vessel pattern objectively and without any bias.

In adults the diagnosis of plethora or ischaemia is often unimportant, other features indicating the haemodynamic situation. In neonates and young babies not only is the preliminary diagnosis of the type of defect more difficult, but so also is the division into those with plethora and those without. If a magnification technique is available (*see* p. 263), it may show the vessels more clearly than a conventional plain radiograph, and thus aid a decision as to whether the vessels are dilated or normal.

Pulmonary plethora in a neonate is of particular importance when it is associated with cyanosis. This combination is seen with transposition of the great vessels and a mixing site at ventricular or ductus level. It can occur in a Fallot situation with gross pulmonary stenosis, or in pulmonary atresia, if there is a very large systemic collateral circulation to the lungs. It is also seen if there is total anomalous pulmonary venous drainage, particularly to a portal vein. This will raise the right atrial pressure and blood will shunt through an A.S.D. from right to left.

Bearing in mind that in a normal person a big increase in cardiac output on exercise may not be demonstrable in the plain radiographs, one cannot equate cardiac output to vessel size without some reserve. Hence in an A.S.D. vessels of similar size may be seen whether the shunt is 2/1 or 7/1. On the whole, vessel size relates better to pulmonary vascular resistance.

CORRELATION OF HEART AND VESSEL CHANGES WITH THE CLINICAL FINDINGS

The radiographic abnormalities should be viewed as a whole, and the balance between changes in heart size and vessel size and other lung changes may give valuable clues concerning the haemodynamic state. The balance of these various changes in relation to the different clinical conditions is considered below.

In Left-to-right Shunts

Atrial septal defect

The classical findings in an A.S.D. in a patient over 15 years of age are as follows. The heart is enlarged particularly to the left, although the hypertrophy and dilatation are of the right atrium and ventricle. The pulmonary artery, the hilar vessels (both upper and lower), arteries and veins, are dilated (Figs. 289 and 294), but the mid-lung vessels are normal (Fig. 294). The left atrium is normal. These findings usually indicate a shunt of 2/1 or more, with the pulmonary artery pressure still normal. Variations of the classical appearance illustrated in Fig. 294, but with similar haemodynamic features, are common, and the cases can be grouped in the following manner by the x-ray appearances.

(1) Classical, as in Fig. 294.
(2) A heart and pulmonary trunk somewhat larger.
(3) A very large heart shadow and pulmonary trunk and hilar vessels (Fig. 295).
(4) A heart very much smaller (Fig. 296).
(5) A moderately large heart but no obvious dilatation of the pulmonary trunk (Fig. 297).

The last-named appearance is quite common. The percentage of each group in a consecutive series of A.S.D.s all with shunts of 2/1 or more, and defects of 3 × 4 cm or more of the secundum type which were closed, are shown in Table 8.

TABLE 8

INCIDENCE OF THE DIFFERENT TYPES OF X-RAY CHANGES FOUND IN ATRIAL SEPTAL DEFECT

	1	2	3	4	5
Age (years)	Classical (Fig. 294)	Heart Larger	Very large (Fig. 295)	Heart small (Fig. 296)	P.A. not large (Fig. 297)
15–35	21	12	7	8	17
Over 35	8	8	5	4	10
Total	29	20	12	12	27

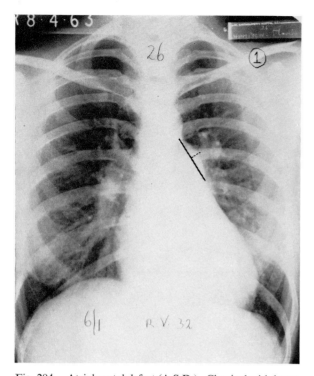

Fig. 294.—Atrial septal defect (A.S.D.). Classical with heart enlarged to left, moderate dilatation of the pulmonary artery and hilar vessels; normal lung vessels. Female aged 26 years. Shunt 6/1; R.V. 32/0.

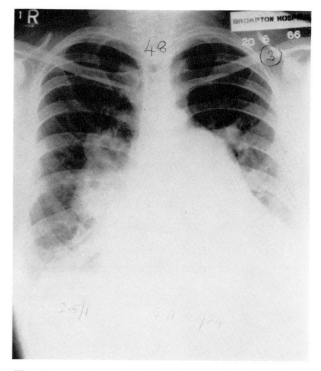

Fig. 295.—Atrial septal defect (configuration 3). Heart, pulmonary artery and hilar vessels much larger than classical Fig. 294. (Configuration 2 between these.) Female aged 48 years. Shunt 2·5/1; P.A. 60/24; P.V.R. 2·4.

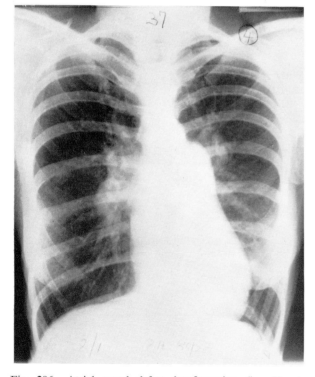

Fig. 296.—Atrial septal defect (configuration 4). Heart smaller than Fig. 294. Female aged 37 years. Shunt 2/1; P.A. 80/25; P.V.R. 9·4 (rising). Most of the other cases with this appearance had normal pressures.

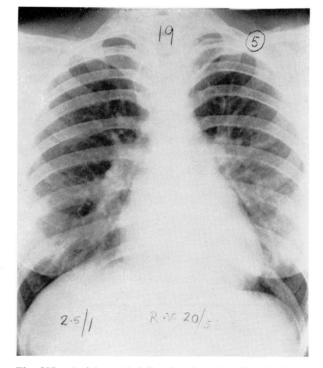

Fig. 297.—Atrial septal defect (configuration 5). Moderate dilatation of heart, but trivial dilatation of the pulmonary artery and hilar vessels. Female aged 19 years. Shunt 2·5/1; R.V. 20/5; P.V.R. 1.

In young children these changes may be much less marked. After the age of 20 years or more, the pulmonary artery pressure may rise and the dilatation of the pulmonary artery and hilar vessels may increase (Fig. 298). Such an appearance will suggest the pulmonary vascular resistance is rising and the Eisenmenger situation is imminent or has already arisen. The actual onset of the Eisenmenger situation with the blood being shunted from right to left, with the consequent onset of cyanosis, may pass undetected in the radiographs. For instance, the x-ray appearances seen in Fig. 298 remained unchanged as the pulmonary vascular resistance rose in a few months from 5 to 20 units. In some cases, as the shunt becomes less or reversed, the mid-lung vessels may become smaller and the heart decrease in size.

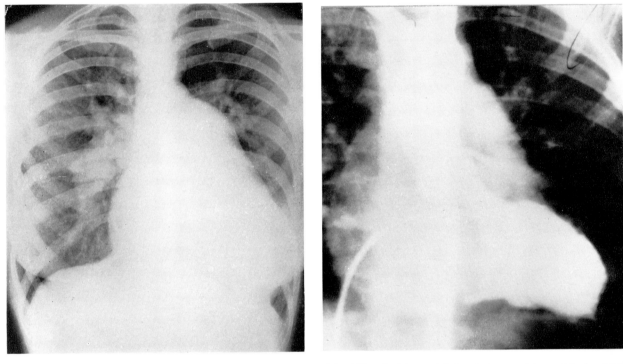

Fig. 298.—Atrial septal defect—Eisenmenger situation. Large heart, pulmonary artery and hilar vessels (usually configuration 3 or 4). Female aged 23 years. Shunt 2·7/1; P.A. 60/20 → 77/44; P.V.R. 5 → 21. During this rise in P.V.R. the radiograph was unchanged. Interval between catheter studies 4 months.

Fig. 299.—Atrial septal defect (primum, atrio-ventricular canal defect). Left ventricular angiogram showing swan neck deformity of outflow tract of left ventricle due to displaced anterior cusp of mitral valve. Male aged 7 years. Asymptomatic. Plain radiograph as Fig. 294. E.C.G. left ventricular hypertrophy.

In a high pressure state of an A.S.D. a greatly dilated hilar vessel when seen end-on gives a 2–3-cm oval shadow which may be mistaken for a tumour.

In some cases the vessel dilatation appears more marked on the right than the left side, an effect which is often an artefact in that the main and left branch and its early divisions are obscured by the enlarged heart shadow, and there is a tendency to compare more peripheral branches in the left lung with more proximal ones in the right. Vigorous pulsation of the dilated hilar vessels may be seen on fluoroscopy (hilar dance), but this observation does not contribute to the assessment.

The x-ray changes may be the same whether the A.S.D. is a secundum type, sinus venosum type or a primum type. In the latter there may be no changes in the lung vessels but dilatation of the left atrium from the mitral regurgitation through a cleft mitral valve. The displaced mitral valve may give rise to the swan neck deformity of the outflow tract of the left ventricle in an angiogram (Fig. 299). Filling of the left or right atrium may also be seen, the right atrium often filling directly through the A.S.D. from the left ventricle.

Ventricular septal defect

If the V.S.D. is trivial the radiograph will be normal, while if the radiograph is abnormal (as in Fig. 292) it will indicate that the defect is relatively large and may need closure.

In a significant defect the heart and pulmonary artery are dilated from an early age, and the dilatation of the heart is less marked to the left than with an A.S.D. The hilar vessels are often rather less dilated and the mid-lung vessels more dilated than in an A.S.D. In about 20 per cent of cases some left atrial dilatation will be seen. In very severe cases peripheral vessels may also be dilated, or there may be local accentuation of vessel dilatation giving a lobar haze in one area, often a right upper lobe, simulating an area of consolidation (Fig. 300). Vessel tortuosity (Fig. 293) means the pulmonary vascular resistance is high and that irreversible damage has occurred to the small vessels as a result of the high pulmonary artery pressure.

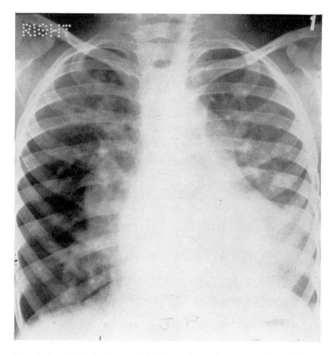

Fig. 300.—Ventricular septal defect. Haze from vascular plethora right upper zone, mistaken for inflammatory lesion. Shunt 1·5/1; R.V. 75/2; P.V.R. 19 units. Same case as Fig. 293.

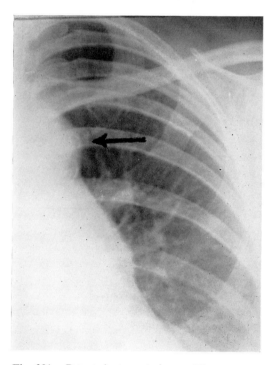

Fig. 301.—Patent ductus arteriosus. Upper prominence (opposite arrow), dilated aorta; lower prominence, dilated pulmonary artery. Line of calcium region of duct. Female aged 39 years.

Patent ductus arteriosus

A patent ductus often gives rise to a loud machinery-like murmur, but if the flow through it is small only a systolic murmur may be heard. If the ductus is wide enough with a considerable flow of blood from the aorta into the pulmonary artery, there will be dilatation of the pulmonary artery (Fig. 302). This will merge above with a somewhat dilated, rather long aortic knuckle (Fig. 301). The hilar vessels and mid-lung vessels may be normal, but will show some dilatation if the flow through the duct is considerable. The appearances tend to be more like a V.S.D. than an A.S.D.

If the pulmonary vascular resistance rises as a result of damage to the peripheral pulmonary arteries by the high pressure and flow, the shunt may become balanced or even reversed, so that the blood flow is from the pulmonary artery to the aorta (the Eisenmenger situation). The pulmonary artery then becomes more dilated while the hilar and lung vessels are small (Fig. 303).

A large duct in infancy will cause a large heart shadow without a local prominence of the pulmonary artery, while there may be blotchy shadows in the lungs from pulmonary oedema.

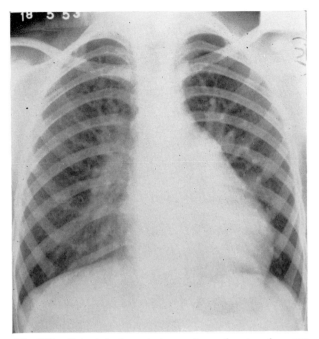

Fig, 302.—Patent ductus arteriosus. Large heart, pulmonary trunk and hilar vessels. Child aged 6 years. Asymptomatic. Following ligation, reduction in size of lung vessels.

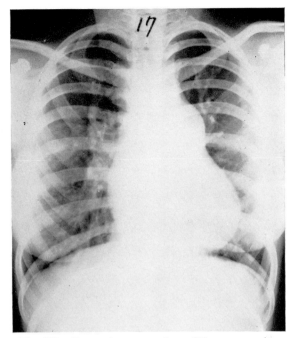

Fig. 303.—Patent ductus arteriosus (Eisenmenger situation). Large heart, very large pulmonary artery, large hilar vessels but small lung vessels. Female aged 17 years. Recent cyanosis. R.V. 100/5; P.V.R. 27. Bi-directional shunt.

IN RIGHT-TO-LEFT SHUNTS

Fallot situation

In many cases with a V.S.D. combined with pulmonary stenosis (the Fallot situation) the heart shadow and the lung vessels may be normal even when the patient is greatly disabled and severely cyanosed. The hilar and lung vessels may appear small but are often within the normal range. If the hypertrophied right ventricle dilates there may be some heart enlargement. The pulmonary artery is not seen except in a few cases when there is some post-stenotic dilatation. In about 20 per cent of cases the aortic arch is right sided and displaces the superior vena cava to the right, so that the two cause a conspicious shadow high up on the right side (Fig. 304). This is quite a useful diagnostic feature. A deep bay in the region of the pulmonary artery giving the heart the shape of the toe of a well-worn boot (Fig. 280) is more characteristic of tricuspid or pulmonary atresia than pulmonary stenosis. In a classical Fallot, evidence of a lung supply from systemic vessels is not often seen, but in pulmonary atresia abnormal vessels may be seen in the region of the hila. Occasionally the collateral circulation from systemic vessels is so well developed that there is even pulmonary plethora.

Pulmonary stenosis with intact septum and no shunt

A somewhat enlarged heart, and obviously dilated pulmonary artery, and normal or small lung vessels are characteristic of pulmonary valve stenosis (Fig. 287). Unfortunately the plain radiograph is of limited value in assessing the severity of the stenosis. A normal sized heart with a dilated pulmonary artery may be present with quite a small pressure gradient between the right ventricle and pulmonary artery. Sometimes the heart enlargement may be too slight to be detected in the radiograph, and the dilated pulmonary artery lies rather medially and thus does not project beyond the left heart border, so that the appearances are within normal limits, and yet the patient may have severe pulmonary stenosis. Obvious heart enlargement, or right ventricular hypertrophy on the electrocardiogram, or the presence of symptoms will all indicate that the gradient is high and the stenosis should be relieved by surgery, after confirmation of the gradient by cardiac catheter studies. Even when the stenosis is severe and the pulmonary artery much dilated, the hilar and lung vessels are often normal, or at any rate within the range of small but normal.

The post-stenotic dilatation is probably due to a turbulence set up by the deformed valve. In some cases the dilatation continues into the left pulmonary artery and down into the left basal artery which will appear larger than the right (Fig. 305). Rarely the stenosis is infundibular and below the valve, when there is no dilatation of the pulmonary artery. In a severe case the high right ventricular pressure may lead to tricuspid incompetence with dilatation of the right atrium so that the heart becomes grossly enlarged and rounded in shape (Fig. 275), as in a pericardial effusion, myopathy or in Ebstein's anomaly.

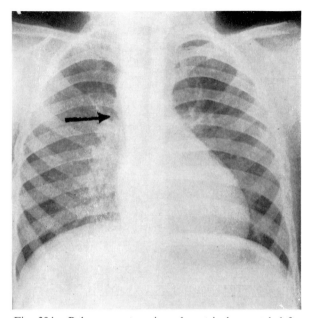

Fig. 304.—Pulmonary stenosis and ventricular septal defect (Fallot situation). Right aortic arch (opposite arrow) otherwise normal. Male aged 5 years. Dyspnoea and cyanosis since birth. R.V. 100/14; P.A. 20/12.

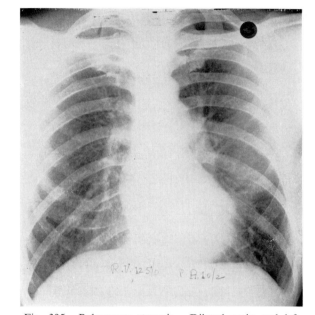

Fig. 305.—Pulmonary stenosis. Dilated main and left pulmonary arteries. Male aged 41 years. Asymptomatic. Pulmonary systolic ejection murmur. R.V. 125/0; P.A. 10/2.

Mitral stenosis

The heart size and vessel pattern in critical mitral stenosis are very variable, but let it be said at once that there is no place for radiology in the diagnosis of mitral stenosis, the diagnosis being made on the clinical findings. Mitral stenosis with a high pulmonary vascular resistance may have no murmur and be diagnosed as primary pulmonary hypertension with an x-ray appearance like Fig. 286. If by chance the typical murmur cannot be heard, a large heart and large left atrium are not sufficient evidence for a diagnosis of mitral stenosis and might equally well be the result of a myopathy.

The classical picture of mitral stenosis is that of a moderately enlarged heart shadow, a moderately enlarged left atrium seen as a double outline on the right border, and a large left atrial appendage seen as a small convex bulge half way down the left border (Fig. 283); there is slight dilatation of the pulmonary artery below a small (normal) aortic knuckle. The hilar vessels are somewhat dilated and there is obvious upper-lobe blood diversion (Figs. 290 and 291), and perhaps at some stage basal horizontal septal line shadows above the costophrenic recesses (Fig. 188).

There are many variations of this appearance. In about 0·5 per cent of cases the heart is normal in size, the left atrium is not dilated and the vessel pattern is normal. Such cases have a tendency to go into severe pulmonary oedema if any extra strain is thrown on the heart (such as a pregnancy), and they are in considerable danger unless the stenosis is relieved. Somewhat less rare is a similar appearance but with slight left atrial dilatation and definite upper-lobe blood diversion. In both these types of response to the stenosis, there is a tendency for the patient to have an incident of fever and cough which is often diagnosed as acute bronchitis, but is really due to pulmonary oedema induced by an upper respiratory tract infection. If a radiograph is available at the time of the incident, blotchy shadows of pulmonary oedema may be seen, and these are an important warning sign that the stenosis needs relieving.

At the other extreme are cases with marked heart enlargement and obvious vessel and lung changes.

The causes of a large heart shadow in mitral stenosis are discussed on page 173.

A very large pulmonary artery indicates pulmonary arterial as well as pulmonary venous hypertension. This will be confirmed if there are also small lung vessels and no septal lines so that the lung fields appear rather empty (Fig. 286). A much dilated pulmonary artery may occur with upper-lobe blood diversion and positive vasoconstriction of the lower-lobe vessels, a change which may be detected with certainty if earlier radiographs showing normal lower-lobe vessels are available.

The hilar vessels are often normal but may be somewhat dilated, and their outlines are indistinct because of perihilar oedema (Fig. 274), the soggy hilar structures being apparent at thoracotomy.

The mid-lung vessels as a whole are rarely dilated, but in upper-lobe blood diversion the vessels beyond segmental level may also be dilated.

Occasionally there is dilatation of the vessels at all levels, and the combination of dilated peripheral vessels and septal lines may give an almost reticular pattern in the lower zones. Septal line shadows with a large heart shadow and perhaps upper-lobe blood diversion are in fact only seen in about 25 per cent of cases and are often transient, whereas upper-lobe blood diversion alone or in combination with other changes is nearly always present and persistent.

Septal line shadows (see also p. 113) may remain static for some time or may disappear with bed rest. They usually disappear rapidly after successful surgery, though if some fibrosis has occurred they may persist for a few weeks before eventually disappearing. Occasionally the septal line shadows are unilateral. This will indicate that the side with no lines is protected from the high pulmonary venous pressure by a low pulmonary artery flow, for instance because of pre-existing lung disease limiting flow, as in emphysema or bronchitis obliterans. If no such cause seems apparent in the radiograph, it will suggest that one side is protected by a lower-lobe vessel thrombosis.

Other changes in the lungs are referred to on pp. 196–198. A summary of the contribution of radiology in mitral stenosis is that it may indicate the haemodynamic consequences of the lesion without the necessity to catheterize the patient, and that any changes present, apart from slight dilatation of the left atrium, will indicate that the stenosis is critical and in need of surgical relief.

Mitral regurgitation

Mitral regurgitation or incompetence may cause some rather non-specific heart enlargement with only slight left atrial enlargement, or there may be gross heart enlargement due mainly to gross dilatation of the left atrium (Fig. 282). Often there are no lung vessel changes, but in some cases mild blood diversion or faint septal line shadows may be seen.

Mitral incompetence may be due to a lesion of the valve cusps, ruptured chordae, stretched chordae from left ventricular disease, particularly ischaemic heart disease or a myopathy.

Mitral stenosis and mitral regurgitation (incompetence)

Since a large heart shadow, dilated upper-lobe vessels, septal lines, perihilar haze and so on can occur in pure mitral stenosis or in pure mitral incompetence (although the vessel changes are much commoner in the former), when both lesions are present it is not possible to tell from the radiographs which is the predominant lesion. Therefore, left ventricular angiography seems the most reliable method for showing the degree and actual site of the regurgitation. Too close a grading is unprofitable, and a grading into none, slight or more than slight, is adequate.

Aortic stenosis

In aortic stenosis the earliest change may be a fullness of the left border just above the apex (Fig. 272) which gives the left border a rather rounded contour. This may be the only change in the radiograph even when the stenosis is severe and there is much left ventricular hypertrophy. The ascending aorta is usually dilated and this may be seen in the anterior-view radiograph, unlesss the aorta happens to lie rather medially, in which case the dilatation may only be detected in the lateral view. If the condition deteriorates further the heart may dilate and will then appear enlarged in the radiograph.

The presence of dilated upper-lobe vessels, even if the heart shadow is not enlarged (Fig. 272), will indicate that the left ventricular end-diastolic pressure is rising and that there is haemodynamic, even if not yet clinical, heart failure. If heart failure is present clinically, there will often be confirmatory evidence of this such as upper-lobe blood diversion, septal line shadows, or the presence of small lower axillary line shadows due to some pleural fluid.

An important feature in an adult will be calcification in the aortic valve area, which may be seen most clearly in the lateral view (Fig. 285) or on fluoroscopy. Failure to detect such calcification will suggest the stenosis is sub-valvar or even supra-valvar, and this should be confirmed on angiography, since it is of great importance to the surgeon.

Aortic incompetence (regurgitation)

A very large heart shadow with protuberance of its border to the left, posteriorly and downwards will suggest aortic incompetence. The heart is usually larger than in aortic stenosis and the dilatation of the ascending aorta more marked. Usually there are no lung changes and often there is no evidence of valve calcification. In multiple valve disease or when there is both aortic stenosis and incompetence an aortogram is often of great value in assessing the degree of aortic incompetence. Even a faint puff of contrast medium through the valve may be significant, and will indicate that difficulties may be anticipated in circulatory by-pass techniques, even if the regurgitation is not severe enough to warrant valve surgery.

Ischaemic heart disease

A large heart shadow may be due to ischaemic heart disease secondary to coronary artery disease, and the diagnosis will be made on clinical grounds. Severe ischaemic heart disease may be present with a normal heart shadow, so that the gravity of the lesion will depend on the clinical assessment rather than the heart size. However, in such cases the heart shadow will usually enlarge in the course of time if the patient survives long enough.

Dilatation of the upper-lobe vessels is common and is an indication of poor left ventricular function.

Acute left ventricular failure

Dilated upper-lobe vessels, or widespread dilatation of the lung vessels whose outline is often blurred from oedema of the vessel sheaths and tissues around, indistinct hilar shadows and a perihilar haze, will suggest a failing left ventricle. This may occur in acute ischaemic heart disease with or without infarction. In many cases there may be dilatation of the peripheral vessels, blotchy lung shadows of pulmonary oedema, or horizontal septal line shadows above the costophrenic recesses. Also, long line shadows in the upper half, independent of the vessel shadows (Kerley "A" lines), or tram line shadows from oedema of the bronchial wall are often seen. Pleural effusions are common in the acute phase but less common later. They are usually bilateral with the effusion on one side being much larger than on the other side, where it may be quite small and pass undetected unless carefully sought. In acute myocardial infarction a pleural effusion is often secondary to an associated pulmonary infarct. An effusion on the left side is sometimes the result of a reaction set up by the adjacent necrotic portion of left ventricular wall.

In the acute phase of a myocardial ischaemia with or without infarction any of the above-mentioned changes may be seen, but owing to the difficulties of radiography of such patients the radiograph is often of indifferent quality. Daily radiographs are not indicated as a routine, but should be done on clinical indications. An isolated area of opacity in a lower zone is often due to a pulmonary infarct, a not uncommon complication of such a condition.

One complication of a myocardial infarct is the formation of a left ventricular aneurysm and consequent local bulge of the left heart border (see p. 178). Another is necrosis of the interventricular septum and the late onset of a ventricular septal defect. This will be suggested in the radiograph if there is sudden dilatation of the pulmonary artery and hilar vessels.

Angina

Anginal pain, whether due to aortic stenosis or ischaemic heart disease, may be the result of coronary artery disease.

In many cases investigation of the state of the coronary arteries by coronary angiography is indicated. This is a safe and painless procedure, and from a study of the radiographs it will be possible to see whether the coronary arteries are normal or whether there are local areas of narrowing (Fig. 306) which might be amenable to local surgical procedures, or if there are widespread occlusions of several branches, the effects of which can only be mitigated by bringing in some other artery to nourish the heart muscle. Anginal pain is common, but the indications for coronary arteriography are still somewhat uncertain, and the long-term results of surgical procedures are also uncertain, especially in older patients with severe and widespread occlusions.

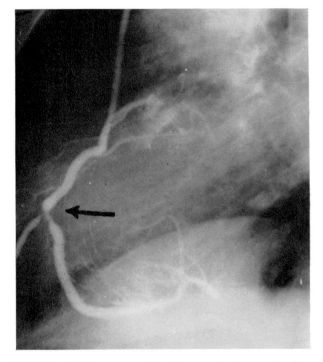

Fig. 306.—Right coronary artery disease. Angiogram showing stenosis of right coronary artery (opposite arrow). Male aged 34 years. Angina. Relief following vein graft.

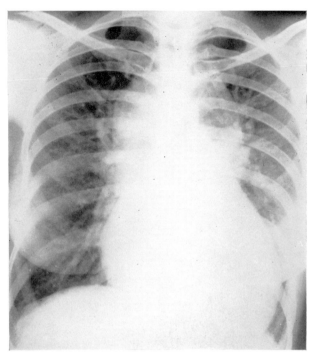

Fig. 307.—Total anomalous pulmonary venous drainage. Cottage-loaf shape of central shadow, the upper right border being formed by a dilated superior vena cava, the left by a persistent left superior vena cava which joins the right and into which drain the pulmonary veins from both lungs. The inevitable atrial septal defect causes the large heart and hilar vessel shadows.

CHANGES IN THE POSITION OF THE HEART CHAMBERS OR GREAT VESSELS

During development the primitive part of the cardiac tube which gives rise to the ventricles, loops to the right to bring the right ventricle anteriorly and to the right, and the left posteriorly and to the left. Occasionally it loops the other way so that the left ventricle ends up on the right; if the rest of development is normal, this will not cause symptoms and can be considered a normal variation. If such an appearance is seen, a sort of mirror transposition of the heart shadow, special attention should be paid to the position of the gastric air bubble. If this is also beneath the right dome, the chamber connections may well be normal. If it is on the left so that it and the left ventricle are on opposite sides, a complicated cardiac situation will probably be present which can only be clarified by catheter studies and angiography. As a rule the liver is on the same side as the morphological and functional right atrium.

The position of the aortic knuckle should also be identified. It lies to the right of the trachea in a right-sided arch. A long, rather flat prominence on the left heart border where the aortic knuckle would normally be seen—perhaps suggesting a dilated pulmonary artery, but in fact due to the ascending aorta coming up on the left side instead of the right—is seen in corrected transposition. The pulmonary artery in an angiogram will be seen to lie centrally instead of on the left. There will be no functional derangement.

Other complex abnormalities will require catheter studies and angiograms to see the sites of the heart chambers and their connections, and the sites of the great vessels.

A bilateral convex shadow placed on the top of the heart shadow and simulating a mediastinal tumour is seen with total anomalous pulmonary venous drainage—the dilated pulmonary trunk running up the left side to join the innominate vein, and the dilated superior vena cava on the right producing a shadow which, with the heart shadow below, is like a cottage loaf (Fig. 307). Since the pulmonary venous blood flows into the right atrium, there will be a large flow through the lungs, and the pulmonary vessels will be dilated, while oxygenated blood will only be able to reach the left atrium through an associated atrial septal defect. In a truncus the pulmonary arteries come off the aorta at various levels.

LUNG CHANGES IN CARDIAC DISEASE

Cardiac disease may not only cause alterations in the pulmonary vessel pattern, but may result in abnormal shadows in the lungs themselves.

HAEMOSIDEROSIS

Small nodular or pin-point shadows mainly in the middle two-thirds of the lungs may be due to haemosiderosis (*see* pp. 95, 97) and are seen in about 5 per cent of patients with mitral stenosis. Such shadows are only seen if the clumps of haemosiderin are 0·5 mm or more in size. The shadows can generally be identified because similar shadows of this small size made up of particles of a lower atomic number would not ordinarily be visible. They are for the most part widely disseminated over the middle third of both lungs, and may be sparse or so numerous that they result in a ground-glass appearance, and the radiograph may appear under-exposed. After successful valvotomy the shadows tend to persist for months or years, though in some cases they eventually become fewer in number and less distinct.

If the shadows are only moderately numerous and of larger size reaching up to 2 mm in diameter, distinction from small areas of oedema or fibrotic nodules without haemosiderin deposits associated with them may be impossible. In addition the shadows of the iron particles may be somewhat obscured by the presence of shadows from engorged peripheral vessels, or even oedematous areas in the lung. They have become less common than in the past, since the advent of mitral valve surgery cuts short the period of high venous pressure.

PULMONARY FIBROSIS

Pulmonary fibrosis may occur in severe long-standing mitral stenosis. It is as a rule associated with engorgement of the pulmonary vessels, and the effect of these superimposed on the shadows of the fibrous tissue is to give a complicated series of shadows which has a reticular or net-like, or even a honeycomb appearance.

ECTOPIC BONE

Several 2–5-mm well-defined circular shadows lying in the lower half of the lungs due to ectopic bone are occasionally seen in a patient with mitral stenosis (Fig. 167). (*see* p. 99). These lesions are probably the result of old foci of rheumatic pneumonia occurring at the time of the original rheumatic fever, and not of the cardiac lesion.

SHORT HORIZONTAL LINE SHADOWS ABOVE THE COSTOPHRENIC RECESSES

Short horizontal line shadows above the costophrenic recesses (*see* p. 113 and Fig. 188), sometimes known as Kerley "B" lines or septal line shadows, are cast more by the oedematous septa than the dilated lymphatics within them. They are fairly common with a rise in pulmonary venous pressure and are seen particularly in mitral stenosis (*see* p. 193), whether at valve level or due to a left atrial myxoma, and in left ventricular failure whatever the cause. They denote interstitial oedema as opposed to the more homogeneous or blotchy shadows of alveolar oedema.

PLEURAL EFFUSION

A small homogeneous shadow with an ill-defined margin concave towards the lung and occupying a costophrenic recess, or a larger shadow with a similar configuration will indicate a pleural effusion (*see* p. 35). Less easily seen is a short line shadow parallel to the lower axilla just above a costophrenic recess, rather like the companion shadow referred to on p. 37. Its appearance or disappearance in serial radiographs or its change with posture (Figs. 48 and 49) will indicate it is a small pleural effusion.

Widening of the line shadow of the horizontal fissure often with variations in width in serial radiographs will also be evidence of fluid in this interlobar septum. Sometimes the widened line of the horizontal fissure remains as a permanent feature after the incident of failure has been treated, suggesting fibrous organization of the fluid. A small effusion may be more readily demonstrated in the radiograph than clinically. In heart failure the effusion is usually bilateral, but is very much smaller on one side than the other, with the result that the smaller one often passes unnoticed.

The mechanism by which these effusions are produced is still uncertain. They are common in acute left ventricular failure, but even a moderate effusion is uncommon in mitral stenosis in spite of the rise in pulmonary venous pressure.

In mitral stenosis during episodes of deterioration, a very small effusion, indicated by a lower axillary line shadow (Fig. 48) or a widening of the line shadow of the horizontal fissure, is seen more often than a moderate effusion. It will disappear as improvement sets in. When a large effusion does occur it is often secondary to a small infarct, the shadow of which may be detected above that of the fluid in an anterior view (Fig. 164), or it may only be seen independently of the effusion in a lateral view. A moderate effusion on the right side is sometimes due to occlusion of the lower-lobe veins either by a thrombus in the left atrium, or in the vein itself. If such an effusion is seen, a left thoracotomy should not be done until the possibility of a venous occlusion on the right has been considered and such a state of affairs perhaps excluded by an angiogram. A left effusion after an acute myocardial infarct may be secondary to the local muscle disintegration, or to an associated pulmonary infarct (Fig. 308) rather than the poor left ventricular function. Small effusions are sometimes present with gross pulmonary oedema, but in acute left ventricular failure either may occur without the other.

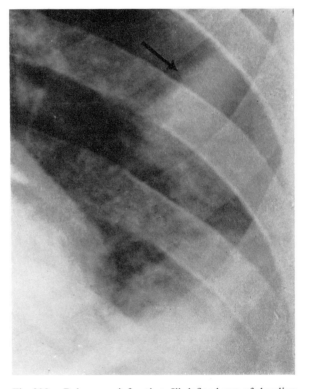

Fig. 308.—Pulmonary infarction. Ill-defined area of clouding (opposite arrow), raised left dome, and shadow of pleural effusion. Acute left chest pain and haemoptysis; embolus apparently from calf vein.

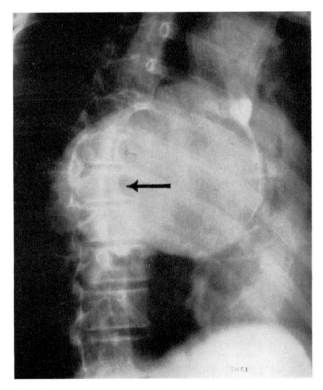

Fig. 309.—Aortic aneurysm. Arrow points to the vertebral erosion caused by the aortic aneurysm, the large circular shadow of which is visible around the arrow. A trace of barium is seen in the oesophagus, which is displaced anteriorly.

PULMONARY OEDEMA

Diffuse opacity of both lungs, a perihilar or bat's wing type of shadow, widespread blotchy or nodular shadows, an upper or lower zone haze or even localized nodular shadows may all be caused by pulmonary oedema (*see* p. 91). Many cases have neither frothy sputum nor basal crepitations; in others the condition is obvious clinically.

Pulmonary oedema may occur with a rise in the pulmonary capillary pressure, which reflects a rise in the left atrial pressure. It is seen in some cases of left ventricular failure from whatever cause. It is commonly found in hypertension with uraemia, but may also occur in hypertension without uraemia, in ischaemic heart disease, in myocarditis or mitral stenosis; it may occur with some bio-chemical disaster, but without a long-standing or irreversible cardiac lesion or a water overload.

In mitral stenosis the pulmonary oedema tends to be very transient, and its detection depends on radiographs being taken during incidents of deterioration. The bat's wing shadow is very uncommon, whereas a lower zone haze is common (Fig. 39). This is often mistaken for the breast shadows, the result of a high position of the diaphragm or a pleural effusion. An upper zone haze can occur, but in spite of the upper lobe blood diversion is very uncommon. There may be a fairly generalized haze (Fig. 39). Coarse blotchy shadowing is found particularly in pulmonary oedema in cases with a small left atrium and small heart. The rapid disappearance of all these types of shadow following successful treatment will confirm the diagnosis.

The shadows of pulmonary oedema are on the whole less radio-opaque than those of an infective consolidation, and they may come and go rapidly, or may persist unchanged for many days. The great variation in the type of shadow seen in pulmonary oedema should be kept in mind, for in many cases the condition is not particularly suspected clinically or its extent is underestimated, or the shadows are mistaken for infective lesions.

THE AORTIC SHADOW

Prominence of the central shadow, particularly the upper half, may be due to unfolding of the aorta, or dilatation due to aortic regurgitation or stenosis, aortitis, or to an aneurysm. The enlargement may be associated with an increase of the transverse diameter of the heart, especially if there is a lesion of the aortic valve, but sometimes there is gross enlargement of the central shadow from an aortic aneurysm and no enlargement of the heart shadow.

UNFOLDING OF THE AORTA

Unfolding of the aorta without actual dilatation is a condition which is often seen in older persons, particularly men over 65 years of age. In the anterior view it causes a lateral convex prominence of the middle third of the central shadow on the right side, and a prominence of the aortic knuckle on the left side, both having well-defined margins. On the right side the upper part of the prominence may be caused by the displaced superior vena cava. On the left the aortic knuckle not only projects out farther but is higher than in a normal younger person. The descending aorta may curve considerably to the left, and the shadow formed by it may be so marked as to simulate a mediastinal tumour projecting out from the region between the aortic knuckle and the left ventricle. A well-exposed anterior-view radiograph will show the continuity of this aortic shadow from the knuckle to the diaphragm, while an oblique or lateral view will confirm the absence of any abnormal mediastinal shadow. The oblique and lateral views will also show that there is no appreciable increase in width of the aortic shadow, the walls of which remain parallel. A considerable kyphosis is often apparent.

SYPHILITIC AORTITIS

In syphilitic aortitis the increase in size of the central shadow is less obvious than in unfolding of the aorta, but in an oblique view, preferably the left anterior-oblique view, a local or general increase in width of the aorta will be apparent. Faint lines of calcification are sometimes seen in the ascending aorta which are much thinner than those seen in atheroma.

AORTIC ANEURYSM

In a routine anterior-view radiograph an aortic aneurysm will often result in a large homogeneous shadow projecting out from the central shadow. If it arises from the ascending aorta, the prominence will be seen on the right side of the central shadow at the level of, or somewhat above, the hilum.

Rarely it extends downwards, when the appearances will be exactly the same as that of the mediastinal effusion illustrated in Figs. 62 and 63, p. 43.

If it arises from the descending aorta it may project to the left behind the hilum shadow. If the aneurysmal dilatation is S-shaped it may project behind the right hilum or lower down on the right border of the central shadow. The posterior position of the shadow will be evident from oblique or lateral views, and the correct diagnosis thus made. If the aneurysm is fusiform and low down just above the diaphragm, the shadow will simulate that of a collapsed lower lobe. There will, however, be none of the other changes such as alteration of the hilar or lung vessel pattern and hypertransradiancy (*see* pp. 57, 67).

Sometimes the routine anterior view appears normal, whereas the aneurysm is either seen clearly in one of the oblique or lateral views in a high-penetration anterior view, or is inferred from oesophageal displacement demonstrated after a barium swallow. Therefore, when an aneurysm is suspected clinically, these further radiological investigations should be carried out, whether the anterior view appears normal or whether it shows a shadow of doubtful nature.

The condition will be excluded if the shadow of the aorta is seen to be independent of, and sufficiently remote from, the abnormal shadow. The shadow of an aortic aneurysm would be in contact with that of the aorta at some point and would usually be obviously continuous with it at both the proximal and distal ends.

Considerable displacement of the oesophagus round the shadow is common if the aneurysm is in the arch or descending aorta. The displacement is usually more marked than with a neoplasm.

Erosion of the sternum is common with an aneurysm of the ascending aorta, and erosion of one or two vertebrae with an aneurysm of the descending part. These vertebral erosions tend to be in the anterior part of the vertebral body, and result in a deep anterior concavity since the intervertebral structures are relatively resistant to the pressure erosion (Fig. 309). Generally there is no reactive sclerosis. Often both sternal and vertebral erosion are most easily seen in a true lateral view. Sometimes the vertebral erosion is at the side of the vertebral body and can then only be seen in a posterior view taken for the bone.

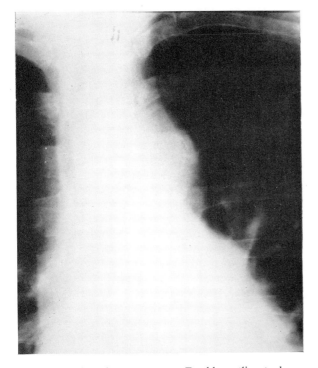

Fig. 310.—Dissecting aneurysm. Double outline to large aortic knuckle. Male aged 59 years. Sudden chest pain. Loud diastolic murmur appeared from aortic incompetence secondary to the aortic lesion.

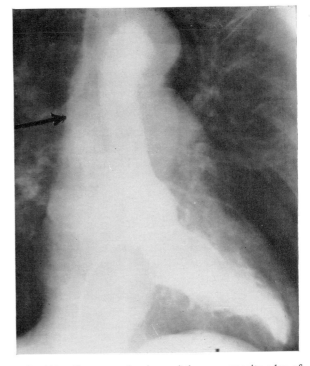

Fig. 311.—Same case (angiogram) (arrow opposite edge of dissection). Contrast medium in main channel does not fill to edge of aortic shadow, nor into aortic knuckle. P.M.: false lumen thin walled.

Sometimes an aneurysm presses on a bronchus and occludes it, and the shadow of the aneurysm may then be obscured by that of the collapsed lung. Often only a single lobe collapses, or distal inflammatory changes result in an area of patchy clouding, the shadow of the aneurysm remaining visible near the hilum.

Sometimes the clinical and radiological findings indicate the diagnosis quite clearly, in others there may be no clinical clues, while radiologically it may be difficult or impossible to distinguish the shadow from that of a mediastinal neoplasm (*see* p. 203). If there is doubt about the diagnosis, it can usually be solved by angiography since most aneurysms will fill with the contrast medium (Fig. 315) even if they contain much clot.

If a double outline is seen to a dilated aortic knuckle, particularly if the outer shadow is somewhat irregular instead of having an even convex curve (Fig. 310), or if there is a sudden increase in size of the aortic knuckle since a previous radiograph, it will suggest a dissecting aneurysm. There may be some leak from the aneurysm into the pleural cavity, when the shadow of a left pleural effusion will be seen, or into the pericardial cavity, which will be suggested if there is a sudden unexplained increase in the size of the heart shadow. In either case, if the leak is not torrential, it may well be detected by either of the above-mentioned changes occurring in serial radiographs.

If surgery is contemplated, angiography should be done not only to confirm the diagnosis (Fig. 311), but also to show whether any of the major vessels arising from the arch are involved and thus what surgical intervention will entail.

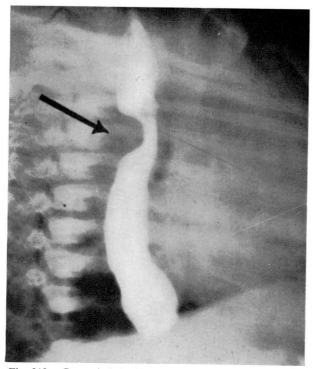

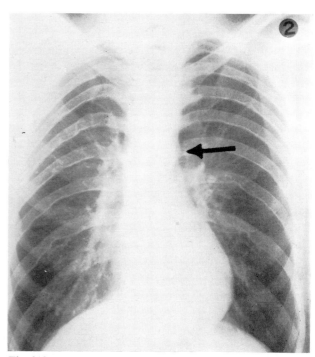

Fig. 312.—Congenital double aortic arch (aortic ring). Note indentation on posterior wall of barium-filled oesophagus from abnormally placed vessel. Child aged 1 year. Recurrent respiratory infections with stridor. Left aortic arch compressed trachea and was tied off. Good recovery.

Fig. 313.—Coarctation of aorta. Indentation of aortic knuckle (opposite arrow). Marked rib notching of posterior part of ribs 4–9. Angiogram showed tortuous intercostal vessels lying under the rib notches. Male aged 34 years. Asymptomatic. Coarctation resected.

TRAUMATIC RUPTURE OF AORTA

Deceleration injuries may include a tear of the intima of the aorta with the adventitia remaining intact so that there is not an immediately fatal haemorrhage. Oedema and minor haemorrhage round the area of injury, which usually is just below the origin of the left subclavian artery, and extends down for some 2 cm into the descending aorta, may result in a shadow adjacent to the aortic knuckle which will appear enlarged. Since there may be multiple rib fractures and a left haemothorax, an aortogram is of great use to confirm the aortic injury, and guide the surgeon in handling the situation. A local prominence of the lumen will mark the site, and the torn ends of the intima may appear as short linear transradiant zones in the shadow of the contrast medium. The risks of the procedure are probably worth the valuable information it may give.

Congenital Anomalies of the Aortic Arch

Aortic ring

In babies or young children stridor may be caused by a persistent aortic ring pressing on and narrowing the trachea. The plain radiographs may appear normal, but a small barium sulphate, hypaque or iodized oil swallow will show a small indentation of the posterior wall of the oesophagus, with some forward displacement at about the level of the third and fourth thoracic vertebrae. The appearances are most easily seen in a right anterior-oblique view (Fig. 316). Sometimes the oesophagus shows a slight narrowing on both sides in the anterior view, that on the left corresponding to the normal aortic indentation, and that on the right corresponding to the right arch of the aortic ring. The tracheal narrowing may be seen in tomograms, but it is not always possible to obtain a clear picture in a restless baby.

Coarctation of the Aorta

A flat aortic knuckle or one showing a shallow lateral concave notch will suggest a coarctation of the aorta (Fig. 313). The shadow above the notch is usually due to a laterally placed subclavian artery rather than a post-stenotic dilatation of the descending aorta. After about the age of 15 years notching of the ribs may be seen due to dilated intercostal vessels taking blood from the subclavian artery to the descending aorta. Notching is most commonly seen along the inferior aspect of the posterior parts of ribs 5–8; though it may be seen at a higher or lower level. If a barium swallow is given there is often a sharp indentation into the posterior wall of the oesophagus, best seen in a lateral view at the level of D6. This is caused by a post-stenotic dilatation of the top of the descending aorta starting just below the coarctation, and is useful evidence that the coarctation is in the classical site at ductus level. If there is inequality of the pulses or some other feature to suggest the coarctation is at a more proximal level, then catheter studies and angiograms will be indicated. They will also be indicated if there is any suspicion of associated aortic stenosis, so that the severity of each lesion can be assessed.

Aortic Window and Truncus Arteriosus

A rather uncommon congenital defect is a communication between the ascending aorta and the pulmonary artery lying just to the left of it. The haemodynamic consequences will be much the same as a V.S.D. with elevation of the pulmonary artery pressure and a left-to-right shunt, so that the plain radiograph may show a dilated pulmonary artery and large hilar vessels.

Another defect of a similar nature is a truncus arteriosus, when there is no pulmonary outflow tract, and the pulmonary artery or the right and left branches come off from the aorta. In the former case there may be a prominence of the artery just below the aortic knuckle. In the latter case the left branch may come off at a higher level than the right, a diagnostic feature which may be apparent in the plain radiograph. If the arteries are small, the plain x-ray may be normal; if large, there will be dilatation of the hilar and perhaps mid-lung vessels. In many cases the diagnosis and exact site of origin of the pulmonary arteries can only be determined from angiocardiograms, an injection into the ascending aorta being the most suitable site.

CHAPTER 7

THE MEDIASTINAL AND DIAPHRAGM SHADOWS

THE BORDERS of the central (mediastinal) shadow which are outlined by the transradiant lung fields on either side, are normally formed by the heart and its pericardial covering, together with the great vessels. An abnormality of the size, shape, or density of this shadow may result from cardiovascular disease as described in Chapter 6. It may also result from enlargement of one of the other contents of the mediastinum which are normally invisible, such as the oesophagus, thymus, lymphatic glands, or part of the vertebral column. Finally, it may be due to the presence of a tumour, hernia, or effusion.

The diaphragm shadow is intimately related to mediastinal lesions lying in the lower part, such as a parapericardial or pleural cyst, a pleural fibroma or a lipoma resting on it. It may itself contribute to the mediastinal shadow, either when a local defect permits a hernia into the mediastinum, or when a portion of one dome of the diaphragm is pushed upwards as a result of a local weakness, allowing the shadow of the liver or spleen to encroach on a lung field.

CONFIRMATION AND LOCALIZATION OF THE ABNORMAL SHADOW

It will usually be possible to make quite sure that a suspected shadow is in fact an abnormal shadow and not just an unusual normal shadow resulting from a minor variation in the size or position of some normal structure, or even an artefact. Tomograms are often of great value to confirm the presence of a small and inconspicuous abnormality, the lateral view being the most suitable in some cases and the posterior in others.

Whether the shadow is small and inconspicuous or large and obvious, its spatial position has to be determined. A plain lateral view will generally suffice to prove that it does in fact lie in or adjacent to one of the mediastinal spaces or is related to the diaphragm; sometimes, however, more elaborate investigations are needed, such as a high-penetration anterior or posterior view, a similar view taken with a clearing grid, tomograms, fluoroscopy, and a barium swallow may be needed in a difficult case.

DIAGNOSIS OF THE ABNORMAL SHADOW

There may be clues to the diagnosis from the clinical side, such as physical signs suggesting an aneurysm, an abnormal blood count indicating leukaemia, or a gland biopsy indicating one of the reticuloses. In the absence of any such clinical clues, not only is differentiation of an aneurysm from a neoplasm or inflammatory mass sometimes difficult, but in many cases a pre-operative opinion as to the nature of the abnormal shadow can only be a hazardous guess.

The size of the shadow, its shape and density should be noted, since certain features may point to one diagnosis rather than another. Examples of this are the small size of the shadow in a parathyroid tumour, the shape of the shadow seen on the right border in a megaoesophagus or achalasia of the cardia, gas transradiancies seen in a hernia, or the presence of teeth or small calcifications in a dermoid. Tomograms are sometimes useful to prove to exclude the presence of small inconspicuous calcifications in the tumour.

Accurate localization of the shadow will also contribute towards the diagnosis if, as is often the case, there is no evidence of disease other than the x-ray findings. Certain lesions are found in one region but not in another, or are more common in certain sites.

Differential diagnosis of any mediastinal shadow may be a problem, and even exact anatomical localization is not always easy. In particular a bronchial carcinoma lying very medially will occupy the same spatial site as mediastinal secondary deposits, and will therefore be indistinguishable from these unless there are other clues such as a bronchostenosis. An encysted effusion of the mediastinal pleura will give rise to a shadow indistinguishable from a mediastinal tumour or an aneurysm.

DIFFERENTIATION OF ANEURYSM FROM TUMOUR

If there is any possibility that a mediastinal shadow is caused by an aneurysm of the aorta or pulmonary artery, and not by a mediastinal tumour, the oesophagus should be outlined with barium sulphate paste and examined by fluoroscopy to see whether it is displaced or encroached upon in any way. In addition, plain right and left anterior-oblique views at 60–70 degrees rotation should be taken to outline the aorta, thus showing the condition of the vessel and the relation of the shadow to it, and to show or exclude vertebral or sternal erosion.

The presence or absence of pulsation of the shadow itself is without significance, since some tumours show vigorous pulsation and some aneurysms very little.

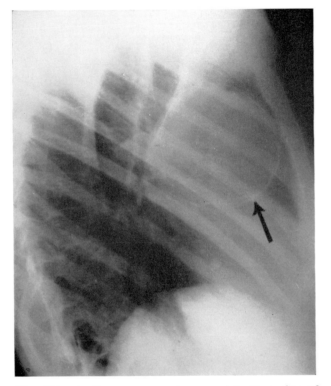

Fig. 314.—Aortic aneurysm. Arrow points to a ring of calcification round the periphery. Female aged 17 years. Mass x-ray finding. No physical signs. At thoracotomy it was some time before it was realized that the "tumour" was in fact an aneurysm.

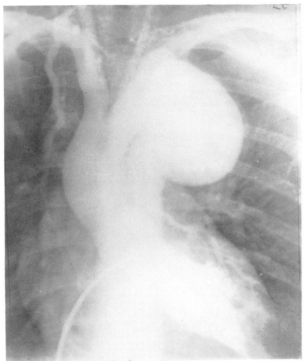

Fig. 315.—Aneurysm of aortic arch (angiogram). Sac to left of arch outlined with contrast medium. Injection into left ventricle (trans-septal). Female aged 26 years. Asymptomatic. Aortic systolic murmur. L.V. 150/5. Aneurysm resected, 8 × 6 cm. Good recovery.

The situation of the shadow should be carefully noted. If it is clearly separated from the aorta, lying for instance well anteriorly on the left side, or posteriorly on the right, it is probably a tumour. Well-defined sternal or vertebral erosion extending from the surface, gross oesophageal displacement, and failure to demonstrate a normal independent aortic shadow will favour the diagnosis of an aneurysm.

It is only fair to say that these criteria are not entirely reliable and that differentiation of an aortic aneurysm from the many other causes of abnormal mediastinal shadows is sometimes impossible by routine radiological examination. Fig. 314 demonstrates such a case. Even at thoracotomy it was some time before it became evident that the well-defined circular shadow with a rim of calcium did in fact represent an aneurysm and not a neoplasm. If there is any doubt, an angiogram is usually decisive though it can on rare occasions be indecisive since these unusual types of aneurysm may fail to fill with the contrast medium either because of a thrombus within it or because of the smallness of the opening.

ANTERIOR MEDIASTINAL SHADOWS

Anterior mediastinal shadows always lie in contact with, or close to, the sternum. They may be further grouped into those lying very high up, those in the upper three-quarters, and those low down reaching to the shadow of the diaphragm. In the anterior view, some are seen to lie centrally and may either be covered by the normal cardiovascular shadow, or project some distance beyond it on one or both sides. Others, such as a paratracheal cyst, lie entirely to one side and even their medial border may be several centimetres to one side of the mid line. Sometimes the shadow is large, wide and rather pear shaped, as in a lymphosarcoma; sometimes it is smaller and has a well-demarcated oval or circular shape, as in a dermoid. Certain of these characteristic appearances may occasionally assist the diagnosis (*see* Table 9 and the following comments).

If the shadow is large and lies anteriorly behind the middle third of the sternum and shows no unusual features, then an anterior and lateral view will suffice, since further radiological investigations are un-likely to help the diagnosis. If on the other hand it lies anteriorly in the lower third then a careful search should be made for abnormal gas transradiancies both above and below the diaphragm. If there is any suspicion of these, confirmation or exclusion of a hernia through the foramen of Morgagni should be sought by a barium meal. Since a hernia in this region usually contains small intestine or colon, the barium meal should be specially timed to outline these parts. To save the patient several journeys to the x-ray department, a double drink is useful. The first drink consisting of 6 ounces of barium sulphate emulsion is given about 24 hours before the x-ray examinations, and the second drink is given in place of breakfast on the day of the examination, the first radiograph or fluoroscopic examina-tion being some 2 hours later. If the parts are not outlined, ordinary meals are then taken, and the progress of the barium through the intestine is followed until it can be proved for certain that no gut lies above the diaphragm, or the transverse colon is drawn upwards towards the diaphragm.

TABLE 9

CAUSES OF ANTERIOR MEDIASTINAL SHADOWS

Position of shadow	Cause
Tending to lie very high up	Retrosternal thyroid Aneurysm of innominate artery. Very high aorta Post-thymectomy haematoma
Tending to lie in upper three-quarters	The reticuloses: Hodgkin's disease; lymphosarcoma, lymphoma; leukaemia Secondary deposit Tuberculous glandular abscess Non-tuberculous inflammatory abscess or glandular enlargement Ectopic thyroid gland Ectopic parathyroid gland Thymic tumour Dermoid (teratoma) Cystic hygroma Lipoma and other rare benign tumour
Tending to lie touching diaphragm	Parapericardial and pleural cyst Hernia through foramen of Morgagni

Retrosternal thyroid

A retrosternal enlarged thyroid is usually partly palpable in the neck and clinically obvious.

The shadow covers the medial half or more of one apex, and is seen to extend well below the clavicle. It tends to lie more to one side than the other. If it lies towards the right side, its well-defined slightly concave lateral margin will simulate that of an obstructive atelectasis of the upper lobe, but there will be no fissure displacement or alteration of the pulmonary vessel pattern.

The trachea is deviated away from the side of maximal shadowing, is often narrowed, and may be seen in the lateral view to be displaced posteriorly.

The shadow may be difficult to identify in the lateral view, but a haziness in the place of the normal retrosternal transradiancy will be seen. The margins of the shadow can be demonstrated in lateral-view tomograms. Sometimes calcifications are visible within it.

Aneurysm of the innominate artery

An aneurysm of the innominate artery can usually be felt with its expansile pulsation in the lower neck region, and can thus be diagnosed clinically. It tends to show vigorous pulsation on fluoroscopy.

There is usually marked unfolding or enlargement of the aortic arch. If the condition were not so uncommon, the difficulties of diagnosis would be more generally appreciated.

The reticuloses

The reticuloses (lymphosarcoma, leukaemia, Hodgkin's disease, and the like) often give rise to a rather large shadow in the upper half (Fig. 316). Commonly this extends either side of the mid line and

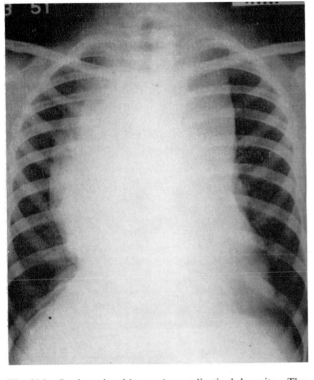

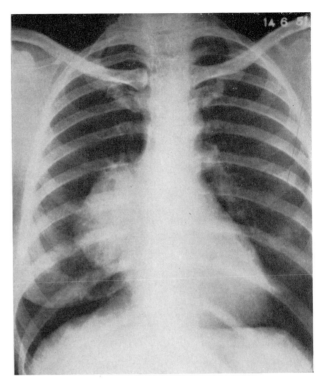

Fig. 316.—Leukaemia with anterior mediastinal deposits. The deposits lay retrosternally, extending posteriorly to surround the trachea, and inferiorly to encase the heart. White blood count 100,000. Blast cells 78 per cent. Male aged 13 years. Six weeks cough, sputum, and difficulty in breathing.

Fig. 317.—Hodgkin's disease with localized shadow lying on the right side. Female aged 53 years. Mass x-ray finding. Large encapsulated solid tumour found lying retrosternally, which was removed. No other mediastinal deposits.

has well-defined slightly convex lateral margins. The superior vena cava is obscured by it. There may be slight compression but there is little or no displacement of the trachea. The normal aortic shadow may be seen through the tumour shadow in a film taken with a grid. If the mass is very large it will surround the upper part of the heart shadow, which because it cannot be separately distinguished may appear to be enlarged. Frequently the lung fields are clear, but the anterior mediastinal shadow may be associated with hilar glandular enlargements, especially in Hodgkin's disease, or there may be small areas of ill-defined clouding in the lungs from additional deposits.

In a lateral view the normal retrosternal transradiant area can no longer be seen and this area appears grey relative to the darker retrocardiac area similar to Fig. 319. The limits of the shadow are often difficult to see in a plain lateral-view radiograph, but will stand out clearly in lateral-view tomograms. If the mass is large it will extend back to and surround the trachea, and may even cause slight posterior displacement of it and the oesophagus.

The nature of such an opacity may be inferred if a white blood count shows leukaemia, or the histology of an enlarged palpable gland after removal shows the characteristic changes of Hodgkin's disease. If on the other hand there are no clinical clues and no gland is available for biopsy, a small dose of therapeutic x-rays may be given, and if this is followed in 2 weeks by a marked decrease in size of the shadow, it would suggest a diagnosis of a highly radio-sensitive tumour such as a lymphosarcoma.

but occasionally one becomes infected, the patient becomes febrile and the outline of the shadow becomes less distinct; occasionally one ruptures as a result of a severe traumatic incident.

Cystic hygroma

A cystic hygroma may cause a well-demarcated 5–10 cm oval shadow in a young child in the lower half of the retrosternal region more or less in the mid line.

Lipoma or other rare benign tumour

A lipoma or other rare benign tumour is usually in the lower half. A lipoma may grow to a very large size and may be lobulated.

Parapericardial cyst and pleural cyst

A parapericardial cyst or pleural cyst usually occupies the angle between the sternum and the diaphragm in the lateral view. In the anterior view it lies in the cardiophrenic recess if it is on the right side, but is usually covered by the heart shadow if it is on the left. It may project beyond the apex and simulate the pericardial pad of fat seen in this region in stout individuals. It is well demarcated and usually some 2–3 cm in diameter though occasionally one may be as large as 10 cm. They do not become infected, nor do they show a rim of calcification. These cysts are the commonest cause of a symptomless shadow in this situation.

Hernia through the foramen of Morgagni

A hernia through the foramen of Morgagni may result in a shadow retrosternally in the mid line or to one side. If it contains only omentum the shadow will be homogeneous, but if some colon or small intestine, gas transradiancies will be seen within it or lying high up well anteriorly just below the diaphragm, a situation in which they are not usually apparent (see also p. 204).

MID-MEDIASTINAL SHADOWS

If the shadow lies in the mid-mediastinal region roughly on a level with the trachea or oesophagus, the oesophagus should be outlined with barium sulphate paste to see whether it is displaced by the abnormal shadow or related to it in any way. If a fluid level or gas transradiancies are seen, the stomach should be examined with a barium sulphate emulsion to exclude a hernia. If the shadow is small and inconspicuous, tomograms will be needed to confirm its presence, and show its relation to nearby structures, such as the trachea. Sometimes it is of help to take the tomograms while the oesophagus is still outlined with the barium paste. Any of the following conditions may give a mid-mediastinal shadow.

Ectopic thyroid gland

The thyroid gland or an accessory gland may lie within the thorax around the trachea. It casts a more or less circular well-defined shadow several centimetres in diameter. It may displace the trachea forwards and the oesophagus backwards or it may be wrapped round the trachea leaving it in its normal position. It is possibly found incidentally in a radiograph, when its nature may not be appreciated, or there may be symptoms of hyperthyroidism.

Oesophageal pouch

An oesophageal pouch large enough to cast a shadow is generally associated with symptoms of a type to suggest the need for a barium swallow, which in its turn will prove the diagnosis. A careful search including a well-exposed film will often show a fluid level within the shadow with a transradiant air bubble above.

The reticuloses

The reticuloses may result in a paratracheal instead of a retrosternal mass. Multiple paratracheal glandular masses fusing to produce a considerable shadow are not uncommon, but more rarely a single circular mass is found 5–10 cm in size, and its nature only discovered after removal.

Enlarged paratracheal and sub-carinal glands

If the paratracheal glands are very enlarged they may be seen in a plain anterior view extending either side of the central shadow, on the right beyond the superior vena cava, on the left above and lateral to the aortic knuckle. The shadow is generally well defined, and tends to have a slightly convex or wavy lateral margin, which will serve to distinguish it from the normal central shadow. Except in the case of one of the reticuloses, the trachea is rarely either narrowed or displaced by the enlarged glands.

If the enlargement is only moderate, the shadow may be difficult to identify in either the anterior or lateral view plain radiograph, but is often clearly visible in tomograms, particularly in the lateral view when it may be seen just in front of the trachea, just behind it, or level with it in a more lateral layer. It nearly always has a clear-cut margin, and is usually distinct from the shadow of the pulmonary artery or the vessels going up into the neck.

Slight enlargement of a paratracheal or more often a sub-carinal gland may be invisible in the plain radiographs but may be presumed if there is a local indentation of the barium-filled oesophagus (Fig. 320). Hence a barium swallow is often used in a case of bronchial carcinoma to prove or exclude secondary deposits in these glands. The value of this examination is however limited since in few of the cases which are suitable for surgery are the glands large enough to cause an indentation of the oesophagus. Moreover it is wrong to reject surgery on the evidence of glandular enlargement alone, since a similar oesophageal indentation may be caused by a gland enlarged by inflammation associated with an inflammatory lesion of the lung distal to the neoplasm. Nor is it possible to predict with certainty whether the gland is stuck to the wall of the oesophagus or quite discrete and merely pressing on it, and therefore perhaps removable. Infiltration of the wall will be suggested if the defect is irregular, or the oesophageal rugae distorted, though such findings are uncommon.

A primary bronchial carcinoma close to the mediastinal pleura on the right side may itself press on the oesophagus, though removal may be quite easy.

The enlarged sub-carinal glands are best shown after a barium swallow in a left anterior oblique view with only 15–20 degrees rotation of the patient.

Enlarged hilar glands

In the anterior view the shadow of an enlarged hilar gland will lie more laterally than the shadow of an enlarged paratracheal or sub-carinal gland, but in a lateral view, since they all three lie in the same plane, they will all be seen in the mid-mediastinal region near or just below the trachea. If the enlargement of the hilar glands is gross, it will be clearly seen in the plain radiographs, but if it is relatively slight it may only be seen, or it may be seen with greater clarity, in hilar level posterior-view tomograms. The enlarged glands tend to lie adjacent to the main bronchi and in the angle between the lobar bronchi (Fig. 348). Each enlarged gland may be well defined and more or less circular with a well-defined lateral and inferior convex margin which will serve to distinguish it from the adjacent vascular shadows.

Sometimes the glands are poorly defined, and the whole hilum appears to be diffusely enlarged but with an ill-defined outer margin. In such cases the enlargement may only be detected in the plain radiographs by comparison with previous radiographs provided these were taken before the enlargement was present.

Bilateral well-defined enlarged hilar glands may be the only radiological abnormality in sarcoidosis, particularly in the early stages, in hyperplastic tuberculous adenitis, in Hodgkin's disease or more rarely in secondary deposits from an extrathoracic carcinoma. The enlargement may not be confined to the hilar glands, and may be associated with enlarged paratracheal or retrosternal glands.

Less well demarcated enlarged hilar glands may be seen in acute inflammatory lesions, particularly measles, whooping cough or bacterial pneumonia, when the clinical condition will indicate the cause.

Unilateral poorly defined enlargement of one hilar shadow with a localized pulmonary shadow on that side, which may be quite small or occupy most of a lobe, will suggest primary tuberculosis in a child, but a bronchial carcinoma in an elderly man.

In sarcoidosis the shadows of the enlarged glands may disappear without any further lesions being seen. In other cases ill-defined 5–8 mm coarse nodular shadows may appear in the middle third of the lungs either concomitantly with the glandular shadows or some weeks after these have resolved. These intrapulmonary shadows may spread further but in the majority of cases resolve within a year or two.

If the lung shadows associated with the enlarged glands are predominantly in the upper third, it would suggest tuberculosis, though the nodules may extend up into the apices in sarcoidosis. Rather better defined and larger nodular shadows with enlarged hilar glands may be seen in Hodgkin's disease or secondary deposits from a carcinoma.

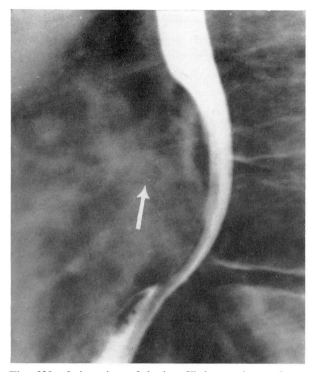

Fig. 320.—Indentation of barium-filled oesophagus from enlarged mediastinal glands with secondary deposits from a bronchial carcinoma. Oesophageal mucosal folds still normal, so no invasion by enlarged lymph nodes. (Arrow opposite carina.) Confirmed at thoracotomy. 15° left anterior-oblique view.

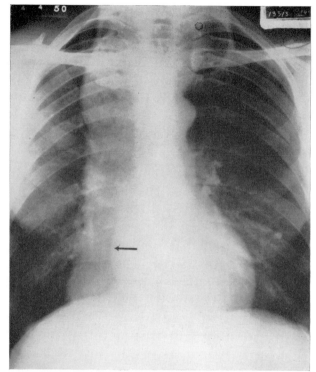

Fig 321.—Achalasia of the cardia and dilated oesophagus, causing enlargement of the mediastinal shadow. Arrow points to the right border of the heart. Small transradiant areas within the shadow are seen below the clavicle, and are due to food and air bubbles contrasted with the fluid in the dilated oesophagus. Male aged 49 years. Inability to cough freely, so chest radiographed. Dilatation of oesophagus confirmed by barium meal, and oesophagoscopy. Heller's operation.

Calcification in hilar and paratracheal glands

Calcification is common in one or more of the hilar or paratracheal glands following a primary tuberculous infection. An associated calcification in the lung in the region of drainage of the gland will substantiate the diagnosis, though similar calcification may follow infection with histoplasmosis in those areas where the condition is endemic.

The shape of the calcification is generally amorphous, and it may range in size from several milli-metres to a small spot best seen by tomography (*see* p. 136).

A peripheral ring of calcification in an enlarged gland, sometimes known as an " egg-shell " calcifi-cation, may be seen in a patient with an industrial pulmonary disease, particularly from pottery working or coal mining. The associated nodular shadowing in the lungs and the industrial history will indicate the cause (*see* p. 136).

Paratracheal and paraoesophageal cysts

Paratracheal and paraoesophageal (foregut) cysts are identical in the radiograph, and the two conditions cannot therefore be differentiated by this means. Either may cause slight indentation of the barium shadow as it fills the oesophagus. The shadow is well defined, oval and homogeneous, measuring about 4–6 cm long, and in the anterior view lying to one side of the mid line, more commonly to the right than to the left. In a lateral view it lies at the same level as the trachea or oesophagus. Attempts to differentiate a fluid-containing cyst from a solid-tumour mass by kymography have not been very successful. In oesophageal reduplication, barium may fill into the shadow. An I.V.P. may also help.

Neurilemmoma

A well-demarcated oval shadow in the paratracheal region to one or other side may be due to a neurilemmoma of the vagus nerve.

Achalasia of the cardia (cardiospasm) and megaoesophagus

The oesophagus may be greatly enlarged as in achalasia or megaoesophagus, and will then project to the right to form a part or the whole of the right border of the central shadow. It may form one continuous slightly convex curve from the clavicle to the diaphragm (Fig. 321) or may project beyond the heart shadow only in the upper or lower third. Sometimes the shadow is homogeneous, sometimes a slightly mottled appearance is seen due to the admixture of fluid, solid-food particles, and air bubbles. The nature of the shadow will be readily appreciated either from the symptoms or after a barium meal examination. The barium will fall through the residual fluid in the dilated oesophagus in a characteristic manner, and will also reveal the degree of enlargement.

In a plain lateral view the shadow is often inconspicuous even when the dilatation is enormous, but careful inspection of the radiograph will show that the retrosternal transradiant area is darker than the retrocardiac area which will appear grey. This, combined with the fact that a barium swallow is indicated in all cases when an abnormal mid-mediastinal shadow of doubtful aetiology is seen, should lead to the correct diagnosis.

An oval shadow superimposed on the heart shadow, or one projecting beyond the right heart border, may be due to a very large oesophageal tumour (such as a leiomyoma) (*see* p. 170). A barium swallow will show a long filling defect in the oesophagus with a smooth concave indentation into the normal column of barium above and below.

Hernia

A hernia, generally of the stomach, may cast a shadow in the lower half of the mid-mediastinal area behind the heart. It usually contains gas and perhaps fluid which, together with the position of the shadow, are indications for a barium meal examination, so that the diagnosis is usually straightforward. Sometimes the hernia contains a solid abdominal organ such as a part of the liver, spleen or a kidney, and the diagnosis may then be more difficult. A pneumoperitoneum will assist the diagnosis in a difficult case, and may indicate the abdominal origin of the contents of the hernia.

A hernia of the stomach, large enough to give a shadow on the plain radiograph, will fill readily with barium if the patient is lying down, and there will be no need to tilt him at an angle, head downwards. It is important however not only to make the diagnosis but to show the type of hernia and any associated features such as regurgitation or ulceration. When the part of the stomach lying in the thorax is outlined with barium, a second drink is given with the patient lying down to outline the oesophagus a second time and show its relation to the stomach and diaphragm. This will also show any shortening of the oesophagus and any secondary oesophageal changes such as dilatation, narrowing, any irregularity of outline indicating oesophagitis, or a projection indicating an ulcer crater.

The presence or absence of regurgitation of the barium from the stomach into the oesophagus should be carefully investigated with the patient lying, standing and stooping down. If regurgitation is very free the possibility of some relationship of the hernia to any abnormal intrapulmonary shadow suggesting an aspiration pneumonia should be considered.

If the oesophagus is full length and pierces the diaphragm, an attempt should be made to measure the size of the defect through which the stomach enters and returns from the thorax. This may be gauged from inspection of anterior and lateral views provided the connection between the thoracic and abdominal parts of the stomach can be outlined with the barium. If the defect is so large that it cannot be defined with certainty, it may be difficult to differentiate a hernia passing through a very large central defect in the diaphragm from a gross elevation of the diaphragm, especially if the stomach is rotated round under this. In the latter condition the upper margin of the shadow tends to be marked by the very even thin bow line of the raised diaphragm, whilst a hernia tends to have a flatter more irregular margin.

If there is some functioning muscle around the defect, contractions of this more or less at the usual level of the left dome may indicate the true state of affairs.

Torsion of the contents in a hernia may result in temporary obstruction of the stomach, which then becomes much distended with air and may occupy the whole of the left thorax and thus simulate a spontaneous pneumothorax or hydropneumothorax should there be some fluid in it (Fig. 221). If the obstruction is not relieved spontaneously the onset of severe clinical symptoms will suggest the diagnosis.

POSTERIOR MEDIASTINAL SHADOWS

If the shadow lies posteriorly an additional view of the posterior part of the ribs nearby may be needed to demonstrate any splaying out or bone erosion. If the shadow extends to the vertebral margin, the vertebrae in its neighbourhood should also be radiographed, and sometimes even demonstrated in tomograms to see whether there is any erosion, or splaying out of a pedicle.

Neurilemmoma (neurofibroma)

An isolated intrathoracic neurilemmoma arising from an intercostal nerve or the sympathetic chain may be found at any level between the first and twelfth ribs, but is most frequently seen in the upper two-thirds. Characteristically it lies posteriorly to one or other side of the mid line, and even when it attains a large size there may be no vertebral or rib changes, or at the most only slight splaying out and pressure erosion of a rib (Fig. 322). The shadow is homogeneous without calcification, oval in shape, and with a well-defined lateral convex margin.

These lesions are for the most part clinically silent and are usually seen only in adults. They are generally single, but occasionally two are seen one below the other giving a dumb-bell shaped shadow (not to be confused with a dumb-bell tumour). In rare instances, a single one is situated peripherally against a rib in the axilla. A fibroma of the visceral pleura gives a similar shadow (*see* p. 78).

Ganglioneuroma

A ganglioneuroma is more likely to cause pressure erosion of a vertebra or rib, and splaying out of the ribs. If there are any clinical indications of intraspinal extension, careful radiography of the vertebra in the neighbourhood of the shadow is indicated, including tomograms. Erosion or broadening of a pedicle may suggest that the intraspinal portion should be removed prior to the intrathoracic part of the tumour. Sometimes deep-seated calcifications are seen in the tumour. They are seen particularly in children.

Dermoid

A dermoid may be situated posteriorly, although it is a very rare tumour in this site, and may show the shadows of bone or teeth within it to indicate its nature.

Meningocoele

Rarely a 2–5-cm well-defined circular shadow with a well demarcated margin, lying adjacent and slightly anterior to the vertebral column, may be due to a meningocoele and will usually be mistaken for a neurilemmoma, its true nature being only revealed at thoracotomy. In one such case, a patient also with multiple neurofibromata, the mengingocoele filled with contrast medium during myelography.

Paravertebral abscess

A paravertebral abscess may be present even in the absence of radiographic changes in the inter-vertebral spaces or in the bones. It may lie in the same position as a neurogenic tumour, but can generally be distinguished from it because the lateral margin is straighter. It is more likely to be mistaken for a collapsed lower lobe than a tumour, but there will of course be no fissure displacement or alteration in the pulmonary vessel pattern (*see* pp. 57–58, 69).

Paravertebral neoplastic deposit

A paravertebral neoplastic deposit, especially in Hodgkin's disease, will result in a shadow indistinguishable from an abscess, but its nature will usually be known from the clinical findings.

Hypertrophy of paravertebral marrow deposits

Hypertrophy of paravertebral marrow deposits may occur in some cases of haemolytic anaemia, and result in a shadow like a neoplastic deposit alongside the lower thoracic vertebrae.

THE DIAPHRAGM SHADOW

A lower zone shadow based on one dome of the diaphragm may be due to a hernia through a large defect in that dome, which may be developmental or the result of trauma. If the hernia contains some gut, the presence of gas transradiancies will often suggest the diagnosis which can then be confirmed by a barium meal. A 1–2 cm defect in the middle third of the right dome may result in herniation of a portion of the liver which may spread out after passing through the diaphragm to produce a 2–3-cm circular shadow with its base on the diaphragm. A similar shadow may be caused by a localized weakness of the muscle, which nevertheless remains intact. The liver bulges up with it, but there is no hernia.

A diagnostic pneumoperitoneum is indicated in some cases to try and determine the exact anatomical site of the abnormal shadow. If after the induction of the pneumoperitoneum air can be seen between the liver and the diaphragm, it will be possible to see whether the shadow encroaches upon the air transradiancy, suggesting a cyst or tumour; whether it is entirely intrathoracic; or whether only a thin band-like shadow separates the lung from the intraperitoneal air transradiancy, indicating a local weakness of the diaphragm, or a small hernia. If the air does not intrude between the diaphragm and the shadow, caution should be observed in the interpretation of the x-ray appearances, since old peritoneal adhesions or an anatomically short peritoneal recess may limit the spread of air, and give a false impression of the position of the diaphragm.

A localized bulge of the diaphragm may be caused by an intra-abdominal lesion such as a sub-phrenic abscess, liver abscess, hydatid cyst, or tumour. Sometimes an intra-abdominal lesion can be seen below a normal diaphragm shadow, such as a clinically unsuspected spontaneous pneumoperitoneum or gut abnormally distended with gas or lying in an unusual position. Gas transradiancies from a loop of gut between the right dome of the diaphragm and the liver are seen occasionally, and are of no importance except that they would make a liver biopsy hazardous for instance in a case with pulmonary shadows suggesting sarcoidosis.

An abnormal low-density shadow such as an unsuspected splenic enlargement or high-density shadows suggesting calcifications in the liver or spleen, associated with abnormal mediastinal or lung opacities, may have importance in the diagnosis of an obscure chest shadow.

At times an intra-abdominal condition presents clinically as an intrathoracic lesion, and the finding of an intrapulmonary or pleural shadow must not distract attention from the inspection of the sub-diaphragmatic region in a chest radiograph. A companion shadow running with that of the right cupola of the diaphragm may be seen when the liver is abnormally radio-opaque, as in such a condition as haemachromatosis.

CHAPTER 8

BONES OF THORAX, SOFT TISSUE COVERING AND REMOTE BONE LESIONS IN CHEST DISEASES

CAREFUL inspection of the bones and extrathoracic soft tissues adds considerably to the time taken to examine a chest radiograph, and is impracticable as a routine. These shadows should at least be given a perfunctory glance in every radiograph, and in all difficult cases they should be inspected with care.

If a rib lesion is suspected, but no abnormality can be seen in the routine anterior-view radiograph, or if an abnormality is present but not clearly seen, then additional radiographs should be taken. More detail of a suspected abnormality in a rib may be obtained by the use of a coned down view, by an oblique view centred on the affected area with the affected part of the rib as nearly as possible parallel to the film, and by using a Potter–Bucky diaphragm. A view on expiration is also useful in some cases to show whether a doubtful shadow does in fact move with the rib, or is independent of it. In many cases tomograms are of value, and may reveal periostitis, erosion, or the presence of a sequestrum which was invisible in the plain radiographs.

PERIOSTITIS OF RIB

Periosteal new bone formation along a rib may result particularly from trauma or infection; it may be the only radiographic evidence of disease, or other changes may also be present. It appears as a hair-line shadow or a shadow 2–3 mm wide running parallel to the rib. In its early stages it is separated from the cortex by a zone of transradiancy 1–2 mm wide, but at a later stage it will tend to merge with the cortical bone.

Where the rib is much curved, it tends to lie or be most easily seen on the medial concave surface, but when situated on the straighter portions of a rib, it is often seen on both sides.

The shadow of periosteal new bone must be distinguished from the various soft tissue companion shadows (*see* p. 27) which are generally bilateral and symmetrical, and from the normal osseous ridge on the under surface of the posterior third of the rib. This latter shadow may be unduly conspicuous if there is slight rotation of the rib as a result of local retraction of the chest wall or of scoliosis, the presence of which should be apparent on the radiograph.

PERIOSTITIS SECONDARY TO EMPYEMA OR ACTINOMYCOSIS

Periosteal new bone should be sought in those ribs adjacent to any large long-standing pleural shadow, or any pulmonary shadow of unknown aetiology. The combination of a shadow suggesting a large area of pulmonary consolidation with periostitis of the overlying ribs will suggest a diagnosis of actinomycosis (Fig. 323).

PERIOSTITIS FROM TRAUMA

Periosteal new bone should also be sought in cases of local chest pain or tenderness, especially if there are no clinical clues as to the cause, and no abnormal lung shadows or transradiancies in the radiograph which might account for it. Careful inspection of the ribs in the general area of the pain is often rewarding. The tell-tale white line of periosteal new bone or the shorter broader half-moon protuberance of a haematoma or of calcifying callus may be the first evidence of a stress or cough fracture, the fracture line itself being seen only on subsequent radiographs at a later date.

PERIOSTITIS IN OSTEOMYELITIS

More rarely a localized area of periostitis may be the first radiological indication of primary osteomyelitis of a rib, the presence of which may have been ushered in a few days previously with a dramatic onset of fever and malaise, but not necessarily with obvious local physical signs. Such an inflammatory lesion may result in an unusual looking shadow over the lung due to the surrounding extrapulmonary abscess, which is easily mistaken for a pleural or lung shadow. Sometimes osteomyelitis of a rib is less acute, and may follow weeks or months after a traumatic incident without any infringement of the skin surface. In such a case, as well as in the more acute manifestations of the disease, the localized areas of periostitis may be associated with bone erosion or even a sequestrum.

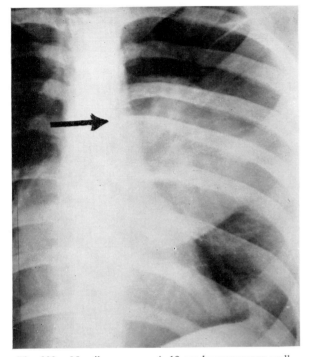

Fig. 322.—Neurilemmoma. A 10-cm homogeneous well-demarcated roughly oval shadow left side (in lateral view it lay posteriorly). Note rib spread and thinning of sixth rib posteriorly (opposite arrow). Female aged 16 years. Asymptomatic. Surgical removal.

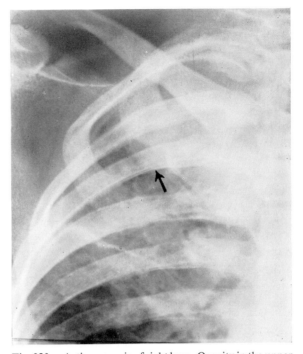

Fig. 323.—Actinomycosis of right lung. Opacity in the upper third due to consolidation. No tracheal displacement. Arrow points to periosteal new bone on the under surface of a rib. The ribs above show a similar change. Female aged 6 years. Febrile illness with cough, and actinomyces in the sputum. Lesion spread to spine and meninges with fatal result. Post-mortem proof of upper-lobe consolidation.

RIB FRACTURE

TRAUMATIC FRACTURE

A fracture of a rib will be quite conspicuous if there is displacement of the fragments. If there is no displacement, the dark transradiancy of the fracture line may not be easy to see unless carefully sought, and may be detected more readily if a magnifying glass is used. It may also be seen if attention is drawn to it by the finding of a ring or half-moon shadow of periosteal new bone bordering on the rib, or if there is any evidence of local disease of the rib. A fracture may be the result of known trauma, the patient being acutely conscious of the incident, or it may be a spontaneous fracture which may also be due to trauma so slight that the patient was unaware when it occurred, as in trauma during a bout of coughing, or a lurch against an object when consciousness was dulled by sleep or alcohol.

STRESS FRACTURE

In another condition, known as a stress fracture, there is an appearance suggesting a fracture line across the bone, usually with a 1-mm rim of dense bone adjacent to it, and a small bulge due to periosteal new bone at the edges. It is possible that the condition is not a fracture at all, but a linear zone of decalcification. It usually occurs in the first rib, but can occur in other ribs, and is usually asymptomatic. Union or reforming of the calcified elements is very slow and may take a year or more.

POST-RADIATION FRACTURE

Following x-ray therapy ribs in the main field of irradiation may become unduly brittle. For instance fractures in a line along the anterior ends of several contiguous ribs are sometimes seen in a patient who has had a glancing field of irradiation in this region for a carcinoma of the breast.

PATHOLOGICAL FRACTURE

A fracture may be seen through an area of abnormal bone, particularly through the small erosion of an early secondary deposit. It may occur of course through an extensive erosion of a more advanced secondary deposit, or an erosion due to any cause, including a myelomatosis.

A spontaneous fracture of a rib may also occur in any general bone disease causing a generalized brittleness of the bones. In fact a routine radiograph showing multiple rib fractures may be the first evidence of such a general condition, for example, Cushing's syndrome. Abundant circular masses of calcified callus in this or a similar condition must not be mistaken for intrapulmonary secondary deposits.

Many patients on long-term steroid therapy show a rib fracture without pain or a history of trauma. The rib otherwise looks normal and healing takes place in the ordinary way with a shadow of calcified callus for a time.

RIB EROSION

DEVELOPMENTAL DEFECT

Erosion and gross expansion of a rib, usually of its anterior end, may be seen in fibrous dysplasia. The expanded end is well demarcated from the normal part of the rib by a rim of dense bone, and from the intercostal transradiancy by a thin and perhaps rather incomplete rim of cortical bone. Strands of bone running across it give it a trabeculated appearance. The appearances are very similar to the sarcoma illustrated in Fig. 324, which was probably originally a fibrous dysplasia, with late sarcomatous change. The condition is often monostotic, though the same rib on the opposite side may show a similar lesion.

CYST AND BENIGN TUMOUR

A well-defined localized area of rib erosion, that is, an area of calcium absorption or actual bone destruction, is seen in a cyst or benign tumour. The transradiant zone is often well demarcated by a white line due to condensed or sclerotic bone, whilst if the lesion causes a local expansion of the bone, the cortex remains intact over it. In a cyst the radiotranslucency is uniform, but in a chondroma small white spots may be seen due to small areas of calcification in the cartilage. In an osteochondroma larger areas of opacity are seen partly due to the formation of bone which will show evidence of trabecular structure, and partly due to calcification in the cartilage. A cyst may be of uncertain origin or the result of hyperparathyroidism, so that a radiograph of the hands should be taken to demonstrate or exclude the characteristic cortical resorption of some of the phalanges which will be seen in hyperparathyroidism by the time a rib cyst develops.

XANTHOMATOSES

A well-demarcated erosion, but often without a complete ring of condensed bone around it, and perhaps even with a breach of the cortex, may be seen in a patient suffering from one of the xanthomatoses, particularly an eosinophil granuloma. A rib erosion in a xanthoma is sometimes associated with xanthomatous alveolar lesions in the lungs, resulting in a fine nodular or honeycomb pattern in the lower two-thirds indistinguishable from an interstitial pulmonary fibrosis as illustrated in Figs. 163 and 169. There may be erosions in other bones—the skull, pelvis, femora or humeri being the most common sites. These bones should therefore be radiographed if a rib erosion or lung nodular and honeycomb shadows are seen of unknown aetiology.

PRIMARY MALIGNANT RIB TUMOUR

The x-ray diagnosis of a primary malignant rib tumour is not always easy or reliable. The erosion may be well demarcated, and this together with a localized well-defined area of bone expansion may suggest a benign tumour; Fig. 324 illustrates such a case. The lesion was found on mass radiography and was asymptomatic. A slight swelling could be felt, and although the radiographic features indicated a benign lesion, the anterior part of that rib together with the tumour were removed. It was then found that the tumour was a sarcoma, with tumour cells invading the nearby intercostal muscle. Other similar cases have emphasized the difficulty of guessing the histology of rib tumours from the radiographic appearances.

In another type of primary malignant tumour of a rib, extensive bone destruction is the predominant change, and differentiation from a secondary deposit is not always possible, while if the tumour has invaded the soft tissues around, producing a 2–5-cm low-density shadow, differentiation from a bronchial carcinoma invading the rib and surrounding tissues of the chest wall may not be possible from the radiographs.

In a few cases some faint line shadows or feathering can be seen at right angles to the cortex, suggesting an osteosarcoma.

RIB SECONDARY DEPOSITS

A secondary deposit in a rib usually causes a poorly demarcated area of erosion without a line of condensed bone around it and without any bone expansion. There is no periosteal reaction, although this may be simulated by the calcifying callus should a spontaneous fracture pass through the area of erosion.

It may be isolated or there may be deposits in several ribs. It is not a very common finding in a bronchial carcinoma, but the presence of such a rib erosion might discourage the performance of a pneumonectomy in some cases. Erosions from secondary deposits may of course be seen in any of the bones included in a chest radiograph. They are not uncommon in the clavicle, or the scapula, particularly in the region of the superior or inferior angle, and may be seen in a vertebra in the lateral view.

TUBERCULOSIS OF A RIB

In a tuberculous lesion of a rib, bone erosion is the predominant feature, extending over an area of 1–2 cm, and generally poorly demarcated. It may be associated with some periosteal new bone, but this is often either absent or of slight extent. The lesion may occur in any part of the rib. A not unusual feature of tuberculosis affecting the anterior end of the rib is the presence of extensive caseation, and clinical evidence of swelling, without any visible changes in the radiographs.

ACUTE OSTEOMYELITIS OF A RIB

A small area or several contiguous small areas of bone destruction may precede the appearance of periosteal new bone deposits in osteomyelitis. This will only last for a few days before the periosteal reaction becomes obvious, so that confusion with a secondary deposit is unlikely to occur.

PRESSURE EROSION OF RIBS (" RIB NOTCHING ")

Small pressure erosions from tortuous dilated intercostal vessels acting as collateral channels are seen in co-arctation of the aorta, and are easily overlooked unless they are suspected. They are seen on the inferior borders of the posterior horizontal parts of the ribs most commonly in the region of the fifth to the eighth ribs. If they are seen in a radiograph they may be the first finding to draw attention to the condition. They are demarcated by a thin layer of compact bone which has a rather wavy outline.

More rarely pressure erosions of the ribs are caused by grossly dilated intercostal veins because of a collateral circulation through them either from superior vena caval obstruction or from a large oesophageal venous flow in cases of portal hypertension with cirrhosis of the liver. A third cause is the presence of multiple intercostal nerve neurofibromata, generally in association with generalized neurofibromatosis.

Unilateral rib notching on the right side only will be seen if the co-arctation of the aorta lies more proximal than usual, so that the left subclavian artery arises from the aorta where the pressure is low. Very rarely the co-arctation is at the usual ductal level, but the left subclavian comes off below the area of narrowing and is thus at a low pressure.

Unilateral rib notching on the left side may follow a Blalock anastomosis (left subclavian to left pulmonary artery). This cuts off the blood supply to the left arm and a collateral circulation develops from the intercostal arteries to supply the distal part of the left subclavian artery.

STERNAL EROSION

Erosion of the sternum is usually due to secondary deposits, but a rather similar erosion is seen as a late manifestation of syphilis. In either condition the erosion may be seen in a lateral view of the chest before a lesion is suspected clinically. Sometimes the erosion is so extensive that no sternal shadow can be seen, and its absence may pass undetected in the radiograph. A more localized erosion may be caused by a smaller secondary deposit or a gumma. Pressure erosion may also occur with an aortic aneurysm, and is generally well demarcated, whilst the shadow of the aneurysm will be obvious. A small sternal lesion is most easily seen in oblique views or in an oblique-view tomogram.

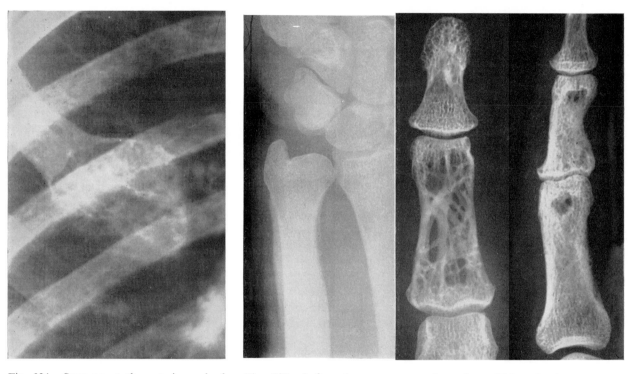

Fig. 324.—Sarcoma at the anterior end of the third right rib. Male aged 30 years. Mass x-ray finding. Removal of rib. Poorly differentiated spindle-celled osteogenic sarcoma destroying bone and infiltrating the muscle.

Fig. 325.—*Left*—pulmonary osteoarthropathy. Wrist showing periosteal new bone lower end of ulna. Male aged 50 years. With joint pains. Three-centimetre bronchial carcinoma. After removal, rapid resolution of bone changes. *Centre*—finger in a case of sarcoidosis with pulmonary shadows. Finger swollen and much pain. *Right*—finger in another case of sarcoidosis with pulmonary shadows. No pain or swelling.

INCREASE IN DENSITY OF RIB

An isolated increase in the density of a rib without any other changes is usually due to a developmental defect, dense bone being substituted for cancellous bone. Such a change is without clinical significance. A localized increase in density with some thickening of the bone and an alteration in the trabecular architecture is seen in Paget's disease. An increase in density of many or all the ribs without an increase in width is seen in marble bones (osteopetrosis). This increase in density is of the trabecular bone which is never formed, and the cortex thus extends into the medullary cavity and may almost occlude it.

An increase in density with loss of the trabecular pattern and its replacement with sclerotic bone may be due to sclerosing secondary deposits, especially from the prostate. In sclerosing secondary deposits there may also be widely disseminated areas of patchy clouding in the lungs, and without tomography it is sometimes difficult to see which shadows are in the lung and which in the ribs. A diffuse increase in density of all the ribs may be seen in myelofibrosis.

DISPLACEMENT OF RIBS

Local rib retraction is frequently seen overlying an area of lung disease, and is usually apparent on clinical inspection of the chest. A severe kyphoscoliosis will result in such crowding together of the ribs that their shadow, together with those of the vertebrae, may make the plain anterior-view radiograph useless for the detection of a chest lesion. In such a case some help may be obtained from oblique views or tomograms.

Local spreading out of the ribs may occur over a large lung or mediastinal tumour, or over a large pleural effusion.

SOFT TISSUE COVERINGS

A tumour or an inflammatory mass in the soft tissue coverings of the thorax may result in a shadow overlying the lungs in one view; a localized tumour in particular may result in a circular shadow simulating an intrapulmonary lesion. Its extrathoracic position will however either be apparent on clinical examination, or radiologically when a lateral view or tomograms are taken to localize the position of the shadow.

Gas transradiancies in the extrapleural spaces are described on pp. 39, 140.

REMOTE BONE CHANGES ASSOCIATED WITH INTRATHORACIC DISEASE
PULMONARY OSTEOARTHROPATHY

Certain lung diseases may be associated with bone lesions outside the thoracic cage. The association of pulmonary osteoarthropathy with a fibroma of the lung or pleura has been referred to on page 78. It is also occasionally seen in association with a bronchial carcinoma squamous cell but not an oat cell bronchial carcinoma, and more rarely with a secondary deposit particularly those associated with a rich fibrous stroma. It is seen in some cases of fibrosing alveolitis, though in such cases it is important to make sure there is not an unsuspected bronchial carcinoma in addition. It may be seen with a mycetoma, or with a long-standing intrathoracic inflammatory condition such as a chronic lung abscess or empyema.

A radiograph of the appropriate bones will show a 1–2-mm wide line shadow parallel to the cortex starting 1–2 cm above or below the joint and extending some distance along the shaft (Fig. 325). The line is usually separated from the cortex by a narrow transradiant zone, but may be fused to it. It may be obvious or only seen with the aid of a magnifying glass. Common sites are the lower end of the radius and ulna, the femora and either end of the tibia and fibula. At an advanced stage the metacarpals and metatarsals may be affected, but it is rare in the phalanges. It may be seen only in one region, for instance the lower end of each radius and ulna, or tibia and fibula. As an isolated site the wrists are most commonly affected, but in most cases all the above-mentioned bones show the tell-tale lines. The lesions are symmetrical on the right and left sides.

Pulmonary osteoarthropathy is sometimes found accidentally when a bone is radiographed for some other purpose, for instance to exclude a fracture after trauma, but it is more often seen because pain or swelling in or near a joint draws attention to the condition. In fact pain and swelling of the forearms and wrists or the ankles may be mistaken for arthritis, which is why a radiograph is requested. Clubbing is invariably present and may be a presenting sign of both the lung lesion and the osteoarthropathy.

If bone lesions are seen, a radiograph of the chest should be taken if this has not already been done and a lung lesion already recognized. If a routine anterior view is normal, further radiographs should be taken in the same manner as when neoplastic cells have been found in the sputum but their site of origin is uncertain (*see* p. 246), and should include a lateral view, fluoroscopy and tomograms of those regions not well seen in either view. In the great majority of cases the lung lesion will be obvious in the initial radiograph, and in the others discovered by a more careful search or by bronchoscopy.

SARCOIDOSIS

Of the many cases of sarcoidosis in which pulmonary shadows are present, very few show any bone changes. When they are present, they are most commonly seen in the metacarpals and phalanges and take the form of well demarcated cyst-like areas (Fig. 325). There is no periosteal reaction and no surrounding decalcification. There may be no clinical evidence of the lesion, or there may be local pain and swelling. Occasionally similar well demarcated erosions are seen in other bones, even including the vault of the skull.

CHAPTER 9

COMBINATIONS OF DIFFERENT SHADOWS

IN THE foregoing sections cases have been described in which a single shadow is seen in the radiograph as in a peripheral neoplasm, or multiple shadows of similar size and density, as in miliary tuberculosis. Sometimes there are several kinds of abnormal shadow together in one radiograph, and the particular combination in each case may be a valuable factor in the diagnosis, or may give a clue to some particular feature of the underlying pathological changes.

SMALL CIRCULAR SHADOWS AND ILL-DEFINED LARGER SHADOW

A case in point where the combination of shadows is an aid to the diagnosis is that of the 2–3-cm ill-defined area of clouding—or the larger shadow with irregular borders and line shadows radiating out from it—of an area of massive fibrosis. The x-ray diagnosis of either of these shadows will only be substantiated if, in addition to the relevant occupational history indicating the possibility of a pneumoconiosis, there are also the small widely disseminated low-density circular shadows of the basic lesion (*see* p. 102).

SMALL CIRCULAR SHADOWS WITH HILAR GLAND ENLARGEMENT

When small circular shadows, or a mixture of circular and line shadows, are seen in the lungs, the demonstration of enlarged hilar glands, if necessary by tomography, will be of value in the diagnosis. This particular combination of shadows, together with a certain clinical picture, will strongly suggest sarcoidosis, although it is not pathognomonic, nor does the absence of glandular enlargement exclude this interpretation. Similar appearances are seen in some cases of tuberculosis, glandular fever, and secondary deposits.

SMALL CIRCULAR SHADOWS WITH SMALL RING SHADOWS

The combination of small circular shadows and small ring (honeycomb) shadows is characteristic of fibrosing alveolitis whether cryptogenic, secondary to inhalation of noxious substances, xanthomatotic, or allergic (bird fancier's lung). In some cases the small circular shadows are the most conspicuous feature; in others it is the honeycomb shadows which may obscure the small circular shadows which have to be carefully sought out amongst them (*see* p. 101).

SHRUNKEN UPPER LOBES WITH SMALL CIRCULAR AND HONEYCOMB SHADOWS

This combination will suggest bird fancier's lung, honeycomb shadows being uncommon in tuberculosis. The diagnosis will depend on the failure to show tubercle bacilli in the sputum, and the finding of immunological responses to the bird's serum (*see* p. 94).

SMALL CIRCULAR SHADOWS AND LINE SHADOWS

A combination of small circular shadows with a few rather long line shadows cutting across the vessel pattern is seen particularly in lymphangitis carcinomatosa. This condition is rarely demonstrable on the radiographs until the terminal stages when only a few weeks of life can be expected. The same radiographic appearances in a relatively fit patient will therefore suggest some other cause, such as lymphatic obstruction in any lesion with nodular lung shadows. Small circular shadows, short line shadows and septal line shadows are a combination frequently seen in fibrosing alveolitis.

LARGE CIRCULAR SHADOW WITH SMALL SATELLITE SHADOWS

The presence of some small circular shadows (satellite shadows) in the neighbourhood of a large circular shadow may be the only pre-operative point in favour of a diagnosis of tuberculosis rather than neoplasm. They are not pathognomonic of either condition, but are found much more commonly

220

in tuberculosis. The satellite shadows near a neoplasm may be due to superadded inflammatory changes, or to small groups of neoplastic cells, possibly the result of a local bronchial dissemination.

AREAS OF CLOUDING AND RING SHADOWS

A combination of 2–5-mm circular shadows or ill-defined areas of clouding with a ring shadow indicating a cavity, together with some line shadows, or a crowding of the vessel pattern is a very common feature in tuberculosis. It is often an expression either of the different dates of origin of the various foci, or of superadded incidents of mechanical rather than bacterial origin, such as a local bronchostenosis producing a tension cavity or airless shrunken lobe. Lung destruction may result in loss of volume, the remnants perhaps being held together by fibrous tissue, the end result being an aerated but shrunken lobe. This combination of shadows is also seen in cases of asthma complicated by bronchopulmonary aspergillosis and eosinophilia, the mechanism of the lobar shrinkage in tuberculosis, bird fancier's lung and this condition being similar.

SMALL CIRCULAR SHADOWS AND TUBULAR SHADOWS

The combination of low-density circular shadows with tubular shadows in the same area will suggest caseous foci associated with bronchiectasis, which itself may be tuberculous, or a simple distension due to local mechanical factors.

PARALLEL LINE, TRAM LINE OR TUBULAR SHADOWS AND PATCHY CLOUDING

A combination of thin parallel line shadows, the distance between the lines being appropriate for a normal bronchus at this level (tram line shadows), wider parallel line shadows with the transradiant zone between them either narrower or wider than a normal bronchial lumen at that level, and areas of ill-defined patchy clouding from a few millimetres to about 1 cm, scattered throughout the lungs or only here and there, will suggest lung complications in a patient with cystic fibrosis (Fig. 326). In some cases small 3–8-mm ring shadows, or a few larger ring shadows about 1 cm in size may be seen in one or two areas. These abnormalities may be seen in a young child, or their development observed in serial

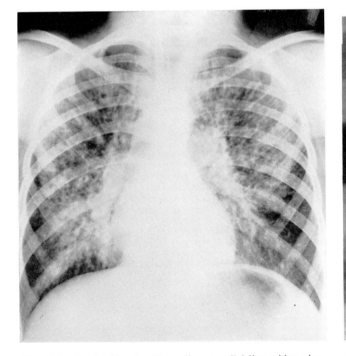

Fig. 326.—Cystic fibrosis. Tram line, parallel line wider, ring shadows and ill-defined small areas of patchy clouding. Large hilar shadows, normal diaphragm. Female aged 14 years. Sweat test + ve. Sputum: *Staph. aureus.*

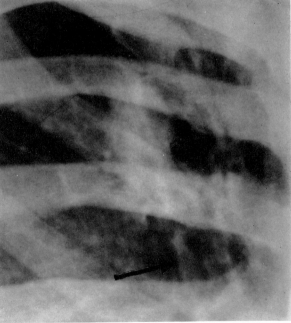

Fig. 327.—Asthma with bronchopulmonary aspergillosis and eosinophilia. Patchy clouding right upper zone. Parallel line (tubular) shadow opposite arrow. Skin tests + ve and serum precipitins to *Aspergillus fumigatus.*

radiographs over a period of years, the child often reaching the age of 15 or more before such gross changes occur. Prior to this the radiographs may have been normal, or show a few such shadows which may have come and gone from time to time. Patchy clouding and tram line shadows particularly may disappear from time to time, but wider spaced parallel line shadows are usually permanent. Bronchograms may show that these are due to bronchiectasis, but they may be seen with an almost normal bronchogram. Pathological studies of the patients are difficult because they often die with a severe pulmonary infection which obscures the earlier lesions, but in one case which showed the parallel line shadows in the radiograph, no pathological basis for these could be found although the actual bronchus with the lines could be identified and studied.

Radiological evidence of widespread emphysema is not often seen in these cases, but a large pulmonary trunk and hilar vessels are sometimes seen, suggesting the onset of pulmonary hypertension.

In most cases the areas of patchy clouding are due to staphylococcal infections, but some cases later show serological evidence of secondary aspergillosis. This is not indicated by any specific additional changes in the radiographs. If the areas of patchy clouding are larger and the patient is over 25 years old, it will suggest asthma complicated by bronchopulmonary aspergillosis and eosinophilia (Fig. 327).

HIGH-DENSITY AND LOW-DENSITY SHADOWS

A combination of shadows of high density due to calcification in the lesions, with shadows of lower density is particularly common in tuberculosis. It will indicate that some of the foci have progressed towards resolution and quiescence, but in general the demonstration of calcification will not appreciably affect the prognosis or influence the plan of treatment. In a series of asymptomatic patients over the age of 30 years with small (minimal) lesions, the percentage of cases in which the disease spread, or in which tubercle bacilli could be isolated, was less when calcification could be seen in the initial radiograph than when no calcification could be seen (see p. 135). Such statistical information is, however, often of little value in handling the individual case.

If the calcium is superimposed on or is near other abnormal shadows, tomography may be indicated to see how it is related to these. Should the calcification be shown to lie within the wall or lumen of a cavity or bronchus, it may influence the decision as to the plan of treatment to be adopted.

There are several conditions other than tuberculosis in which calcified lesions are seen in combination with neighbouring low-density shadows such as an old abscess or empyema, a blood clot in the pleura or a lung cyst, histoplasmosis, or even some pneumoconioses—particularly asbestosis. Even assuming calcifications represent long-standing regressed tuberculous foci, they will not always assist a comprehensive diagnosis, for the associated low-density shadows may represent sarcoidosis or a neoplasm, either of which can occur even in the presence of calcified foci.

Since tubercle bacilli may be found in the sputum when a neoplasm is present as well, the hazards of x-ray diagnosis need no stressing, especially when a combination of shadows is present. It is wise to study each type of abnormal shadow and consider it separately in its possible relation to the clinical picture, and not to take into consideration only the most obvious or most diagnostic looking shadow.

SHADOW OF NEOPLASM AND OF COMPLICATING LESION

In a bronchial carcinoma the shadow of the neoplastic mass is frequently associated with other more distally situated shadows, which are the result of a bronchostenosis or vascular occlusion caused by it. If the bronchostenosis is severe, there will be a shadow due to the shrunken airless atelectatic segment or lobe, the appearances of which are described on pp. 57–71. Usually the oval or circular shadow of the neoplasm is merged into that of the shrunken lobe, but the former can sometimes be separately identified if it causes a local prominence of the proximal end of the opacity.

If the bronchostenosis is incomplete, it will commonly result in distal inflammatory changes without atelectasis. Small areas of consolidation will result in a group of small poorly defined circular shadows in a single segment or lobe, which may be indistinguishable from tuberculous foci (Fig. 153). Such shadows may be seen together with the shadow of the neoplasm, but the latter is often invisible on the plain radiographs, although it may be seen in tomograms. More severe distal inflammatory changes will produce consolidation of the whole lobe, the appearances then being similar to those described on pp. 45–55.

Another frequent result of bronchostenosis is bronchiectasis, which will give rise to tubular shadows if the dilated bronchi contain air, or to gloved-finger, and band-like shadows if they are full of secretions which cannot be expectorated. Again the shadow of the neoplasm may be invisible in the routine radiographs, but may be seen in a film with more exposure, or in tomograms.

If the neoplasm is rather peripheral and occludes bronchi of the fourth or fifth generation, a lobulated shadow may be seen, resulting partly from the neoplasm, partly from an adjacent dilated bronchus filled with secretion, and partly from an area of pneumonia.

Finally the distal inflammatory changes may develop into a lung abscess. This will show as a trans-radiant zone in the area of opacity, usually about 1–2 cm in size, though it may be much larger, or as a well-defined ring shadow with or without a fluid level. Again the shadow of the neoplasm may be clearly visible nearer the hilum or it may only be seen in tomograms, or the bronchial stenosis may only be demonstrated on bronchoscopy or in bronchograms.

A neoplasm may press on or invade a branch of the pulmonary artery producing an area of infarction, or this may arise without the vessel narrowing being demonstrated. The shadow of the infarction may be merged with that of the neoplasm or the distal atelectatic or inflammatory changes, or it may cast a separate 1–2-cm circular shadow remote from the neoplasm, or a larger wedge-shaped shadow with its base in the axilla and its apex towards the hilum where the shadow of the neoplasm will also be seen.

Sometimes the shadow of the neoplasm is associated with the shadow of a complicating pleural effusion. The combination of a shadow suggesting a neoplasm and pleural effusion does not necessarily indicate that the neoplasm is involving the pleura and is therefore perhaps unsuitable for resection, since the effusion may be secondary to the distal inflammatory changes.

The shadow of a neoplasm may be seen combined with an abnormal appearance of the vascular pattern such as that seen in emphysema, and this may indicate the double diagnosis and influence the line of treatment.

The shadow of a neoplasm may be combined with local rib erosion suggesting direct involvement, or with erosion of a rib in some other part indicating a secondary deposit. In either case such a finding will indicate a poor prognosis.

LUNG SHADOW WITH PERIOSTITIS OF RIB

A lung shadow indicating an area of consolidation together with some periosteal new bone formation of several adjacent ribs overlying the shadow will suggest actinomycosis (Fig. 323).

CHAPTER 10

BRONCHOGRAPHY

TECHNIQUE OF BRONCHOGRAPHY

BEFORE introducing the contrast medium for bronchography the operator should see that suitable and recent plain radiographs are available, and should inspect them carefully. From these and from the clinical picture he will be able to decide which parts need filling, and in what order this should be done.

The contrast medium

Excellent bronchograms can be obtained with an absorbable non-toxic contrast medium of the propyliodone type. No preliminary tests for iodine sensitivity are necessary, partly because there is no free iodine in these compounds, and partly because they are so rapidly excreted by the kidneys, that the concentration in the blood is very small.

For adults the opaque material can be suspended in an oil such as arachis oil, but for very young children a watery suspension is preferable since it is less likely to cause a temporary bronchial obstruction.

PREPARATION OF THE PATIENT

Whatever method or medium is used, careful preparation of the patient will be an important factor in obtaining satisfactory bronchograms.

Excessive secretions should be reduced as much as possible by preliminary chemotherapy and postural drainage. Normal secretion may be reduced by an injection of atropine, $\frac{1}{100}$ grain (0·65 mg), 1 hour before the examination, but is rarely effective in patients with excessive secretion.

Reassurance and sufficient explanation of the procedure as is suitable should be given to the patient to gain his co-operation and confidence. He should be shown the position of the cassettes, and trained to take up the positions in which he will be required to stand or lie, especially if the radiography is to be carried out in a room with which he is not familiar. If the examination is to be carried out under a general anaesthetic, this will not be necessary, but the appropriate preparation for the anaesthesia will be needed.

In an adult when no general anaesthetic is used, a mild tranquillizer such as Sodium Amytal 90–180 mg can be used.

ORDER OF FILLING OF BRONCHI

If both sides are to be filled at one session, it is best to fill the right side first, and take a right lateral view as well as an anterior (or posterior) view. This will ensure that a satisfactory view of the middle lobe and apical lower lobe bronchi is obtained without obscuration by shadows from the left side. Later when the left side is filled, a left posterior-oblique view is taken instead of the lateral and in this view the lingula will be displayed, and the orientation of the other branches can thus be determined. If after a rapid inspection of the films it is felt that a left lateral view would be of help, the bronchi of the left side can still be shown in a left lateral view, in spite of the right-sided filling, by taking a left lateral tomogram with a multisection box (see p. 267).

INTRODUCTION OF CONTRAST MEDIUM

The technique for the introduction of the contrast medium is best learned under the supervision of someone who has already acquired the necessary skill and experience.

There are several methods of injecting the contrast medium, and the choice will depend in the first place on the age and condition of the patient. In the case of a co-operative adult requiring neither a general anaesthetic nor selective filling of one lobar bronchus, the method chosen should be that which the operator finds easiest.

Whichever method is used, the patient must be persuaded to breathe evenly but not deeply during and after the injection, and must try not to cough until after the radiographs have been taken, and seen to be satisfactory. All patients should be told not to eat or drink anything for 4 hours after the injection, as the anaesthetized larynx may permit food or drink to pass into the trachea.

Crico-thyroid route

A small area of the skin and subcutaneous tissue in the front of the neck is anaesthetized with 2 per cent procaine. The trachea is then anaesthetized by the injection of 1 ml of 4 per cent lignocaine (Xylocaine) down a needle or down the cannula passed through the crico-thyroid membrane, followed in 1 minute by a similar injection.

The contrast medium is then injected through the needle or cannula, with the patient reclining backwards at an angle of 30 degrees and slightly towards the side it is desired to fill. A sufficient dosage for one side is 10–15 ml, and it should not be warmed or it will be too fluid, and run too rapidly into the smaller bronchi.

Intubation via the larynx under general anaesthesia

Intubation via the larynx under general anaesthesia is the method of choice when the patient is a young child. The following technique has given consistently satisfactory results in the hands of experienced anaesthetists. Premedication, given 1 hour prior to induction, is measured in minims drawn from a standard 1-ml ampoule containing $\frac{1}{3}$ grain (20 mg) of papaveretum and $\frac{1}{150}$ grain (0·4 mg) of scopolamine. The dose is 1 minim per year of age. This amount seldom causes sleep, but the child is calm and co-operative.

Anaesthesia is induced with nitrous oxide, oxygen and halothane using a Boyle's type of machine. When the jaw is relaxed laryngoscopy is performed and the trachea sprayed with 1–2 ml of 4 per cent Xylocaine (lignocaine) via a long straight spray inserted through the cords. Such topical analgesia tends to prevent bronchospasm which is prone to occur in patients with chronic chest disease. The analgesic usually causes some coughing, and the nitrous oxide, oxygen and halothane are again administered until breathing is regular. Laryngoscopy is repeated and an endotracheal tube, fitted with a Magill or Cobb suction union, inserted.

Aspiration of secretions via a catheter is then carried out, for in cases of bronchiectasis much secretion can often be removed by this procedure even in cases which appeared to be dry following preliminary chemotherapy and postural drainage.

A soft rubber or gum-elastic catheter is then passed down the Magill suction union and endotracheal tube, and should be of such a size that it does not fit the latter tightly. The catheter is marked so that it is possible to see when the tip lies just distal to the end of the endotracheal tube. This is important, since if the tip of the catheter lies in the tube, the contrast medium may block the lumen and thus the airway, whilst if inserted too far it may enter the right main bronchus and prevent filling of the left side. If a radio-opaque catheter is used, the tip can be positioned just above the carina under fluoroscopic control. The head of the table is then raised 20 degrees and the patient rotated towards the side it is desired to fill. The medium is then injected rapidly and will be sucked in on each inspiration, aided if necessary by slight pressure on the anaesthetist's bag. By this technique no special posturing will be needed. If possible, filling should be watched on the fluoroscopic screen, and radiographs taken as soon as satisfactory peripheral filling is seen.

Since the radiographs are taken while the patient is unconscious, co-operation with the anaesthetist is essential to ensure freedom from excessive respiratory movement. Controlled respiration enables the exposure to be made during apnoea, but also involves a tendency for the contrast medium to be blown too far down the bronchial tree into the peripheral bronchioles. Perfectly adequate radiographs can be obtained during quiet spontaneous respiration. The exposure is made towards the end of inspiration or of expiration, the latter being the longer period without chest movement. If respiration is quiet, an adequately sharp image of the filled bronchi will be obtained with an exposure of 0·04 second. If the patient develops a rapid respiratory rate during trichlorethylene anaesthesia, intravenous thiopentone is given prior to exposing the films; 0·1 g (4 ml of a 2·5 per cent solution) is injected into a dorsal vein of the hand and repeated if necessary. If apnoea develops, intermittent compression of the reservoir bag is carried out until breathing returns.

If after inspection of the first series of radiographs, tomograms are indicated, it may be necessary to inject a further small dose of thiopentone to ensure very quiet respiration during the 2-second exposure which will be needed.

At the conclusion of the examination, a thorough tracheo-bronchial toilet is performed, an artificial airway inserted, and the child returned to the ward in the lateral position with the head low.

Intubation via the larynx without general anaesthesia

This is the best method in a co-operative adult patient. The mucosa of the upper respiratory passages is anaesthetized by spraying on a local anaesthetic such as Xylocaine 4 per cent. Two millilitres are used for the tongue, pharynx, and nostril, and another 2 ml are then sprayed into the opening of the larynx. A few minutes later a catheter is passed through the larynx into the trachea. If a radio-opaque catheter is used (a grey Odman catheter, as for cardiac catheterization, is suitable), the position of its tip can be seen with the aid of image intensifier fluoroscopy. The patient sits or stands opposite the x-ray screen, and the tip of the catheter is seen in a lateral view of the pharynx. The catheter is manipulated so that it lies with its end curved forwards just above the larynx, and is then pushed onwards once or twice until it can be seen to have passed down into the trachea, 2 ml of the local anaesthetic are injected down it and the patient allowed to cough. The tilting couch is then lowered until the head end is raised about 45 degrees from the horizontal. The patient is then inclined towards the side it is necessary to fill, and the tip of the catheter is positioned 2 cm above the carina. Then 20 ml of the contrast medium are injected rapidly down the catheter, and the patient is instructed to breathe deeply. As soon as the contrast medium reaches the lobar bronchi it will be seen to be sucked out to the periphery on each inspiration, and after 3–4 breaths filling of all areas will be complete. Since it is sucked into the bronchi, gravity plays no part and no special posturing is necessary. If by chance some area is not filled, the patient should then be positioned so that the bronchus to this area is dependent, and another 5–10 ml injected. The radiographs are then taken. The catheter is kept in position during posturing and radiography so that it can be used as a channel for filling the other side a few minutes later.

A variant of this method can be used to obtain highly selective filling of a single lobar or segmental bronchus. The tip of the catheter is placed under bronchoscopic or fluoroscopic control in or just opposite the lumen of the bronchus it is intended to outline, and 5 ml are then injected into it, or rather less if only a segment is being outlined. In most cases it is necessary to prove that the surrounding regions are normal even if the disease on the plain radiographs appears to be confined to a single segment, and there are therefore few indications for such very selective filling.

Nose drip method

In the nose drip method the patient sits on the x-ray couch with his head tilted backwards and 2 ml of 4 per cent Xylocaine are run into the nostril, and from there some travels down the pharynx causing some coughing. Another 2 ml of local anaesthetic are then instilled into the nostril, and the tongue is held well forward with a swab to encourage some of the solution to enter the larynx. The contrast medium is then injected into the nostril, and if the tongue is held well forward it too will pass down the anaesthetized pharynx and larynx into the trachea. With this method some of the medium will be swallowed, but this is without adverse effects. To allow for this loss some 15 ml should be instilled for each side.

Transoral method

The mouth and throat are sprayed with 2 ml of 4 per cent Xylocaine. A further 2 ml are then sprayed on the larynx and the patient asked to breathe deeply in order that some of the spray is inhaled into the larynx and upper trachea.

The patient sits and the tongue is gripped with a piece of gauze and pulled well forward to prevent the patient swallowing. The contrast medium is then tipped from a teaspoon on to the back of the tongue whence it will flow down over and into the larynx and down the trachea.

POSTURING OF THE PATIENT DURING BRONCHOGRAPHY

If the medium is introduced rapidly down a translaryngeal catheter as described above, and the patient then breathes in deeply, the medium will be sucked into the various segments without any special manoeuvres. In all the other methods some postural manoeuvres are necessary to ensure filling of all the segments, and the following is a suggested routine.

The right side

When the medium is injected the patient should be reclining with head raised and inclined 30 degrees towards the right side. After about 10 seconds, during which time the medium descends to the right main bronchus, the patient (still inclined to the right) should lean forwards 30 degrees past the vertical position to fill the anterior basal and middle lobe branches; then backwards 30 degrees to fill the lateral and posterior basal and apical lower lobe branches. He then lies on his right side to fill the axillary branches.

In order to get good filling of the upper lobe, especially if an intratracheal catheter is not being used, it is helpful to inject the contrast medium in two parts starting with 10 ml and after the lower lobe has been filled, injecting a further 5 ml with the patient still lying on his side. Whether this is done, or only a single injection is made, the patient is then turned to lie in the prone oblique and finally the supine oblique positions to fill respectively the anterior, apical and posterior branches of the upper lobe.

When all the major bronchi of the right side have thus been filled, the patient should lie on his right side on the cassette and a right lateral-view radiograph of the chest should be taken. He then turns and lies prone or supine or stands up and an anterior (or posterior) view is taken.

Sometimes an additional right anterior-oblique view is indicated; finally an anterior view may be taken with the patient standing, if this has not already been done, for the purpose of showing an opaque oil level in any partly filled cystic bronchiectasis, as well as ensuring satisfactory distal filling of the basal bronchi.

Timing of postural manoeuvres

The timing of the posturing will depend on the speed with which the contrast medium runs down. At average room temperature it should reach the main bronchus about 30 seconds after it has been instilled into a nostril, or less if it has been injected down a needle through the crico-thyroid membrane.

The various postural manoeuvres generally occupy 1–2 minutes, after which time the more proximal bronchi should all be filled. To ensure that one radiograph at least will show more distal filling a delayed radiograph taken about 15 minutes later is often valuable, especially if the distal penetration of the contrast medium does not seem adequate in the first series of radiographs.

Check-up on filling

Directly the first series of radiographs has been taken, a rapid fluoroscopic survey may be made to ensure that all the bronchi are adequately filled. Alternatively the radiographs should be inspected as soon as they are cleared by the fixing solution, and a check-up made on the filling and any blurring due to movement or faults of exposure. With the advent of 90-second processing units, early inspection of the radiographs is much easier. If any bronchopulmonary segments are seen to be incompletely outlined and there is no positive evidence that this is due to bronchostenosis, it may be necessary to inject more of the medium and make further attempts to fill these segments by suitable posturing.

The left side

If filling of the right side was satisfactory, the examination of the left side can be undertaken at the same sitting. For this purpose a further 10–15 ml of the contrast medium is introduced into the trachea, this time with the patient inclined to the left. The first radiograph will be a left posterior-oblique view at about 45 degrees rotation, followed by an anterior (or posterior) view. If the left side only is filled, an additional left lateral view should be taken. The adequacy of the filling should be checked as described above.

X-RAY TECHNIQUE

The x-ray technique will in general be the responsibility of the radiologist. It is desirable that the x-ray tube column will rise high enough to give a tube-film distance of not less than 4 feet for the films taken lying down. The radiographs taken standing up should be taken at a tube-film distance of 5 or 6 feet.

The exposure will be roughly of the same magnitude as that used for the plain radiographs but 5–7 kVp higher. The film should be exposed during suspended inspiration of only moderate depth. Full inspiration is unnecessary and likely to precipitate a bout of coughing. The patient should therefore be asked to take a breath in gently and then to hold it in.

In a case showing only slight dilatation in one part, it may be useful to take a pair of radiographs, one in rather full inspiration, the other in full expiration, so that any excessive calibre changes with respiration can be seen.

AFTER-CARE AND DRAINAGE AFTER BRONCHOGRAPHY

Once the patient has coughed up any contrast medium in the trachea and main bronchi neither further coughing, posturing, nor physiotherapy will drain it out further from normal bronchi. Contrast medium in dilated bronchi can be cleared by posture but, since it has no access to lung tissue because of the occlusions, drainage is not urgent.

It is most important to warn the patient not to eat or drink for 4 hours afterwards, that is, until the effects of the local anaesthetic have worn off and the risk of accidental inhalation of food or drink has gone.

THE NORMAL BRONCHOGRAM

Figures 328 and 329 are diagrammatic tracings from normal bronchograms, together with the terminology accepted by the Thoracic Society (1950) and approved by an international committee.

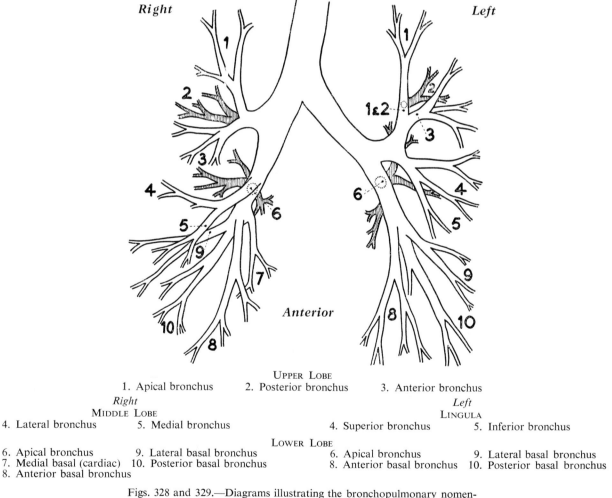

Right   _Left_

Anterior

UPPER LOBE

1. Apical bronchus   2. Posterior bronchus   3. Anterior bronchus

Right		_Left_	
MIDDLE LOBE		LINGULA	
4. Lateral bronchus	5. Medial bronchus	4. Superior bronchus	5. Inferior bronchus

LOWER LOBE

6. Apical bronchus	9. Lateral basal bronchus	6. Apical bronchus	9. Lateral basal bronchus
7. Medial basal (cardiac)	10. Posterior basal bronchus	8. Anterior basal bronchus	10. Posterior basal bronchus
8. Anterior basal bronchus			

Figs. 328 and 329.—Diagrams illustrating the bronchopulmonary nomenclature approved by the Thoracic Society. (_Reproduced by permission of the Editors of " Thorax "._)

When studying a bronchogram it is necessary to identify and name all the various segmental branches outlined even if their position is altered by pathological processes, or if some are not seen because they are occluded or have been removed.

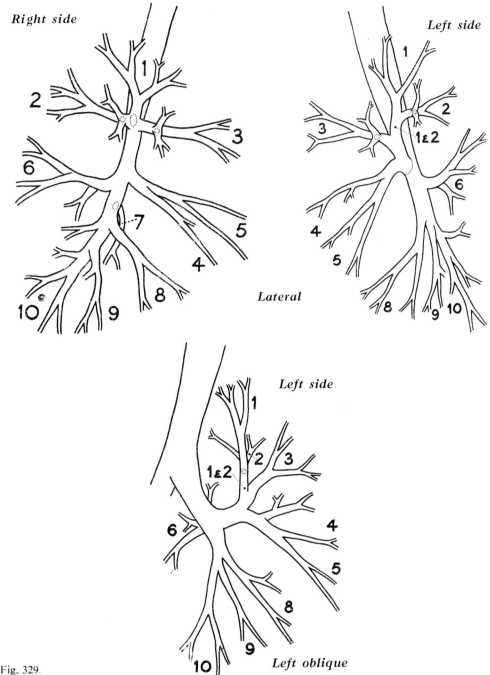

Fig. 329.

The anterior (or posterior) view should be inspected first, and the outline of the trachea noted. Then the right or left main bronchi should be traced down to their first divisions into the upper and lower lobe branches. Absence of either an upper or lower lobe will thus be noted. If bronchoscopy has not been performed recently the lower trachea and main bronchi must also be carefully inspected for filling defects or areas of narrowing. A filling defect in this region is sometimes caused by a large mucous plug, and it may be necessary to repeat the radiograph after gentle coughing to see whether the filling defect is transient or permanent.

The branches of the anterior and posterior segments of the upper lobe in particular, and those of the middle and lower lobe are usually partly superimposed in an anterior view, and can only be properly identified in the lateral or oblique view.

RIGHT BRONCHOGRAM

Starting with the bronchogram taken after filling the right side only, inspection of the anterior view will reveal the presence or absence of an upper and of a lower lobe group, and any premature filling of the left side which might cause confusion in the lateral view.

The right lateral view is then inspected and the origin of the middle lobe bronchus sought. If filled, it will be the first anterior branch after the 2-cm bare area of the intermediate bronchus lying below the uppermost branches which are normally of the upper lobe. Its identity is confirmed if it runs almost parallel to the intermediate bronchus before joining it, and if the apical lower lobe bronchus (6) can be seen passing directly posteriorly just below its origin.

If the middle and apical lower-lobe bronchi are thus confidently identified, then the three upper-lobe bronchi (apical (1), posterior (2) and anterior (3)) should be seen above, and the three basal bronchi (8, 9, 10) below.

Although the cardiac branch (7) is quite large, it is often inconspicuous and distinguished with difficulty from the anterior basal branch (8). It is perhaps more easily identified in the anterior than the lateral view, being the first branch coming off on the medial side below the middle lobe and apical lower lobe bronchi.

The early lateral divisions of the middle lobe (4) tend to lie below the medial division (5) in a lateral view. This relationship will alter if there is shrinkage of one segment, and identification of these two branches may then only be possible by reference back to the anterior view.

A large branch is often seen arising from the posterior basal bronchus (10) passing directly backwards parallel to and 2 cm below the apical lower-lobe bronchus (6). This is often known unofficially as the sub-apical bronchus.

LEFT BRONCHOGRAM

In the same manner, after the left side has been filled, careful identification of the lingular bronchus in the left lateral or left posterior-oblique view will make identification of the other branches much easier. The lingular bronchus is the lowest division of the short upper-lobe stem. It commonly has a large axillary branch passing directly laterally, which must not be confused with the anterior bronchus (3). The superior division (4) passes downwards and forwards, whilst the inferior division (5) is the most medial branch and is further identified by a particularly even-forked division after it has coursed downwards and slightly forwards for 2–3 cm.

If there is any difficulty in identification of the lingular bronchus, identification of the apical lower-lobe bronchus (6) may be of some assistance. It arises immediately after the origin of the lower-lobe stem. Care must be taken to separate the lateral division of this from the inferior division of the lingular bronchus whose path it crosses in the anterior view.

VARIATIONS IN THE MANNER OF ORIGIN OF THE SEGMENTAL BRONCHI

Variations of the manner in which the bronchi arise from the upper-lobe stem or from each other are common (Brock, 1954; Boyden, 1955). If the lingular bronchus is identified on the left or the middle-lobe bronchus on the right, such variations (or displacements) rarely cause confusion.

On the right side the apical bronchus may be displaced posteriorly to come off a short common stem with the posterior bronchus, or anteriorly to come off with the anterior bronchus, or it may as it were be split, one branch coming off the posterior the other off the anterior bronchus. Similarly the axillary branches of the anterior and posterior bronchi may come off more medially and therefore closer to the main bronchus than illustrated in Fig. 329. These variations are usually best seen in the lateral view and some of the commoner ones are shown diagrammatically in Fig. 330.

On the left side the anterior bronchus commonly comes off a common stem with the apico-posterior bronchus as illustrated, but it may be displaced downwards, so that the main upper-lobe stem divides into three branches of equal size, or it may be displaced still farther downwards and come off a common stem with the lingular bronchus. It too may be split, one branch coming off with the apico-posterior, the other with the lingular bronchus. Occasionally, the right apical lower bronchus (6) is displaced downwards so that it comes off 2 cm below the origin of the middle-lobe bronchus.

On the left side a branch corresponding to the cardiac bronchus may be seen. Returning to the more proximal branches, the right apical bronchus (1) may come off separately either close to the origin of the upper-lobe bronchus, the right main bronchus, or even as high as the lower end of the trachea.

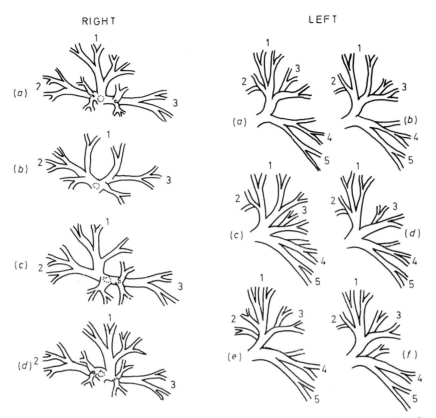

RIGHT   LEFT

Fig. 330.—Diagram showing some of the variations in the pattern of branching of the segmental bronchi.
(*a*) Common pattern.
(*b*) Split apical bronchus (28%).
(*c*) Apical and posterior together (14%).
(*d*) Apical and anterior together (10%).

(*a*) Common pattern.
(*b*) Split apical (38%).
(*c*) Split apical. Part of anterior down. Trifurcate pattern (21%).
(*d*) Whole anterior displaced down. Trifurcate pattern (6%).
(*e*) Lateral branch of posterior displaced down (48%).
(*f*) Lateral branch of superior lingula displaced posterior (15%).

These variations in the site of origin of the segmental bronchi may be quite normal, or they may be associated with other developmental defects suggesting a local growth pattern instability. A tracheal bronchus may supply an otherwise normal apical segment, or there may be some developmental defects in the part of the lung which it supplies. The severity of such a defect ranges from almost total agenesis of the segment to short wide bronchi with blind endings in lung supplied by collateral air drift from a nearby segment. Atresia of an upper-lobe segmental bronchus may be present with variations in the position or pattern of branching of the lower-lobe bronchi on that side (*see* p. 147).

INDICATIONS FOR BRONCHOGRAPHY

Although bronchography is relatively safe and not very unpleasant for the patient, it should not be undertaken without a definite objective. It will not, for instance, be justified in bronchiectasis for diagnosis alone if there is reasonably clear evidence of the condition in the plain radiographs or tomograms, nor for exact localization if, owing to age or other factors, neither surgery nor postural drainage is under consideration.

Once the objective has been defined, every effort should be made to obtain the requisite information. Adequate recent plain radiographs and when necessary tomographs should be available, and in many cases bronchoscopy should precede bronchography, even though this may entail transfer of the patient to a special unit.

The main indications for bronchography are as follows.

For correct x-ray diagnosis

(1) To confirm a diagnosis of bronchiectasis if this is suspected clinically but the plain radiographs (and perhaps the tomograms) are normal, or if changes are present but these are too slight or not sufficiently characteristic for a diagnosis of bronchiectasis.

(2) In cases of unexplained haemoptysis which might be due to bronchiectasis or a neoplasm amenable to treatment, but in which no lesion was seen on bronchoscopy or in the plain radiographs.

(3) To obtain further x-ray evidence concerning the possible nature of a lesion visible in the plain radiographs and tomograms.

(4) To investigate a patient with dyspnoea and airways obstruction if the cause is not obvious, but might be due to bronchial occlusive lesions.

Exact anatomical localization of lesion

(1) To define the exact anatomical extent and segmental distribution of the bronchiectasis, of which there is some definite evidence in the plain radiographs or tomograms, especially if surgical treatment is under consideration, or if accurate postural drainage is likely to be an important feature of medical treatment.

(2) To define the exact segmental localization and bronchial anatomy in relation to a lesion visible in the plain radiographs, if this information cannot be obtained from the lateral-view tomograms, and surgical treatment is under consideration.

For research purposes

Bronchograms may be indicated for the purpose of research provided that the research project is well planned and executed, for example to see the extent and type of bronchial abnormalities in the early stages of chronic bronchitis, or to see if there are bronchial occlusive lesions in cases of unilateral transradiancy with air trapping.

PATHOLOGICAL APPEARANCES IN BRONCHOGRAMS

BRONCHIAL OCCLUSION AND BRONCHOSTENOSIS

Occlusion of large bronchus

Occlusion of one of the larger bronchi may be obvious at the first inspection of the bronchogram, or it may only be detected after careful identification of all the filled larger bronchi. For instance, the occlusion of the medial division of the middle lobe shown in Figs. 129 and 130 was not detected until all the other branches were enumerated and the missing one thus identified.

It may not be easy to decide whether the occlusion is organic, due to a temporary mucous plug, or to a technical fault. Any irregularity of the contrast medium at the site of the block particularly an irregular " rat tail " narrowing, or a lung opacity distal to it (Fig. 331), perhaps only visible on tomograms, will indicate an organic cause.

Proximal bronchostenosis

Bronchostenosis without complete occlusion at the proximal end of a bronchiectasis may easily pass undetected if attention is concentrated on the distal and often obviously dilated bronchi. The whole of the filled bronchial tree should be carefully examined and such a filling defect will then not be so easily overlooked.

The cause of the filling defect is best discovered by means of bronchoscopy, provided the lesion is within range. If not, the shape of the stenosis in the radiograph may give a clue. An irregular narrowing is often seen with a carcinoma, a smoother narrowing with fibrosis following tuberculous endobronchitis, or sarcoidosis. A small local filling defect caused by a mass of tuberculous granulation tissue may be indistinguishable in the radiograph from one caused by a small carcinoma.

An air bubble or mucous plug may simulate either of these conditions, but is unlikely to maintain its position unchanged in all the radiographs of the series, especially if a delayed radiograph is taken 10–15 minutes after the first series.

A temporary local bronchial spasm may be difficult to distinguish from an organic narrowing. It is unlikely to occur except in a patient known to suffer from chronic bronchitis or asthma, and tends to appear as a smooth concentric narrowing without gross distal changes.

Bronchostenosis in area of dilatation

Some bronchial narrowing may be seen just proximal to a dilatation, or between two dilatations, and only one or several bronchi may show such a change. Sometimes there are several areas of narrowing between dilatations along a single pathway giving it a beaded appearance.

DILATATION OF BRONCHI

Dilatation of the lobar and proximal segmental bronchi, that is, of the first five generations along an axial pathway as shown in Fig. 332, is the common appearance of the condition known as bronchiectasis. In this site the dilatations are usually fairly even and tubular, and are perhaps the most striking change in the bronchogram. On pathological examination the walls of such bronchi may be thickened with granulation tissue and inflammatory cells, but if the inflammation dies out, or there is none, the walls may become atrophic and paper thin. The reason why there are dilatations of the first five generations and no filling beyond, is that these proximal bronchi have virtually complete cartilage rings and the walls will therefore not be able to approximate if there is occlusion of the lobar bronchus and consequent distal atelectasis. Beyond the fifth to sixth generation the cartilage is less complete and these bronchi will also collapse with the rest of the lobe. Should inflammatory changes occur, they may thus be permanently sealed off.

Another type of dilatation commonly seen is circular, and is often referred to as cystic. This change can occur in an axial pathway but is more commonly seen in dilatation of a side branch (Fig. 339).

A third type of dilatation is spindle shaped, or fusiform. These fusiform dilatations are usually the result of local damage to the bronchial wall. The damage may be infective but more commonly is due to an allergic response to an antigen as in asthmatics with bronchopulmonary aspergillosis and eosinophilia. The aspergillus alighting on the bronchial wall produces an intense allergic response with local ulceration of the bronchus and surrounding eosinophilic lung consolidation. Almost specific to this condition is a dilated area from the local ulceration without distal bronchial occlusion. There will thus be filling of normal bronchi beyond the dilatation (Fig. 333). Not all the dilated bronchi will show this phenomenon, and many will have obliterations with no filling beyond the tubular dilatation as in ordinary infective bronchitis obliterans (bronchiectasis). The two types of change may be found in two adjacent branches in the same patient.

Tubular bronchiectasis is often the result of a proximal bronchostenosis, and if the stenosis is relieved the dilatations may disappear. Stenosis may be due to a neoplasm, an inhaled foreign body or pressure from enlarged or healing lymph nodes. In these examples treatment of the causative lesion is often more important than the secondary bronchiectasis. Frequently by the time the bronchogram is done the causative lesion is no longer present, as in a temporary proximal occlusion or old inflammatory damage during a suppurative pneumonia.

In an atelectatic lobe whatever the cause, the proximal bronchi beyond the stenosis will always be dilated because of alterations in the local mechanical forces which determine the size of the lumen of a bronchus. Should the proximal occlusion causing the atelectasis disappear and the lobe become re-aerated, the dilated bronchi will return to a normal calibre if there is no residual infective damage. It is therefore impossible to tell for certain from a given bronchogram whether the dilated bronchi in an airless lobe will always be dilated, or whether they will return to normal if the lobe re-aerates (Figs. 341 and 342). Dilated bronchi may be seen in an atelectatic lobe or in an aerated lobe and this may show some reduction in volume or may be of normal size.

BRONCHIAL OCCLUSIONS IN RELATION TO THE DILATATIONS

Inspection of Fig. 332 shows that there is no filling of bronchi beyond the fifth generation, and that the dilated bronchi are occluded and have rounded endings. In addition, there are no side branches. In other words, those branches with incomplete cartilage rings have become occluded, and if inflammation occurs they may become permanently sealed off by fibrous tissue. These occlusions are in fact more important than the dilatations, for they are responsible for the symptoms. Because of the occlusions, no air can reach the dilated bronchi from the more distal areas which it used to supply, or from other areas nearby which may ventilate the alveoli near the dilated bronchi by collateral air drift. There

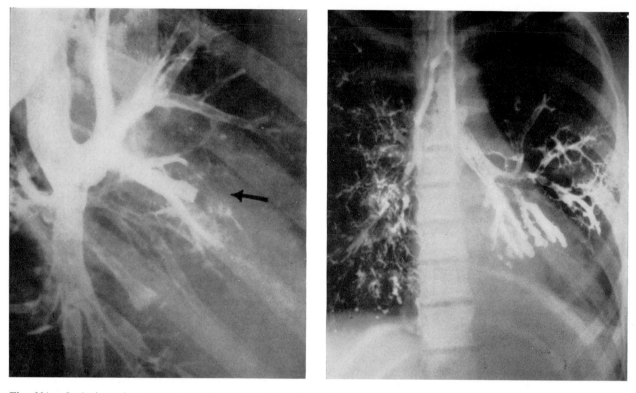

Fig. 331.—Occlusion of the superior division of the lingula (marked by arrow). Left posterior oblique-view broncho-gram. The small shadow below the tip of the arrow is an intrapulmonary calcification suggesting that the occlusion is due to a tuberculous lesion. Female aged 33 years. Small haemoptyses. Tubercle bacilli in sputum. Broncho-tomo-gram showed calcification at the same level as the occluded bronchus. Pathological confirmation.

Fig. 332.—Tubular bronchiectasis of the left lower lobe and lingula. Anterior-view bronchogram. Note the absence of filling of all the side branches and the occlusion of the dilated larger ones which terminate half-way down towards the diaphragm at the fifth generation. Male aged 14 years with cough, sputum, and haemoptyses. Specimen showed much fibrosis in the surrounding alveolar tissue. Normal filling to the periphery in part of the upper lobe.

is therefore no puff of air from below to aid expectoration of any excess of secretions. These secretions whether mucus, infected mucus or inflammatory products from an infected bronchial wall will therefore accumulate in the dilated bronchus, and are only coughed up in due course either because the bronchus overflows into a more normal airway, with a puff of alveolar air behind it to eject the bolus of secretion, or because the secretions reach more normal airways as a result of some postural change which will aid flow out of the dilated bronchus by gravity. The disturbed aeration around the bronchus may also keep it unduly wide during coughing. Upper-lobe dilated bronchi tend to drain by gravity and are therefore often seen in patients without cough and sputum, and are only rarely the site of a haemoptysis.

In the lower parts retained secretions may encourage local areas of inflammation and hence haemoptyses. The haemoptysis consists of red or arterial blood, and seems to arise from ulceration of a peripheral branch of one of the bronchial arteries which, because of the inflammatory changes in the bronchial wall, are usually greatly dilated in bronchiectasis.

Since the occlusions are the predominant cause of the symptoms, the term "bronchitis obliterans" would really be more appropriate than bronchiectasis.

The obliterative lesions will interfere with aeration and may cause atelectasis of the lobe, as well as the dilatations being the result of the collapse. If the lobe is aerated it must be by collateral air drift from nearby unoccluded pathways, and this may lead to emphysema (*see* pp. 149, 237). If the obliterations occur in childhood, they will lead to emphysema and hypoplasia (*see* p. 148).

The functional derangement from patchy airways obstruction if sufficiently widespread may lead to dyspnoea, or cor pulmonale, which complicates some cases of bronchiectasis, though it may be the result of an incidental but associated chronic bronchitis. Another consequence of the occlusions is that there is no fear of obscuring the dilatations by excessive peripheral filling. In fact, if excessive peripheral filling is seen in all lobes in the anterior and lateral views, it will exclude bronchiectasis.

Circular (cystic) dilatation

Circular or cystic dilatations (Fig. 334) are usually dilatations of small proximally situated side branch bronchi or small distal bronchi.

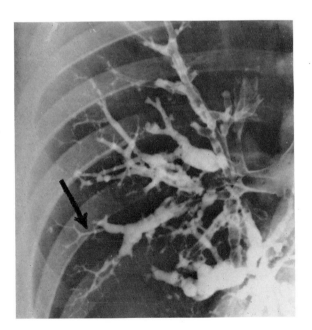

Fig. 333.—Asthma and bronchopulmonary aspergillosis with eosinophilia (bronchogram). Note tubular dilatations here and there, with filling continuing beyond dilatation into a normal bronchus (opposite arrow). Male aged 20 years. Asthma since infancy.

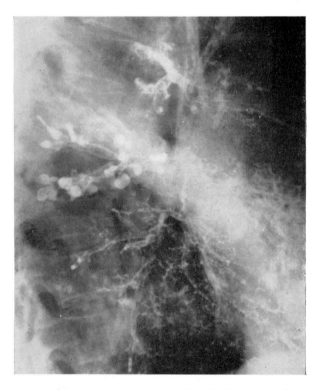

Fig. 334.—Cystic bronchiectasis in the apical segment of the right lower lobe. Right lateral bronchogram. Male aged 46 years. Twelve years cough and a little sputum; one year ago pneumonia developed and much more sputum. One haemoptysis. Basal segments normal.

Fine ring shadows may be seen in the plain radiograph, but sometimes widespread 1–2-cm saccular dilatations are found unexpectedly in the bronchogram when there are minimal changes in the plain x-ray. In some cases the dilatations may be developmental, but a similar radiographic appearance may be found following an inflammatory episode such as a staphylococcal pneumonia. In some cases, saccular, tubular and fusiform dilatations coexist in the same affected lobe.

Another form of cystic dilatation is seen when a whole lobe or segment is more or less destroyed and occupied by large cystic bronchiectatic spaces; these will be formed for the most part by gross dilatations of the larger bronchi.

A rare anomaly is one in which the bronchi lead into very large cystic spaces, and on resection the histology of the lung around these spaces is quite abnormal and suggestive of an angiomatoid developmental defect. Rather more common is a bronchus leading into dilated bronchi in an intralobar sequestrated segment (*see* p. 67) which has become infected and thus communicates with the bronchial tree in the normal part of the lobe.

CLASSIFICATION OF BRONCHIECTASIS

The shapes of the dilatations

A classification of bronchiectasis can be based on the shapes of dilatations shown in the bronchograms, but has the disadvantage that this does not sufficiently take into account aetiological factors such as whether the infection is with tubercle bacilli or other organisms, or what is the morbid histological state of the bronchial walls and surrounding lung.

1. Tubular (affecting larger bronchi)
   - Normal spacing
   - Crowding with lung shrinkage
   - Atelectatic lobe
     - Proximal bronchostenotic cause still present
     - No cause seen now

2. Fusiform
   - With occlusions
   - Without occlusions
     - Frequently end result of a local allergic inflammatory episode

3. Circular (cystic)
   - Smaller bronchi, especially side branches, affected
     - Possibly developmental (improbable)
     - Acquired post-inflammatory
   - Gross destruction in larger bronchi

Its value is further diminished by the fact that there is no close relation between these radiographic appearances and the clinical picture. Extensive bilateral cystic bronchiectasis may be present with insignificant symptoms, whilst the bronchi in a single segment or a single diseased bronchus exhibiting any of the above-mentioned shapes of dilatation may be a source of much cough and foul sputum or of repeated severe haemoptyses.

The extent of the lesion

A more useful grouping perhaps would be one based on the exact anatomical extent of the lesions which can be accurately judged from bronchograms, rather than on the shape of the dilatations. This, combined with the clinical picture, could be tabulated under types of treatment indicated (provided there is no progressive local bronchostenotic cause such as a neoplasm still present) as shown in Table 10.

TABLE 10

Treatment	Bronchogram	Clinical picture
No local treatment indicated	Lesions too widespread or slight	Symptoms absent or slight
Possible need for postural drainage or chemotherapy	Extent of lesion contra-indicates resection	Symptoms present. Clinical state contra-indicates resection
Consideration of resection of affected area	Lesion localized	Symptoms present. Clinical state satisfactory

Associated lung changes in the plain radiograph

Any detailed classification could usefully include associated changes seen in the plain radiograph.

Atelectasis

The presence of the shadow of an airless shrunken lobe in some cases has already been referred to above. If the shadow persists for months and there is no longer a proximal sited bronchostenosis, the change is usually irreversible.

Inflammatory changes

Sometimes small areas of ill-defined clouding are seen between the tubular or honeycomb shadows indicating inflammatory changes in the surrounding lung parenchyma. If such shadows persist for many months they would suggest irreversible lung damage.

Hypertransradiancy

Another change sometimes seen between the tubular shadows is a small area of hypertransradiancy with absence of vessel shadows. This indicates an irreversible localized emphysematous or bullous area and is found distal to the bronchial occlusion in many cases. The emphysema may be secondary to destruction of alveoli in the original infective incident, or to a check-valve effect from the damaged bronchi, or to the occlusions associated with the dilatations interfering with direct aeration. This part of the lung is thus aerated only by collateral air drift, and this may eventually lead to emphysema (*see* pp. 148 and 149).

Changes due to underlying cause

Finally local lung changes producing local associated bronchiectasis may dominate the picture in the plain radiograph. For instance the massive opacity of a chronic suppurative pneumonia with or without lung abscesses is usually accompanied by bronchiectasis in the affected area. Again in most cases of fibro-cavernous tuberculosis some dilated bronchi will be seen in the affected area if a bronchogram is performed.

In many cases of primary tuberculosis, following the disappearance of a massive lobar opacity (with or without shrinkage), a bronchogram will show a residue of dilated bronchi, even if the plain radiograph is by then normal or almost normal. In an upper lobe such a lesion is usually clinically silent.

The plain radiograph in bronchitis obliterans (bronchiectasis)

Whenever dilated bronchi and the associated occlusions have been seen in a bronchogram or in the specimen, a retrospective survey of the plain radiographs, including a lateral view, has shown some abnormality suggesting the condition in nearly all instances (certainly over 90 per cent). In over half of the radiographs the evidence is direct, for instance when tubular, tooth paste, gloved-finger or ring shadows can be seen, or a shrunken lobe with the dilated bronchi being outlined by the transradiant air within the lumen. Bronchiectasis, even if reversible, can be presumed to be present in an atelectatic lobe, and is often due to the altered mechanical factors and not necessarily to structural changes. In other cases the evidence for a bronchial lesion will be indirect.

A shrunken but aerated lobe for which no cause can be found will suggest that there are bronchial or bronchiolar occlusive lesions from infection in childhood, and these have resulted in slowing down the growth of the lobe. Too small a lobe may result in slight elevation of the diaphragm on that side, or displacement of the heart towards the affected lobe. A localized relatively transradiant area will suggest local emphysema, which may be unilateral, lobar or quite local; and when no other cause such as a scar can be seen for this, it will suggest the possibility of an underlying bronchial occlusive lesion with or without dilatation. Evidence of local air trapping in a radiograph on expiration will also indicate a bronchial occlusive lesion.

EXCESSIVE CHANGES IN THE CALIBRE OF A BRONCHUS

The larger bronchi in a normal person appear rather wider in a bronchogram taken in full-suspended inspiration than one in expiration, and in some subjects a local exaggeration of this phenomenon is seen in one or two branches only. It is usually assumed that bronchograms are taken in inspiration, but owing to the patient's fear of coughing, general distress, or perhaps because he is too young to co-operate or is under a general anaesthetic, this is not always the case. If therefore minimal dilatation is suspected, it is worth while trying to obtain one radiograph in deep-suspended inspiration and one in expiration.

Excessive local calibre change indicates local damage either to the bronchial wall or to the surrounding lung parenchyma, and is seen in a few cases of chronic bronchitis when it presumably indicates a past inflammatory episode with local complications and residual alveolar scars.

bronchitis or just a localized bronchiectasis. There is no evidence that such a calibre change is progressive and a precursor of clinical bronchiectasis. In a few cases where the clinical picture is solely that of chronic bronchitis, a bronchogram unexpectedly reveals an area of gross bronchiectasis, which again underlines the necessity for a clinical rather than a radiological diagnosis in these conditions.

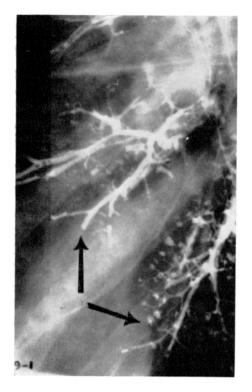

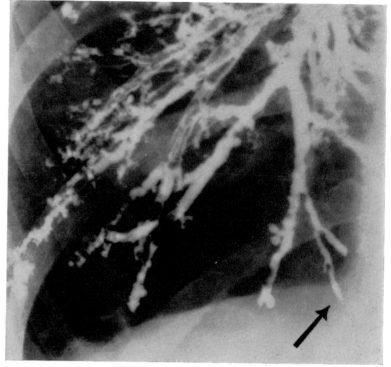

Fig. 337.—Chronic bronchitis. (Right bronchogram, lateral view.) Broken bough appearance above vertical arrow; " pools " or bronchiolar dilatations opposite horizontal arrow. Male aged 64 years. Many years cough and mucoid sputum.

Fig. 338.—Chronic bronchitis. Peripheral bronchial occlusions, with tapering ending (opposite arrow) and an irregular ending more lateral. Passing upwards areas of narrowing are seen. The next division laterally shows a beaded appearance proximally, pools half way down and a bulbous expansion at the distal ending. A similar range of changes is seen in other branches. Female aged 50 years; 20 years recurrent winter cough and sputum, recent dyspnoea.

THE BRONCHIAL ANATOMY AS AN AID TO LOCALIZATION OF LESION

Because the bronchial anatomy can be clearly demonstrated in a bronchogram, the relation of any abnormal shadow to a particular bronchus can be shown, and therefore its exact lobar or segmental distribution or position can be determined.

It may be useful to do a tomogram or simultaneous multisection tomograms of the outlined bronchi if the shadow is small and difficult to see in plain bronchograms.

ABNORMALITIES OF THE BRONCHIAL ANATOMY

Small normal variations in the manner in which the segmental bronchi divide are common, and are easily recognized in bronchograms (see p. 230). Such information may be of value to the surgeon in the execution of a segmental resection.

Whenever such a variation is present, it is still possible to identify all the normal segmental divisions.

In partial agenesis of the lung the changes are more severe, and not only is the lung very small with gross displacement of the heart, trachea and the opposite lung to that side, but it is not longer possible to identify all the segments. This feature will serve to distinguish the condition from an acquired bronchiectasis with lung shrinkage. In partial agenesis the shape of the bronchi is also abnormal, and they may be thin, long and poorly developed (Fig. 344), or they may be short and end with a glove-finger type of dilatation.

CHAPTER 11

TOMOGRAPHY

TOMOGRAPHY should only be undertaken when there is a specific indication for it and when the purpose of the investigation can be defined so that the correct area can be tomographed in the appropriate view with the correct exposure.

A study of the plain radiographs and the clinical features will help in this decision. If the plain radiograph shows a shadow, tomograms may be indicated to show additional features such as cavitation or vascular connections. If it is normal, certain clinical features, such as tubercle bacilli or malignant cells in the sputum, will be an indication for a further search for a lesion by tomography, and this could then be confined to those areas where a small lesion might easily be missed (*see* p. 246).

A detailed list giving all the indications for tomography in chest diseases would be very long. The following abbreviated list is based on cases within the author's experience in which tomograms have provided evidence helpful to the clinician in choosing the correct treatment. There is no doubt that other indications will arise from time to time whenever the evidence of the plain radiograph is inconclusive.

(1) Demonstration or exclusion of a pulmonary cavity in an area where shadows can be seen in the plain radiograph.

(2) Proof or exclusion of a lung lesion when the plain radiograph is normal, but the sputum is positive for infection or a neoplasm.

(3) Extent and segmental localization of shadows.

(4) Further evidence concerning the nature of an abnormal shadow.

(5) To supplement the plain lateral-view radiograph when the evidence from this is uncertain.

(6) Demonstration of the lumen of the trachea and larger bronchi.

(7) Demonstration or exclusion of enlarged hilar glands.

(8) Demonstration of the main vessels in the hilar regions (*a*) in heart disease or (*b*) in obstructive airways disease.

(9) Extent and nature of abnormal mediastinal shadows.

(10) Additional view in lesions of the thoracic cage.

For technique, *see* pp. 265–269.

For technique, *see* pp. 265–269.

PRELIMINARY INSPECTION OF THE TOMOGRAMS

A preliminary inspection of the tomograms to ensure that the technique has been adequate is an important factor which contributes largely to the reliability of the method, particularly in the diagnosis of a pulmonary cavity.

Order of films for viewing

The films should first be arranged on the viewing box in their correct layer order according to the numbers marked on each film. The order should then be checked by observation of some obvious landmark such as the ribs. If, in a posterior-view series, the visible part of the ribs does not become more anterior as the layers progress, the films may have been wrongly marked or an error may have been made in the setting of the layer selector. Alternatively, and more commonly, the patient may have moved in the interval between two exposures, or his respiration may have been of a different depth. If a discrepancy is observed and cannot be corrected with certainty, it may be advisable to repeat the series.

Checking up on the area covered

Assuming that the order of the layers appears to be satisfactory, it is then necessary to make sure that the correct area has been covered. Inspection of the previous plain radiographs or tomographs and the clinical picture will have given a clear idea of the object of the examination, and it will be possible to judge whether the series includes a sufficiently large area. It is important to remember that owing to the relatively short tube-film distance used, the shadow of a lesion near the edge of the tomogram will be some distance from the centre of the x-ray beam and may therefore be considerably displaced from the position it occupied in the plain radiograph. Care should therefore be taken to see that the suspected region is in fact on the tomogram and not displaced beyond the film.

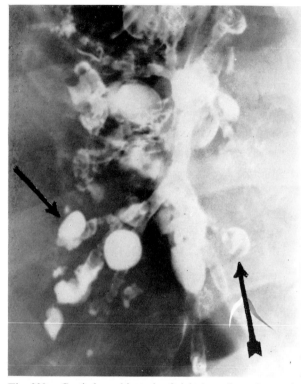

Fig. 339.—Cystic bronchiectasis of right lung (bronchogram). Upward-pointing arrow to cystic dilatation at the end of a pathway. Downward-pointing arrow to cystic dilatation of a side branch.

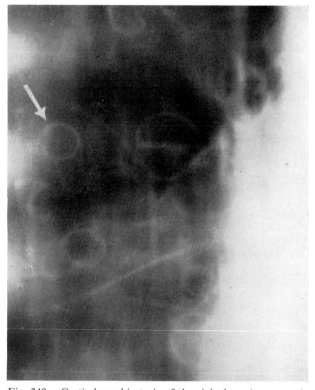

Fig. 340.—Cystic bronchiectasis of the right lung (tomogram). Arrow points to one of the well-defined ring shadows. They were inconspicuous in the plain radiograph but filled with Lipiodol on bronchography. Male aged 40 years. Ten years cough and sputum.

The range in depth of the layers

The range of the layers should then be noted to ensure that it extends sufficiently backwards or forwards, or, in the case of a lateral-view tomogram, medially and laterally. It is safest to judge this by the visible anatomical landmarks rather than by the depths recorded on the films. In a posterior view one layer at least should show the posterior parts of the ribs quite clearly, since only then will it be certain that the whole of the posterior part of the lung has been included in the series. If abnormal shadows are visible in the plain radiographs, care must be taken to identify these in the tomograms. Similarly if previous tomograms are available, any vessels, calcifications or other landmarks in the old series should be identified in the new, to ensure that comparable layers have been taken. Many errors have resulted from a failure to take these precautions.

In comparative tomograms it is particularly important not to place too much reliance on the layer-depth identification numbers marked on the films. Apart from being subject to a radiographer's error, these numbers are often misleading because of differences of calibration on different sets. In some departments the depths are measured from the table top, in others, from the film, which is 2–4-cm lower. Even if the film layer depths are correctly understood, the abnormal shadow may really lie at a different depth from the table top in the two series either because the patient is lying in a different position, if for instance there is an additional pillow under his head, or because the lesion has changed its position in the chest as a result of other intrathoracic pathological conditions, such as nearby scarring, or bronchostenosis, or as a result of a pneumothorax or other therapeutic procedure.

Spacing of layers

The spacing between the tomographic layers should not in general exceed 1 cm. This is the maximum thickness in which poorly contrasted shadows such as those of small cavities or normal vessels are clearly visible. Beyond this limit such shadows are blurred out by diffusion if an arc of swing of 25 degrees or more is used.

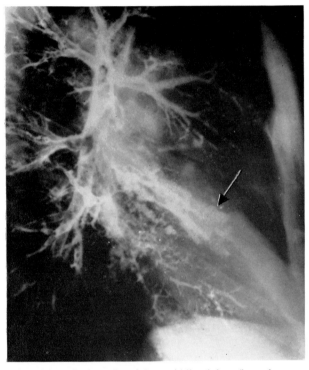

Fig. 341.—Atelectasis right middle lobe (bronchogram; right lateral view). Only first five generations filled, and these are dilated. Arrow points to atelectatic middle lobe.

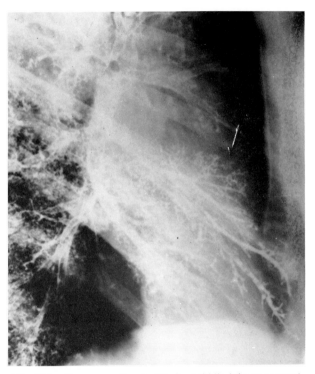

Fig. 342.—Same case (1 year later). Middle lobe re-aerated. Middle lobe bronchi now normal. Female aged 33 years. Cough and sputum for 6 months, became symptom free.

THE DEMONSTRATION OR EXCLUSION OF A PULMONARY CAVITY

THE INDICATIONS

Tuberculous cavity and lung abscess

The demonstration or exclusion of a cavity by tomography is particularly indicated in tuberculosis and many other types of lesion when an abnormal shadow is seen but there is doubt after inspection of the plain radiographs whether a cavity is present or not. With the advent of effective chemotherapy the detection of a tuberculous cavity is less important than it was some years ago, for if tubercle bacilli are found in the sputum the chances of eliminating the disease is high. However, chemotherapy fails in a few cases for one reason or another, and resection may be contemplated, especially if persistent cavitation is seen. Tomography is also important if some shadows are seen in the plain radiograph, but no bacilli are found in the sputum, because the demonstration of a cavity may by itself be an indication for a more thorough search for the organism, which may then be found.

If a cavity has once been seen in a case of tuberculosis or lung abscess, but is no longer visible on the plain radiographs, tomography may be indicated to see whether it has closed or not.

Bronchiectasis

Using the expression " cavity " in the sense of any abnormal intrapulmonary air space, tomography is indicated to prove or exclude gross bronchiectasis in cases where tubular or honeycomb shadowing is suspected in the plain radiographs but it is indistinct or obscured by overlying and surrounding shadows.

Cystic dilatations usually stand out very clearly (Fig. 340), while tubular dilatations can be seen in most cases, especially if a view can be taken with them more or less parallel to the film. The method is of course not as reliable or informative as bronchography, but if the objective is only diagnosis and not to discover the extent and character of the dilatation, the demonstration of any dilatation by tomography may make bronchography unnecessary. This is particularly true in cases of bronchiectasis where surgery is not contemplated.

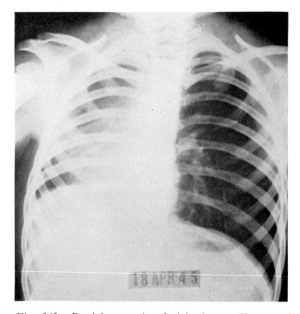

Fig. 343.—Partial agenesis of right lung. Heart and trachea displaced to the right. Somewhat opaque right lung, with small hilar vessels, and small lung vessels taking an abnormal course. Bronchoscopy shows a right main bronchus, but narrow. Female aged 8 years. Asymptomatic.

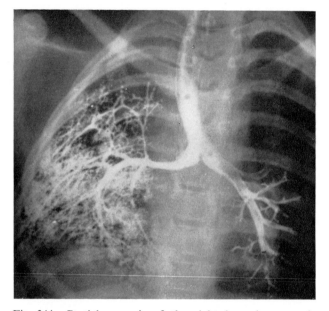

Fig 344.—Partial agenesis of the right lung (same case). Posterior-view bronchogram. The abnormal shape and distribution of the bronchi in the small right lung is clearly seen. There is no distal dilatation of the bronchi. The left side shows a normal pattern.

DIAGNOSIS OF THE RING SHADOW (CAVITY)

Identifying the ring

A clearly defined ring shadow seen for the first time in a series of tomograms is not likely to cause difficulties of interpretation (Fig. 355). Nor is a less well-defined shadow which has already been seen in previous plain radiographs or tomograms. On the other hand in a great many cases, an indistinct appearance giving the impression of a ring shadow is seen for the first time in the tomograms; in such circumstances particular care should be taken to confirm its identity and avoid a false impression.

The wall of the supposed ring should first be examined. If the ring is incomplete, so that an imaginary tiger placed in the central transradiant zone could walk out because of a gap in the ring (excluding walking down the bronchus) then a cavity is not present. If any part of the ring shadow is seen to continue into a vessel shadow, this part should be considered to be a vessel and not a contribution to the cavity wall. Similarly, if the apparent wall is of uneven thickness, close inspection may reveal that some of it is formed by a separate nearby circular shadow. An indrawn tag of thickened pleura may also simulate the lateral wall or roof of a cavity. If all such irrelevant shadows are removed in imagination, what is left may provide no case for the diagnosis of a cavity. On the other hand a complete ring shadow may still be present even after the nearby irrelevant shadows have been ignored, and then a cavity can be diagnosed with confidence.

In a case of doubt valuable and decisive evidence may be obtained from lateral-view tomograms in addition to the posterior ones, or from some additional intermediate layers giving a 0·5 cm spacing.

A ring shadow still seen after such stringent analysis and careful technique will nearly always turn out to be a cavity if the piece of lung becomes available for pathological investigation.

Identification in serial tomograms as the cavity alters

A cavity which has been demonstrated in previous radiographs or tomograms may become much less distinct because it decreases in size or becomes filled with secretions, or because the contrast between its wall and the surrounding lung decreases as treatment progresses. Because of the exact anatomical localization which can be achieved by tomography when vessels or other shadows in the proximity of the cavity can be identified in both series, it is possible to be certain of the continued existence of such a cavity in spite of the alterations in its appearance. If no ring is seen, closure can be assumed.

Shadow within a cavity

Tomograms may throw some light on the nature or state of the pathological process if they demonstrate abnormal shadows within the cavity. A large opacity with a hair-line transradiant zone between it and the cavity wall will suggest a mycetoma (p. 126 and Fig. 139). A similar appearance may be seen if there has been a recent haemorrhage into the cavity, and the blood retained in it, clotted and somewhat shrunken, so that it neither occupies the whole of the air space nor forms a fluid level.

An air space between a hydatid cyst and the adventitia may give a similar appearance.

Small dense opacities will indicate calcified loose bodies within the cavity or stuck to its wall, and may be an indication for resection, since they act as foreign bodies and may result in haemorrhages.

Differential diagnosis

It may not be possible to distinguish radiologically between the different types of cavity or air-containing spaces. The "cavity" for instance may be a distended bronchus (Fig. 204) or a bulla (Fig. 245). Distinction between a small thin-walled tuberculous cavity or a bulla is often difficult. A ring shadow, particularly at the extreme apex of the lung, is more likely to be a tuberculous cavity if the wall is thicker than a hair line (0·5 mm), and if there is any evidence of a linear or tubular shadow extending from it towards the hilum. It is more likely to be a bulla if the wall is very regular and of hair-line thickness (Fig. 345), and if there are linear or stellate shadows, or thicker-walled ring shadow nearby, and if there is a suggestion of vessel atrophy in proximity to it. These two conditions however cannot always be distinguished from each other in the tomograms. For instance in one patient suffering from tuberculosis the tomograms showed three similar ring shadows in the right upper zone, but after resection the specimen showed that one of these was a tuberculous cavity, and the other two bullae.

Reliability of the method

It is a common experience to see a ring shadow indicating a cavity in a tomogram which either could not be seen at all or could not be seen with any certainty in the plain radiographs. If such evidence can be shown to be reliable, the importance of tomography as a method of investigation needs no emphasis.

With care in the technique and interpretation it is possible to find that the diagnosis or exclusion of an air-containing space is confirmed in over 90 per cent of cases when the resection specimen is examined. Disagreement between the radiological and pathological findings is sometimes found if the cavity is full, or almost full, of caseous material.

Sometimes no cavity is found on macroscopic examination of the specimen either because the tomograms are not sufficiently recent and the cavity has apparently closed in the interval, or because the distortion of vessels, thickened pleura, or the position of nearby pathological foci have led to an unavoidable error in interpretation. Such errors are few and are rarely of serious consequence to the patient.

The objection might be raised that the material available for histological confirmation is highly selective, resection being most commonly adopted as a method of treatment if the diagnosis of cavitation is beyond doubt; in the cases from which the present conclusions have been drawn, however, this has not been so, because they have included quite a high proportion of non-cavitated resected lesions.

In addition a careful clinical and tomographic follow-up of cases not treated by resection has also tended to confirm the high degree of accuracy found in the demonstration or exclusion of cavities by tomography.

PROOF OR EXCLUSION OF A LESION WHEN THE PLAIN RADIOGRAPHS ARE NORMAL

Sometimes malignant cells or tubercle bacilli are found in the sputum, or pulmonary osteoarthropathy is present clinically or in the radiographs of the bones of the wrists, knees or ankles, but no abnormality can be seen in the plain radiographs of the chest or on fluoroscopy and bronchoscopy is also normal. Tomograms are then indicated to supplement the plain radiographs.

For this purpose posterior-view tomograms should be taken of the upper half of the lungs in case the lesion is hidden by the clavicle, a rib or a particularly heavily calcified first or second costal cartilage. If no lesion is seen in these tomograms, lateral-view tomograms should be taken of both the right and the left side to show clearly the regions behind or adjacent to the hilar vessel shadows, or the region behind the heart shadow.

Another indication is when a single shadow is in fact seen in the plain radiographs and is considered to represent a secondary deposit. It may then be necessary to know, prior to resection, whether it is really isolated or not. Under these circumstances posterior-view tomograms of the whole of both lung fields with the layers spaced no more than 1 cm apart should be taken to exclude other small secondary deposits. Lateral-view tomograms should also be taken for the region behind the heart shadow and in the posterior recess on both sides which would be hidden in the anterior view by the diaphragm.

EXTENT AND SEGMENTAL POSITION OF LUNG LESION

EXTENT OF LESION

In many cases of pulmonary tuberculosis, tomograms should be taken as soon as it has been decided to undertake treatment. By this method additional small foci are frequently seen which are invisible in the plain radiographs.

Tomography of both lungs is not indicated as a routine, but tomograms should be taken of the lung in the region of any localized group of shadows. If the shadows lie in the region above the clavicle, posterior-view tomograms will suffice; if the shadows are lower down, however, lateral-view tomograms may be most useful. Lateral-view tomograms may also be indicated to prove or exclude the presence of small lesions in some special region, such as the apex of the lower lobe in a case with visible lesions in the upper lobe.

Correlation of lateral-view tomograms with resection specimens shows a very high degree of accuracy of the method in demonstrating or excluding cavities and small solid foci, as well as in their segmental localization. It is however apparent that a lesion smaller than 0·5 cm is usually invisible, whilst a somewhat larger lesion may pass undetected in a large patient if it lies at the extreme apex, posteriorly overlying the vertebral column, or adjacent to the heart shadow. In such a case a higher standard of accuracy will be obtained if the lateral view is supplemented by an oblique-view series of the more medial layers opposite the vertebral column. Small shadows in the posterior part of the apex of the left lower lobe may be seen more clearly if they are thrown clear of the shadow of the vertebral column by rotating the patient until the right shoulder is 10–15 degrees forwards.

On the whole there is a tendency to " under read " the shadows in a lateral-view tomogram, and it is uncommon to see shadows and not find corresponding pathological foci in the specimen; whilst foci seen in the specimen are often not very conspicuous in the tomograms. On this account even faint abnormal shadows seen in lateral-view tomograms should be given more emphasis than they might have received had they been seen in other views.

EXACT SEGMENTAL LOCALIZATION OF LESION

The exact segmental localization of a lesion is obviously of great value to the surgeon. Using lateral-view tomograms the great majority of cavities or solid lesions larger than 0·5 cm can be localized to a particular segment with certainty. The localization is relatively easy if the fine white hair line of an interlobar fissure can be identified. This is commonly so, but even if the fissure is invisible or much displaced by lobar shrinkage, localization will still be possible by identification of the vessels (Fig. 346) or even the segmental bronchus.

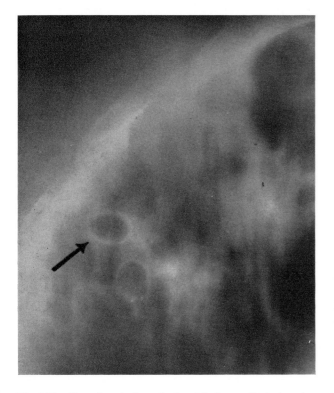

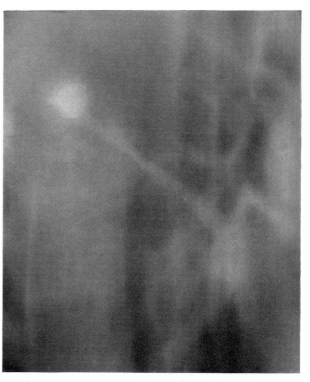

Fig. 345.—Two ring shadows in the right lung. Posterior-view tomogram. The ring shadow with the rather thicker wall (opposite arrow) is due to a tuberculous cavity. The ring shadow medially and below it with a thinner wall is a bulla.

Fig. 346.—Two-centimetre tuberculous focus (tomogram). The band-like shadow is the vessel with surrounding thickened tissue passing from the focus to join inferior pulmonary vein. Shadow is therefore in the apex of the right lower lobe.

FURTHER EVIDENCE TO FACILITATE THE DIAGNOSIS OF AN ABNORMAL SHADOW

The interpretation in terms of morbid histology of almost any shadow seen in the plain radiographs is a hazardous business, and in cases where there are no clues from the clinical and pathological findings, any additional evidence may be of help. In this respect tomograms are often very useful, giving further evidence more certainly and at an earlier stage than the plain radiograph or early clinical investigation.

Tomograms may show any of the following features. The presence of multiple line shadows radiating out from a circular shadow will suggest a bronchial carcinoma (*see* p. 86). The presence of a concave notch in the shadow facing towards the hilum, will also suggest that the shadow represents a neoplasm. The significance of small satellite shadows near a 2-cm circular shadow is less certain, though they are rather more common in tuberculosis than in a neoplasm. Linear shadows along the line of the broncho-vascular bundle between the shadow and the neoplasm are much more common in inflammatory lesions than in a neoplasm. A single vessel shadow from a 2-cm circular shadow, especially when it can be identified as a vein by joining the shadow of another vein leading to the left atrium, will suggest the shadow is an infarct (Fig. 140). Two wide vascular shadows, one an artery and one a vein, passing to or from the circular shadow to the hilum will indicate the lesion is an arterio-venous fistula (*see* p. 78).

Cavitation is more common in a tuberculous lesion than in a neoplasm but it can occur in either condition, and is rarely of value in differentiating one from the other. A very thin-walled cavity will be against a neoplasm, and a thick-walled cavity in favour of a neoplasm, but neither finding is conclusive.

247

Calcifications within a shadow are suggestive of old tuberculous lesions, but occasionally a neoplasm may over-run an old tuberculous lesion or, more rarely, may show intrinsic calcifications. A single spot of calcification in the centre of a very well-demarcated circular shadow will suggest a hamartoma. More diffuse calcifications can also occur in a hamartoma. As a rule the soft tissue surround is less well demarcated in a tuberculous lesion than a hamartoma.

The presence of narrow band-like branching transradiancies indicating air-containing bronchi within a massive shadow will prove the shadow is pulmonary and not pleural (Fig. 89). The presence of a thin " halo " transradiant zone round the edge of a large circular shadow will suggest a mycetoma (Fig. 139).

Adjacent pleural thickening may by its shape and position indicate that the shadow is pleural, as in an interlobar effusion; or that it has a pulmonary and pleural component. If the shadow is near the surface, rib changes such as erosion or periosteal new bone may be seen in a tomogram before they are visible in the plain radiograph. The presence of hilar glandular enlargement in association with small circular shadows will suggest sarcoidosis rather than ordinary tuberculosis.

Tomo-bronchogram

Tomography of the chest during bronchography is sometimes of great value. It is best done using the simultaneous multisection method (*see* p. 267), in which only a single swing and exposure are necessary and the examination is easy and rapid. The box containing the films and screens may be placed ready in position under the couch, protected from the x-rays while the conventional bronchograms are being taken and developed. These will indicate the need for the additional examination, the most appropriate view, the centring point, and the range of layers required.

If both sides have been filled at the bronchography a tomo-bronchogram is the only means of obtaining a satisfactory lateral view of one side. If only one side has been filled it will help to distinguish certain branches, especially if they are superimposed in the routine radiographs or if their position is altered by lung shrinkage. It is also indicated to show the relationship of a particular bronchus to an abnormal nearby shadow. (This was a great help in the case illustrated in Fig. 331.)

TO SUPPLEMENT THE PLAIN LATERAL-VIEW RADIOGRAPH

The great value of the plain lateral-view radiograph in many cases is beyond dispute, but its limitations are not always appreciated. Because of the large number of superimposed normal shadows, the difficulties of interpretation are great even when satisfactory films are available, and almost insuperable when the films are of poor quality, as is too often the case. A lateral-view series of tomograms will usually show an individual shadow so much more clearly that it is often indicated to supplement the plain lateral view.

Figs. 109 and 110 illustrate how much more clearly the spindle shadow of an atelectatic middle lobe is seen in the tomogram than in the plain radiograph. Even a large homogeneous 2–3 cm shadow situated higher up may be equally difficult to see in the plain radiograph because of the overlying shadows of the shoulder girdle, vertebrae, or aorta; it will be seen quite clearly, however, when these structures are " blurred out " by diffusion in a tomogram (Figs. 349 and 350).

The presence of abnormal shadows on the contralateral side, such as may result from an effusion, an old thoracoplasty or other surgical procedure, a pneumothorax, or even much contralateral lung disease, will also result in superimposed and confusing shadows in the plain lateral view. Lateral-view tomograms may be the only satisfactory method of showing the exact position of a lesion in such circumstances.

DEMONSTRATION OF THE LUMEN OF THE TRACHEA AND LARGER BRONCHI

The trachea and proximal bronchi are as a general rule best inspected by bronchoscopy, but in certain circumstances the demonstration of the tracheal and bronchial air transradiancies in a tomogram is a useful supplement and occasionally a substitute for this method of investigation.

Tomograms may precede bronchoscopy in some cases in which tubercle bacilli have been found in the sputum, but no lesion has been seen in the plain radiographs of the lungs. The demonstration of a narrow area in the transradiancy of the trachea or a main bronchus will suggest the possibility of a tuberculous bronchitis, and such a finding may accelerate or delay bronchoscopy.

Tomograms may follow bronchoscopy in some cases in which the lower limits of the affected area have not been seen because of the stenosis. Fig. 347 is a supplementary tomogram of this kind. It shows the whole length of the stricture, with the normal part of the tracheal transradiancy above and below it; proves the stricture to be related to a nearby calcified gland and obviously short; and thus indicates that surgical reconstruction would not be too formidable. This was in fact undertaken in the case illustrated, with complete relief of the near strangulation. The clinical picture and post-operative tomograms showed a good airway, and made further bronchoscopy unnecessary.

If a patient is too old or ill for radical treatment, the demonstration of a bronchostenosis on a tomogram may be a substitute for bronchoscopy. The tomogram will show the relation of the narrowing to any nearby opacity, but will not give any indication of the histology of the lesion.

Finally bronchoscopy may have been performed with a negative result, and yet a tumour may still be suspected. This is apt to occur with a small neoplasm causing narrowing of a segmental upper-lobe bronchus, or of the main middle-lobe stem 1–2 cm beyond its origin, and in such a case tomograms may demonstrate an area of narrowing.

ACCURACY OF THE METHOD

The left and right main bronchus, the right upper-lobe bronchus, and the intermediate bronchus can nearly always be clearly shown in posterior-view tomograms, but distal to these bronchostenosis must be diagnosed with caution. The x-ray diagnosis will be fairly certain if the narrowing or occlusion is related to an adjacent abnormal shadow, or if the narrowing is irregular or tapering. If an apparent narrowing is smooth and rounded or oval, it may in reality be caused by the disappearance of the normal bronchial transradiancy from the clear tomographic layer, as the bronchus is rarely parallel to this. The continuity may be traced into the next tomographic layer, but as the bronchus passes distally it tapers and becomes difficult to see in any case, so that inability to visualize it further does not always prove occlusion.

In certain regions suspected narrowing can often be confirmed or excluded by tomograms taken in other views. The right middle-lobe bronchus is seen most clearly in a right posterior-oblique view tomogram, the left lower-lobe bronchus in a left lateral view, and the left upper lobe and the proximal parts of its segmental divisions in a left posterior-oblique view.

In spite of the difficulties and limitations, the demonstration of the bronchial air transradiancies by tomography is often of great value. The method can be supplemented when necessary by bronchography if no lesion has been seen at bronchoscopy.

DEMONSTRATION OR EXCLUSION OF ENLARGED HILAR GLANDS

DISTINCTION FROM VESSEL SHADOWS

The hilar glands, when they are normal or only slightly enlarged, cannot be seen in the plain radiographs, and even when they are considerably enlarged it may not be possible to say whether the resulting abnormal shadow is an enlarged gland or a prominent or enlarged vessel. Tomograms are particularly useful for making these distinctions. If the enlargement is due to a vessel shadow, the tomogram will reveal continuity between it and other unmistakably vascular shadows. If it is due to some structure independent of the vessels, such as an enlarged lymphatic gland (Fig. 348), the shadow may be found to be most conspicuous in a different tomographic layer to that in which the main vessels are most conspicuous, and its margins will not taper out here and there into the vessel shadows.

The site of the enlargement will also be a factor in the diagnosis. Enlarged glands frequently lie between the tranradiancies of the main upper-lobe and lower-lobe bronchi, and cast a shadow in this situation with a well-defined lateral convex margin. If in addition the shadow has a well-defined inferior margin, or lies at a slightly lower level, the diagnosis will be even more certain; for at this level the vessels cast a continuous shadow down towards the diaphragm.

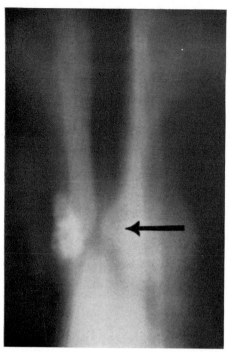

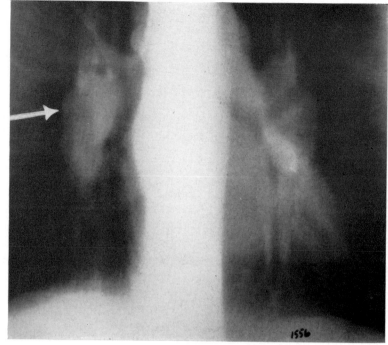

Fig. 347.—Stenosis of lower end of trachea (tomogram). Stricture, with shadow of a calcified gland just to the right, is seen opposite arrow. Male aged 36 years. Five years increasing dyspnoea. Admitted as an emergency. Upper limit of stricture visible on bronchoscopy. Plastic repair. Post-operative tomogram showed good airway.

Fig. 348.—Enlarged hilar glands (tomogram). Arrow points to the lateral convex border of the abnormal glandular shadow, which is demarcated above by the transradiancy of the upper-lobe bronchus, and medially by that of the intermediate bronchus. It has a well-defined convex inferior margin. Oval shadow of azygos vein above upper-lobe bronchus. On left shadow with lateral convexity just below upper-lobe bronchus is also an enlarged gland. Lower-lobe veins to left atrium are seen on both sides. There are enlarged glands around the left lobar bronchial transradiancies. Male aged 32 years. Sarcoidosis.

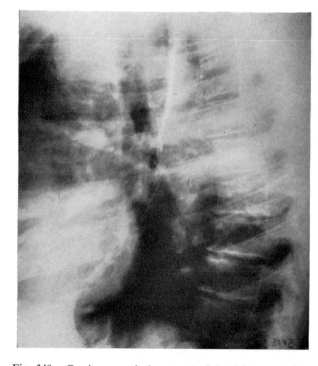

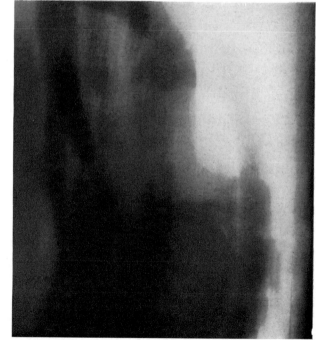

Fig. 349.—Carcinoma apical segment of the left lower lobe. Plain lateral view. Indistinct opacity superimposed on the shadow of inferior part of the scapulae. Anterior view normal, though suggestion of slight enlargement of left hilum.

Fig. 350.—Same case (left lateral-view tomogram). The shadow of the neoplasm can now be clearly seen. Male aged 57 years. Recently a small haemoptysis. Bronchoscopy and biopsy revealed a poorly differentiated bronchial carcinoma.

Greatly enlarged subcarinal glands may be seen as a subcarinal shadow in a posterior-view tomogram with sufficient exposure to see through the heart shadow. The tomogram may also show a medial concave curve of the right main bronchus, which normally has a straight medial border, or even some narrowing of its lumen or that of the left main bronchus by pressure from the enlarged glands. In a mid-line lateral-view tomogram, enlarged subcarinal glands will show a 2–3 cm shadow just below the tracheal transradiancy.

LATERAL-VIEW TOMOGRAMS

A careful inspection of the posterior-view tomograms will generally show whether there is an abnormal shadow at all, and whether it is vascular or independent of the vessels, but in a difficult case, lateral-view tomograms are indicated. These will generally give further evidence, especially on the left side where the sweep of the pulmonary artery round the bronchus gives such a characteristic shadow that it is easily identified and distinguished from any additional shadows close to, but separate from it representing pathological tissue. On the right side, enlarged hilar glands tend to be lateral to the vessels in a posterior view and below the main vessel shadow in a lateral view.

VALUE OF THE METHOD

Bearing the difficulties of interpretation in mind, there is no doubt that hilar glandular enlargements can be detected earlier and with greater certainty in tomograms than in plain radiographs.

If the hilar regions are much obscured by overlying pathological lung shadows, as in some cases of sarcoidosis, the tomograms may be the only reliable radiographic method of showing or excluding hilar glandular enlargement.

Tomograms will show the presence or absence of calcifications in the hilar glands with greater certainty than the plain radiographs, and at the same time will reveal the relationship of these to the larger bronchi.

DEMONSTRATION OF THE MAIN VESSELS IN THE HILAR REGIONS OR LUNGS

The demonstration in tomograms of the main vessels in the hilar regions or lungs is rarely required in cardiac conditions now that increasing familiarity of the vessel patterns in the plain radiographs of normal persons and those suffering from cardiac disease enables the observer to recognize with some assurance upper-lobe blood diversion or general vessel dilatation. However, when an abnormal band-like shadow is seen, as in the scimitar syndrome (Fig. 197), or in other types of anomalous pulmonary venous drainage, tomograms are of value to confirm the vascular nature of the shadow and, if possible, to define its course. They are also indicated when an abnormally large hilar shadow is seen, but there is some doubt whether this is due to vessels or to glandular enlargements.

In obstructive airways disease with bullae it is possible in some cases to see whether a large transradiant area represents an empty air space and thus a type I or II bulla, or whether there are vessels within it (indicating a type III bulla), or an area of emphysematous lung (see p. 130). In unilateral transradiancy with air trapping tomograms may be needed to confirm that the small hilar vessels have a normal pattern with a lobar distribution. They may be indicated to measure the size of the azygos vein which can be seen in a posterior-view tomogram adjacent to the distal end of the right main bronchus. The azygos vein may be dilated because the inferior vena cava is draining into it, or because there is increased flow as in portal hypertension, or because it is obstructed just before joining the superior vena cava. A circular shadow near the hilum can be caused by an aneurysm of a branch of the pulmonary artery, and tomograms may show its close relation to a vessel shadow, but confirmation of the condition by angiography is nearly always needed.

EXTENT AND POSSIBLE NATURE OF ABNORMAL MEDIASTINAL SHADOWS

The exact extent of an abnormal mediastinal shadow can often be seen in the plain radiographs, but sometimes the shadow is so small and indistinct that confirmation of its existence and a demonstration of its exact extent by tomography are indicated. In a suspected thymic tumour associated with myasthenia gravis, the confirmation and exact delineation of the shadow will influence the decision whether to remove the normal thymus or irradiate the tumour. In such a case the tomograms should be taken as lateral views.

When the shadow is obvious there may still be doubt as to whether it represents a tumour or an aneurysm, and before resorting to angiography the evidence from tomograms should be carefully considered. An aneurysm can usually be excluded if the aortic outline is seen independent of the tumour shadow; or if abnormal high-density shadows are detected within the shadow, such as bone or teeth, suggesting a dermoid cyst; or if deep central calcification is seen, calcification being only occasionally present in an aneurysm, and then nearly always peripheral.

In these difficult cases both lateral-view and posterior-view tomograms are desirable. They may be taken simultaneously with a barium swallow, or with an associated pneumomediastinum. A pneumomediastinum can be produced by the presacral introduction of oxygen as used to outline the suprarenal, or it may be injected direct through a cannula inserted via the suprasternal route. If the patient is kept sitting up, some of the gas will diffuse around the mediastinal structures. In retrosternal tumours the demonstration of the posterior limit of the shadow by tomograms may be of help to the radiotherapist if the posterior margin is not clearly seen in the plain lateral view.

DEMONSTRATION OF CALCIFICATIONS IN THE HEART VALVES

Calcification of the heart valves is often difficult to see by conventional fluoroscopy, though is easy to see with image intensification. If this equipment is not available, there is still a place for tomography. The left posterior-oblique view is the most satisfactory for this purpose, and the tomograms should be very well exposed. Owing to unavoidable heart movement the image will be blurred to some extent, but the intracardiac position of the calcification can be firmly established from the layer identification.

ADDITIONAL VIEWS IN SUSPECTED LESION OF THE BONES OF THE THORAX

Tomograms of a rib, the sternum, or the thoracic spine are indicated if a local lesion is suspected in one of these parts but no abnormality can be seen in the plain radiographs; or if a lesion is seen in the plain radiographs, but is rather indistinct, so that there is an element of doubt concerning either the presence or the nature of the lesion.

Tomograms may sometimes show erosion of bone from a nearby peripheral bronchial carcinoma or secondary deposit before these can be seen in the plain radiographs. Similarly early erosion and periosteal new bone due to an inflammatory lesion may also be shown at an early stage by this method. Details of the bone changes may be more clearly seen in tomograms which may aid the diagnosis in a difficult case.

Sometimes an opacity is suspected of being in the lung, but is unexpectedly found on tomography to be associated with a rib or vertebral lesion.

CHAPTER 12

THE TIME FACTOR IN X-RAY DIAGNOSIS AND COMPARISON OF RADIOGRAPHS OF DIFFERENT DATES

THE TIMING OF INITIAL RADIOGRAPHS

AN INITIAL radiograph is rarely premature in chest disease and in an adult may be taken as soon as convenient. This allays the patient's anxiety, avoids any later procrastination, which in a bronchial carcinoma might be disastrous, and at worst produces a normal radiograph by comparison with which even slight abnormalities may be detected at a later date.

In babies and children rather more discretion is advisable. For instance in suspected pulmonary tuberculosis there is usually a time interval of some 6 weeks between the contact with a known case and the appearance of a shadow in the radiograph due to primary tuberculosis, and it is not necessary in these circumstances to take a radiograph until at least 6 weeks after the initial contact, or until the Mantoux reaction has become positive.

The state of the patient and availability of the x-ray apparatus must of course be taken into account. A pleural effusion occurring in a patient who is being treated at home or in a ward remote from x-ray facilities would not justify moving the patient at an early stage to the x-ray department or summoning an external mobile unit. On the other hand if a ward mobile unit is easily available, then the radiograph may be taken with this. Following a severe but controlled haemoptysis, disturbance of the patient for the sake of an early initial radiograph would not be justified even if good radiographic facilities were available.

THE TIME FACTOR AS A HELP IN DIAGNOSIS

In some cases when the diagnosis of the nature of the shadow in the initial radiograph is in doubt, the time interval before changes can be seen in serial radiographs may be of some help. When a large homogeneous shadow is seen indicating a lobar consolidation, there may at first be doubt on clinical grounds whether it represents a tuberculous lesion or some other infective lesion. In the absence of therapy directed towards healing a tuberculous focus, rapid resolution would suggest a non-tuberculous consolidation. Sometimes, however, an untreated relatively asymptomatic coccal consolidation in a child may persist for some weeks, only to resolve rapidly following antibiotic therapy.

Unfortunately the time interval does not help in differentiating the circular shadow of a circumscribed tuberculous focus from a small bronchial carcinoma or other type of neoplasm. Either may grow relatively rapidly or comparatively slowly, and a period of observation is not justified in order to make the diagnosis if resection is contemplated.

Whether a radiograph is an original one or a follow up of a previous one, its date must be given due weight when the x-ray appearances are correlated with the clinical and pathological findings. The date interval between comparative radiographs is often of importance and may either reveal, within a certain range, the date of origin of a new shadow, or give some indication of the time taken for an existing shadow to enlarge or decrease in size.

THE TIME FACTOR IN TUBERCULOUS LESIONS

DIFFICULTIES OF JUDGING DATE OF ORIGIN FROM INITIAL RADIOGRAPH

In most tuberculous lesions the initial or first radiograph cannot indicate the probable date of origin of the lesion. A woolly looking ill-defined shadow suggesting a lesion of recent origin may nevertheless have been present for many months, and may already have begun to regress; while a better-defined shadow may have been present for years, or may just as well be of quite recent origin.

Even the presence of calcifications may be an uncertain pointer to the age of the lesion. It is unusual to see calcification in a lesion much under a year after the appearance of a low-density shadow, and it may be delayed as much as 2 or 3 years.

Evidence of lobar shrinkage, line shadows, or stellate shadows will suggest that some of the lesions are long standing, but one of the features of tuberculosis is that foci of quite different dates of origin may coexist in close proximity, so that the presence of some shadows suggesting long-standing foci will not exclude the presence of adjacent shadows of much more recent foci. Sometimes the more recent foci may be invisible in the radiograph either because they are too small, or because they are obscured by superimposed shadows of the denser older lesions.

DIFFICULTIES OF ASSESSING STATE OF ACTIVITY FROM THE INITIAL RADIOGRAPH

That the initial radiograph is of value in drawing attention to a clinically unsuspected tuberculous lesion is well recognized; it is also of great value in showing the extent, character, and distribution of the lesions, and forms a base line from which subsequent progress can be observed.

The initial radiograph is usually of no value in assessing the activity of the lesion, which can only be revealed by the clinical and pathological findings, and by changes in subsequent radiographs taken at suitable intervals. Even the word " active " is rarely justified in the x-ray report on the initial radiograph. Obvious cavities may be present, and yet the disease may be stabilized for the present. Occasionally, in fact, a cavity is seen in the radiograph, which on resection is found to be epithelialized and without any histological evidence of active tuberculosis. Such a finding however is generally only seen after prolonged chemotherapy.

A calcified and apparently healed lesion may one day discharge into a bronchus or a vessel, so that the demonstration in an initial radiograph of a dense shadow suggesting quiescence may nevertheless be the immediate prelude to an acute spread. Such a shadow may also represent a broncholith, the tuberculous bronchiectasis being demonstrated only in subsequent bronchograms or tomograms.

The finding of tubercle bacilli in the sputum is not uncommon in cases where the appearance of the shadows has led to an x-ray report saying " old healed tuberculous foci ".

It is therefore apparent that any conclusions based on the initial radiograph about whether the shadow represents an active, stationary, or healed lesion are at best only guesses based on probability, and will therefore be found to have a high propensity to observer error if the patient's progress is followed up. Particular caution should be observed if the radiograph shows some shadows of doubtful significance and the patient is being put on steroid therapy. In such a case a second radiograph after 6–12 weeks should be a routine procedure.

RATE OF PROGRESS OR REGRESSION OF TUBERCULOUS FOCI

A curious feature of many tuberculous lesions is the uneven manner in which they progress or regress. It is a common experience to observe a lesion at monthly intervals for a long period during which there is no change, and then, sometimes without any obvious alteration in the clinical picture, to find that the existing shadow has enlarged, or a new shadow has appeared. After this incident there may be no further change in the radiographs for several months. It is sometimes possible to witness the exact onset of this period of activity if by chance, or because of a clinical suspicion of spread, radiographs are taken within a few days of each other. In one example a second radiograph was taken owing to a clerical error only 4 days after the first, and showed extensive new shadowing in the right upper zone due to a local spread from pre-existing tuberculous lesions in this region.

The same uneven rate of progression may occur with a small circular shadow, with a large circular shadow, with a group of shadows, and with or without the demonstration of a cavity.

This timetable so frequently seen in tuberculosis, in which there is an incident with spread occupying a day or two followed by a very much longer period when the lesion is stabilized, is an important factor in the diagnosis or assessment of the lesion in many cases.

TIMING OF SERIAL RADIOGRAPHS IN TUBERCULOSIS

In fixing the time interval between serial radiographs in tuberculosis two principles should be rigorously followed. First that it is better to have too short than too long an interval between radiographs, and second that if the symptoms or signs change, the indications will be the same as for an initial radiograph, and a new one should be taken soon—regardless of when the next serial radiograph had been planned.

Take, for example, a patient with tuberculosis, whose lesion is apparently under control, shadows unchanged and radiographs being taken at 3–6-monthly intervals. A fortnight after the last radiograph, he develops a cold which persists for some days, perhaps with a trace of sputum. This would justify putting forward the next radiograph from 3 months to 3 weeks after the last one.

These remarks are only relevant to the pre-chemotherapeutic era and nowadays most cases of tuberculosis will be given chemotherapy; if this is the case a further radiograph need not be taken until 3 months after treatment has been started, unless in the interval there is clinical evidence of deterioration. If all goes well, further radiographs at 6, 12 and 24 months will be adequate. Thereafter, if resolution was satisfactory, further radiographs need not be taken unless there is some clinical evidence to indicate the need for them.

Persistent cavitation with a negative sputum may be an indication for an annual radiograph for a few years in case a mycetoma develops in the cavity (see pp. 81 and 127).

In an adult the length of time during which to watch a symptomless small (minimal) lesion presumed to be tuberculous is difficult to fix. It should not be less than 3 years, for in a series of such patients observed by Springett (1956) enlargement or local spread of the shadows was observed in a large proportion of cases in radiographs taken during the third year of observation, the appearances having been unchanged during the previous 2 years. Of the patients who still showed no changes in the radiographs after the third year of observation, roughly 2 per cent showed evidence of activity as late as the fifth year, a figure which is not greatly above that which could have been expected had the initial radiograph been normal.

After a tuberculous pleural effusion with no x-ray evidence of underlying lung foci, observation by serial radiographs should be carried out for 5 years (Thompson, 1947), unless chemotherapy has been given, when routine observation beyond 2 years is unnecessary.

TIMING OF RADIOGRAPHS AFTER BACTERIAL OR VIRAL PNEUMONIA

In a patient with a bacterial or viral pneumonia, a posterior and lateral view should be taken as soon as it can be arranged, if necessary with the mobile ward unit. This may not be practicable with a patient being treated at home, but if the patient is in hospital, then the radiographs should be taken soon after admission. These initial radiographs will confirm the site and extent of any consolidation, and will act as a base line which will be useful in revealing the degree of resolution or, if things are not going well, will aid in the detection of complications such as an empyema or lung abscess.

If the clinical response following antibiotics is good, no further radiograph is necessary immediately, but in a young person a further radiograph should be taken in about 3 weeks to confirm resolution is complete. In a patient aged over 40 years, especially if a male and a heavy smoker, the interval before the second radiograph is taken should be extended to 6 weeks. The reason for this is that there may be an underlying carcinoma of the bronchus. Between weeks 2 and 4 the antibiotic therapy for the acute incident will have caused resolution of any distal inflammatory changes, while by week 6 these will usually return, and the presence of residual shadowing will be an indication for bronchoscopy.

If the clinical response is poor, then earlier radiographs will be indicated. Persistent consolidation in spite of antibiotics will suggest a viral pneumonia or even tuberculosis. A transradiant area, perhaps with a fluid level below will indicate a lung abscess.

A pleural effusion will cast a shadow as described on page 35. This will usually be additional to any shadows seen in the initial radiograph, unless the patient has been ill for some days before it was taken.

TIMING OF RADIOGRAPHS AFTER SURGICAL PROCEDURES

The timing of radiographs after the various surgical procedures used in the treatment of chest diseases depends on the wishes of the surgeon in charge. The reason for taking such radiographs should be made known to those concerned with the immediate post-operative care of the patient, so that in the absence of the surgeon, his deputy will know when it will be necessary to alter the fixed routine of the thoracic unit in this respect.

A rough guide to the timing and indications for radiographs in the immediate post-operative period is shown in Tables 11 and 12.

After exploratory thoracotomy, and many operations on the heart and great vessels, the indications are much the same as after lobectomy. Care should be taken to ensure that the final pre-discharge post-operative radiograph is a standard anterior view, so that the heart size can be compared with the pre-operative radiographs, and with later post-operative ones.

TABLE 11

Radiology after Some Surgical Procedures; Clinical Condition Satisfactory

Operation	Timing of radiographs	Purpose of radiograph	Clinical significance of x-ray findings, and possible action indicated
Pneumonectomy	24–28 hours	To show quantity of fluid	If on tube drainage, should be no fluid. If not, fluid should be below bronchial stump.
		To show mediastinal displacement	If excess, introduce air into pneumonectomy space.
	4th or 5th day	Similar	Similar.
	10th day	Similar	Similar.
	3rd week	Similar	Preferably no air, or very little. Mediastinal displacement probably considerable by now.
Lobectomy	24 hours	To show re-expansion of remaining lobe(s)	If poor, increase suction drainage. Measures to clear bronchus such as expectoration. Radiograph next day to see if effective. Physiotherapist.
		To show quantity of pleural fluid	If much, aspiration.
	4th or 5th day	Similar (special watch for contralateral spread)	Similar.
	10th day	Similar, but also take lateral view	Ensure no anterior or posterior pockets of fluid.
	No immediate further x-rays unless re-expansion incomplete, or residual fluid or complications present		
Mediastinal lesions	24 hours	To exclude pneumothorax	
	3 days	To exclude pleural or mediastinal effusion	
	Before discharge	Routine radiograph	Base line for future comparison.
Cardiac surgery	24 hours	To exclude pneumothorax; good lung re-expansion	
	48 hours	To exclude enlarging heart shadow	Might cause tamponade.
	72 hours	Similar	
	3rd–5th day	To exclude pulmonary oedema	Improve respiration, avoid excessive O_2 concentration.
	About 10 days or before discharge	To confirm lungs clear	

TABLE 12

SOME COMPLICATIONS OCCURRING AFTER SOME SURGICAL PROCEDURES, AND THE X-RAY CHANGES
LIKELY TO BE SEEN WITH THEM

Operation	Clinical findings	Possible x-ray findings
Pneumonectomy	High fever, rapid pulse and distress	Too much fluid.
		Contralateral lesion, such as atelectasis.
Lobectomy	Fever, rapid pulse and distress	To much fluid. Atelectasis of remaining lobe.
	Restriction of movement, rapid pulse and distress —usually on the 2nd or 3rd day. (Less likely in tuberculosis than in bronchiectasis, as there is less secretion in the upper respiratory tract or bronchi)	Contralateral lesion.
Cardiac surgery	Poor state of patient	Pulmonary oedema.
		Enlarging heart.
	Drop in Hb level	Fluid (blood): extrapleural, mediastinal. Enlarging heart.

COMPARISON OF RADIOGRAPHS TAKEN ON DIFFERENT DATES

Serial observation of lesions being one of the most important uses of radiology in chest diseases, it is important to make full use of the method and not to undermine its validity with avoidable mistakes.

All the radiographs should be of first-rate quality or, if a difference in quality is unavoidable, at least amenable to accurate comparison. If possible, and in the absence of unavoidable alterations, the shadows should bear the same orientation to each other in each film. Ideally the radiographs should be inspected, and a careful assessment of any change made by at least two observers.

CAUSES OF OBSERVER ERRORS

The comparison of shadows in two radiographs taken of the same chest at different times is often considered a simple matter, and the interpretation is often perfunctory and hurried. The fact that it is not easy is shown by observer-error tests carried out recently with two series of comparative radiographs. It was found that there was a considerable difference of opinion when it came to deciding whether the condition was better, unchanged, or worse, not only between the different observers, but between the same observer re-reading the radiographs on another occasion.

One of the series consisted of a very large number of radiographs showing small (minimal) non-cavitated symptomless tuberculous foci. A conference between the observers was held after the test to discuss the considerable number of radiographs about which there had been a difference of opinion. It was decided that there were not many errors due to shadows being missed either locally or in another zone, but that there were a great number of disagreements (10 per cent) about whether shadows which had been seen by all observers had become smaller or larger between one radiograph and another. These disagreements were in the main put down to differences, from one comparative radiograph to the next, in the orientation of the shadows in relation to each other and the (posterior) ribs. There were practically no disagreements which could be attributed to differences in exposure or dark-room technique, although the differences in the quality of the radiographs were sometimes very considerable. It was agreed that where some shadows had resolved but new ones had appeared, the condition should be considered to have deteriorated, but even with this help there was a small residue of cases in which the disagreement could not be resolved.

In the second series, the comparative radiographs showed a more complicated pattern of shadows, and the same persistent disagreement was found on an even larger scale.

A SUGGESTED ROUTINE METHOD FOR COMPARING SERIAL RADIOGRAPHS

If it is done in a careful systematic manner, comparison of shadows though not always easy may yet be consistent and fairly accurate. It is essential that the radiographs should be viewed together side by side, and for this purpose a suitable viewing box, or two such boxes, should be available giving an even illumination of both radiographs. A routine inspection can then be made on the following lines.

Identity of patient

The identity of the patient should be confirmed not only by checking the name and number on both radiographs but by observation of some obvious anatomical landmark such as a cervical rib, bifurcated rib, unusual shape or notch on any rib, degree of calcification of the costal cartilages, and the size of any extrathoracic soft-tissue shadows, particularly breast shadows.

Dates of radiographs

The dates should be noted, and the radiographs arranged in their date order.

Gross discrepancy in quality

Any gross discrepancy in the general density or contrast of the films should be noted and taken into account when interpreting the films. If it is such that it is likely to make comparison difficult, it may be possible to reject the last radiograph and take another of more appropriate quality to replace it, or if the more recent previous ones showed no change, choose a more appropriate one from amongst these to match the last radiograph.

Orientation of subject

The lateral orientation of the subject in the two radiographs should be compared by noting the position of the sternal ends of the clavicles in relation to the vertebral margins (*see* p. 15).

Centring

Finally the centring should be compared by noting the distance of the top of the apical transradiancy from the clavicle on one side, any difference indicating either that the x-ray beam is centred higher in one film than the other, or that the patient is leaning farther forwards. A more delicate test is to count the number of posterior parts of the rib shadows lying above the level of the clavicle and noting any difference in the two radiographs. Here again it may be necessary to take further radiographs so that comparison can be made between radiographs in which the orientation of the shadow to the x-ray beam is similar.

CONFIRMATION OF DIFFERENCES SEEN

When changes are seen which may be an important factor in deciding on the next phase of treatment, it is often wise to confirm the appearances with different views, perhaps a posterior view and a lateral view, and if necessary a tomogram.

When the differences are slight, it is often useful to compare the last radiograph not only with the previous one, but with another one taken some time before that, so that a slowly progressive rather insidious increase in shadowing may be seen more easily.

It is not uncommon to find that a shadow has increased from 1 to 4 cm, the x-ray reports stating the appearances are unchanged throughout a large series of radiographs over a period of time. This is because the increase in size of the shadow between successive pairs of radiographs was so slight it was not noticed. However, if any one of these radiographs after the first pair had been compared with the initial radiograph, the increase in size of the lesion would have been detected.

APPENDIX

SOME HINTS ON X-RAY TECHNIQUE

THE ANTERIOR VIEW

EXPOSURE FACTORS

THE STANDARD technique for the anterior view chest radiograph for the past 33 years has been that of using a 4-valve generator, a rotating anode tube with a focal spot some 2 mm in size, 300–400 mA, 60–70 kVp, and a time of 0·04–0·08 second, at a tube film distance of 6 feet or 2 metres, the patient standing with the breath suspended in deep inspiration.

There were of course many minor variations of this technique, and in some cases a shorter time was used. The time clock in many of the older sets did not allow of an exposure time of less than 0·04 second, being inaccurate at a greater speed, but with the modern type of electronic and other timers, much shorter exposures can be used, and thus advantage taken of the improvement in screen speed and so on.

Using 120–140 kVp, 300 mA, high-speed tungstate intensifying screens and fast films, it is possible to cut the exposure time down to 0·01–0·003 second. On comparing the resultant radiographs with radiographs of the same adult patient taken with the old standard technique, the margins of the heart shadow were sharper using the short time and high kVp, but the clarity or sharpness of outline of the vessels and other shadows showed very little difference. Since the vessel shadows were visible through the heart shadow in the majority of those taken at the lower kVp there was no great advantage in this respect in the use of the high kVp, while the general greyness of the radiographs taken with the high kVp made detection of small shadows somewhat more difficult. Each radiologist will no doubt make up his own mind on this issue as the modern sets become available, bearing in mind the particular features it is necessary to see with clarity for the x-ray diagnosis, and making a practical rather than a theoretical decision.

USE OF FINE-FOCUS X-RAY TUBES AND CLEARING GRIDS

In thin persons and those of medium build, the vessels and other shadows will stand out more clearly if the effective focal spot of the x-ray tube is 1 instead of 2 mm, even though this will mean a reduction in the maximum milliamperes which can be used, and thus an increase in time. With the high-speed tungstate screens and fast films, exposures of 0·04 second will still be possible. The use of an even smaller focal spot does not seem to be helpful in routine chest radiography owing to the further increase in time which is needed. If an x-ray tube is available with a focal spot of 0·3 mm, a radiograph may be taken with this for the confirmation or exclusion of a few pin-point or nodular shadows in a doubtful case (*see also* magnification technique).

For very large or obese patients it is helpful to mitigate the effects of scatter radiation. This may be done by means of a clearing grid which if given a reciprocating motion will produce no grid lines even with exposures of 0·04 second or less. When using a grid, a kVp of 100–120 will give satisfactory radiographs provided that the grid is designed to work at these kilovoltages. The use of a fixed grid is of doubtful value since in many chest radiographs examination of the image with a magnifying glass is necessary, and the magnified grid lines may cause too much interference with the lung shadows.

If no clearing grid is available, reasonably clear vessel shadows will be seen in an obese patient if the tube film distance is increased to 3 metres, and the patient placed 15 cm away from the cassette. Much of the scatter will be absorbed in the layer of air between the two. The best results will be obtained with a kVp of between 90 and 110.

TECHNIQUE FOR USE WITH LOW-COST EQUIPMENT

In some countries the amount of money available for the medical services is limited, and an undue proportion cannot be spent on elaborate x-ray equipment in all clinics if simpler apparatus will suffice in some. For many purposes an adequate chest radiograph can be obtained with a less expensive low output unit, giving 60–100 mA unrectified, at 60–70 kVp. With fast screens, an exposure of 0·1 second will then suffice for an average adult. A fine-focus rotating anode tube should be used. It may be necessary to send a few patients elsewhere for radiography with more powerful units, but the quality of the radiographs will be adequate in most cases.

POSITION OF PATIENT WHEN STANDING

The body should above all be in an unstrained position, otherwise slight movement may occur and the vertebral borders of the scapulae are likely to be superimposed on the lung fields. In order to encourage a relaxed position, the distance between the top of the x-ray film and the bar on which the chin rests should be kept as short as possible, and should not exceed 2 cm, otherwise the neck will either be hyperextended when the chin is over the top of the bar, or the apices will be too far from the film because the chin cannot be placed well forwards. There should be a free space of at least 10 cm above and behind the cassette so that the chin and head can be placed well forwards.

If the backs of the hands rest lightly on the postero-lateral parts of the iliac crests, the elbows can be placed well forwards so as to bring the scapulae laterally and well forward. This position ensures more relaxation than if the thumb and index finger are separated and grip round the sides of the iliac crests.

CENTRING OF THE X-RAY BEAM

The x-ray beam should in theory be centred on the fourth thoracic vertebra, but in practice centring on a fixed level of the cassette (usually a third of its length from the top) is much easier and saves time. Such a mark, though not as accurate in relation to the patient as an anatomical landmark (assuming one can be easily felt) is nevertheless reasonably consistent, being a fixed distance from the patient's chin which rests on the top of the cassette.

The correct orientation of the x-ray tube in relation to the cassette can be obtained if suitable scales giving distances from floor level are available on or near the cassette holder and the column supporting the tube. A second method is the use of a simple sighting device fixed on to the tube, by means of which the tube is aimed at the correct level on the cassette. A third method is to have the cassette holder connected to the tube by a " link cable " which ensures that the two retain their relation to each other when moved up or down. The design of the link cable must be such that it can be rapidly disconnected or neutralized if another relationship between cassette and tube is required, as in radiography of children when a smaller film is used lower down in the cassette holder, or for a standard lateral view when the tube is directed towards the middle of the cassette, or for some special view taken with the tube at an angle.

TECHNIQUE WITH CHILDREN

Children can generally co-operate as well as adults especially if a little time is spent gaining their confidence and giving them practice in taking a deep breath and holding it for a few seconds. If they are so young that they cannot do this, quite satisfactory radiographs can be obtained even while they are breathing quietly provided the exposure time is kept short (not longer than 0·04 second).

The time of exposure for a given milliamperage can be shortened by raising the kilovolts, but it is best to use a value of kilovolts which will give the degree of contrast in the radiograph best suited to the particular observer. A satisfactory radiograph can be obtained in 0·003 seconds, 300–600 mA at a kVp in the region of 90–100.

There is no great objection to shortening the time by reducing the distance and keeping the kilovoltage in the region of 60, the milliamperes 300–400, and the time as short as the set will do with accuracy. A reduction from 2 to 1·5 metres will allow the exposure time to be halved. In small children a shadow even near the back of the chest is not very far from the film, so that it is not likely to be indistinct on this account.

Very young children are best radiographed sitting on a small seat and holding on to a bar fitted just behind and projecting to either side of the cassette. The breathing should be watched and the exposure made towards the end of the inspiratory phase.

TECHNIQUE WITH BABIES

A baby is best radiographed sitting with its back to the cassette on a suitably padded seat. An anterior view is often not impossible, but the baby is more easily controlled and kept in a straight position when sitting with its back to the cassette. The mother, if available, can hold the baby's arms up against the sides of the head and thus control both the body and head. It is an advantage to have a restraining band over the knees and thighs, so that the mother can exert a gentle upward pull against it to straighten the back and diminish the tendency of the body to fold forwards with a kyphotic curve.

Restraint of babies should not be undertaken by nurses or assistants working regularly in the x-ray department owing to the possibility that they might receive an excessive dose of x-rays if they were to hold many babies during a week. Done only occasionally, the support or restraint of a patient is of course quite harmless.

If a baby is very restless when sitting up, a supine view should be taken, with the cassette covered with a warm soft towel and the baby lying on it. With this view special care must be taken to position the baby so that the clavicles are symmetrical. Slight rotation results in considerable displacement of the mediastinal contents, giving a confusingly wide mediastinal shadow—a feature which is further accentuated if the diaphragm is high because the exposure is taken during forced expiration, often with the child crying (Fig. 353). In such circumstances a more normal appearance may be seen in a subsequent radiograph taken a few seconds later with less rotation and during inspiration (Fig. 354).

Fluoroscopy is of value when examining babies because a normal mediastinal shadow may be seen during the brief moment of full inspiration.

ANTERIOR VIEW TAKEN WITH PATIENT LYING DOWN

A radiograph taken with an adult patient lying down is often useful to displace the breast and nipple shadow or to show the disappearance of a suspected fluid level. The patient may be supine, but an anterior view taken with the patient prone will be more comparable with the routine anterior view taken standing. One end of the cassette should be raised 3 cm by means of a small sand bag, towel or block so that the patient's chin can lie comfortably above the cassette (Fig. 352). The position of

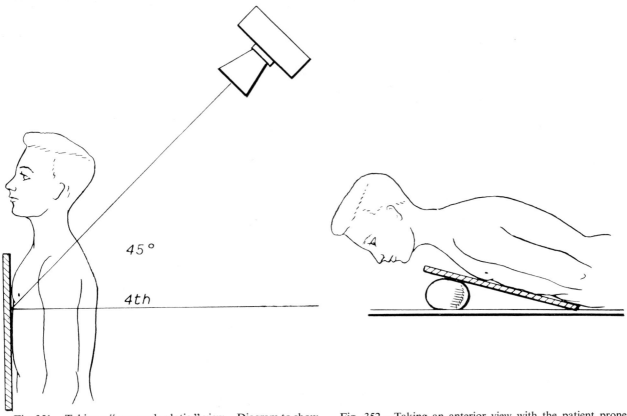

45°

4th

Fig. 351.—Taking a " reverse lordotic " view. Diagram to show the position of the cassette and the patient, and the 45 degree downward angulation of the x-ray tube.

Fig. 352.—Taking an anterior view with the patient prone. Diagram to show how slight elevation of one end of the cassette makes the patient's position comparable to that of a standing patient during routine anterior-view radiography.

the patient's chin, arms and hands can thus be the same as in the standing view. Unless a low table is available, the tube-film distance may have to be less—if a distance of at least 1·5 metres cannot be obtained in any other way, it may be necessary in some cases to put a rug on the floor, and place the cassette on this.

An anterior (P-A) view with the x-ray beam horizontal to the floor, and the patient lying on one side with his back to it, is useful at times, particularly to show the shift of the shadow if a small effusion (Fig. 49) or intracavitary loose body is suspected.

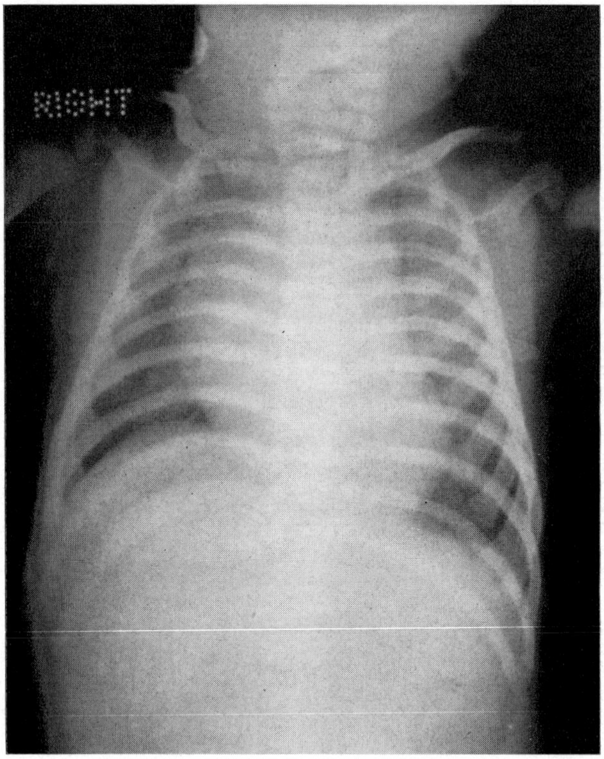

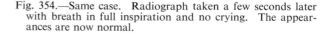

Fig. 353.—Radiograph of a normal child taken during expiration and crying. High position of diaphragm and wide central shadow.

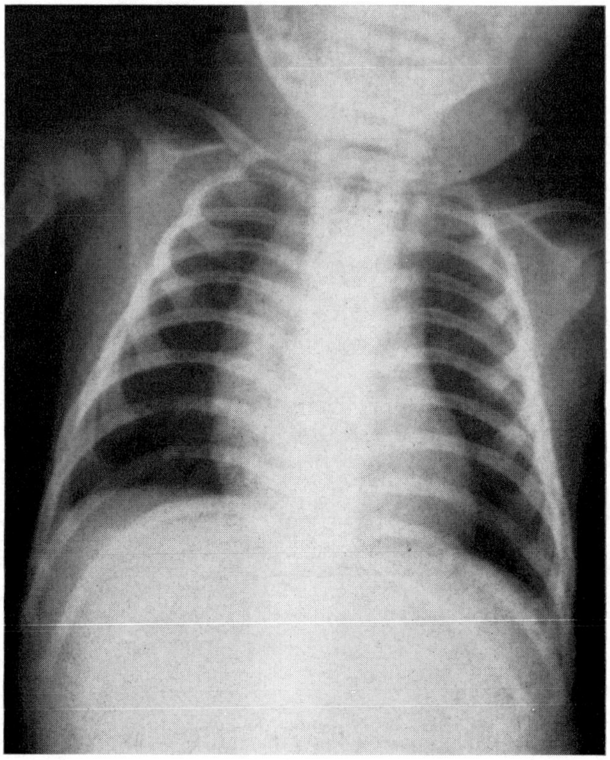

Fig. 354.—Same case. Radiograph taken a few seconds later with breath in full inspiration and no crying. The appearances are now normal.

LORDOTIC AND SIMILAR VIEWS

A lordotic view is taken with the x-ray beam horizontal and the patient sitting and leaning backwards towards the cassette at an angle of some 30 degrees, if possible with the back arched—hence the name lordotic view. The position is uncomfortable, and difficult to hold, while the more the back is arched the greater the tendency for the scapulae to move medially and be superimposed on the lung fields.

A much more satisfactory procedure giving an almost identical projection is for the patient to stand facing the cassette as in a standard anterior view, and the x-ray tube to be raised and angled downwards 45 degrees and centred over the spine of the second thoracic vertebra (Fig. 351). It is usually necessary to reduce the distance between the film and tube column to 1·5 metres since the vertical elevation of the tube may not otherwise be sufficient. This view not only serves to show the shadow of a shrunken middle lobe as clearly as a lordotic view, but is also satisfactory as an additional view of the apices which are projected below the shadow of the clavicles.

If the patient cannot sit or stand, a reverse view may be obtained with the patient supine and the x-ray beam angled 45 degrees towards the head and centred just above the xiphisternum.

APICAL VIEWS

An apical view may be taken as described above with the x-ray beam tilted 45 degrees towards the feet, or it may be taken with the tube angled 30 degrees upwards towards the head and centred on the spine of the sixth thoracic vertebra, thus throwing the shadow of the lung apex well above the clavicle.

ANTERO-POSTERIOR VIEW

An antero-posterior view may at times show shadows invisible in a postero-anterior view. If possible it should be taken with the hands and arms in the same position as the standard view to keep the shadow of the scapula as far as possible clear of the lung field.

This view will often confirm the presence of very small or indistinct shadows better than a magnification technique, or the use of a very low kilovoltage.

THE LATERAL VIEW

A lateral view with a fit patient presents no particular problems. There is a tendency to over-expose the film and then under-develop it, thus producing a radiograph with poor contrast, or to under-expose and produce a radiograph with insufficient blackening. Assuming standard development, a well-exposed radiograph will be easier to interpret than an under-exposed one.

An average patient will require 300 mA, 70 kVp, 0·1 second at a tube-film distance of 1·5–2 metres. An old or ill patient may be rather unsteady but will tend to sway less if radiographed sitting instead of standing. A fit patient can be radiographed with the arms held almost vertically, but an ill patient may find it easier to raise them only to a right angle, and clasp the hands behind the head with the elbows parallel. In this position or with the help of a bar fixed at a suitable level in front of and above the cassette which the patient can grasp, radiographs free from avoidable movement can be obtained.

In fat subjects a Potter–Bucky diaphragm or fixed grid will result in a radiograph with more contrast, but with many kinds of grid there is a slight loss of sharpness of the image, which tends to diminish the advantages of the increased contrast.

THE OBLIQUE VIEW

For an oblique view the patient should be positioned at an angle of rotation most suitable for the purpose in hand. A collapsed lower lobe or calcified heart valve is best seen at 45 degrees rotation, whilst the left oblique view for a bronchogram, or for the heart and aorta, is best taken at 60–70 degrees (that is, biased towards a lateral view). Frequently the most appropriate angle can only be determined by preliminary fluoroscopy.

MAGNIFICATION OF THE IMAGE

Magnification of the image is very helpful when there is doubt whether some very small circular shadows are present or not, as in a doubtful case of pneumoconiosis, small tuberculous lesions, sarcoidosis, or any other lung lesion likely to give small indistinct shadows. It is also useful for the identification of the hair line of a fissure.

It is most easily done with a suitable magnifying glass giving an image 2–4 times the natural size. Only a limited degree of magnification is possible before the inherently granular appearance of the film emulsion becomes indistinguishable from possible pathological shadows.

Direct enlargement of the shadows can be achieved by placing the film 30–45 cm from the patient and by working with a fine-focus x-ray tube at a short tube-film distance of 1·5 metres or less, but this is accompanied by considerable unsharpness or blurring of outline of the shadows. Using a standard x-ray tube with a fine focus of about 1 mm the enlarged image of a small 0·5–2-mm lesion is no easier to see than one in a standard radiograph viewed through a magnifying glass. By using an x-ray tube with a very fine focal spot of 0·3 mm, a more satisfactory image may be obtained by direct enlargement. In neonates or very young children magnification can be obtained using a 0·3 mm focal spot x-ray tube, a tube-film distance of 90 cm (36 inches), with the baby lying on a thin support 45 cm (18 inches) from the film. Factors such as 55 kVp, 160 mA, 0·03 second fast screens may be suitable. Using this technique the lung vessels can be seen much more clearly and certainly than in the conventional radiograph taken at the same time.

IDENTIFICATION MARKS ON FILMS AND SEPARATION OF KEY FILMS

It is worth while giving some thought to the details of dating and marking films, and also to the separation of key films out of the large quantity of chest x-rays often taken of one patient. These things enable the radiological features of a particular case to be grasped with ease and comfort without irritating distractions.

RADIOGRAPHING OF LEAD NUMERAL DATES

The dating of chest radiographs should be bold and clear, so that the time interval between each of a series can be readily appreciated. Lead dating numerals (1–2 cm high) can be radiographed on to the film at the same time as the patient's chest (Fig. 86). If these numerals are placed in a fixed position to one side and in front of the cassette, they will also serve to show in a case of doubt whether the view taken was antero-posterior or postero-anterior, right or left lateral, and, in a known standard postero-anterior view whether there is any transposition of the thoracic viscera. The radiographed lead lettering is on the whole easier to read than lettering made on the film with a pin-point perforating machine or written on by hand.

PHOTOGRAPHIC PRINTING OF PATIENT'S NAME AND NUMBER

The patient's name and number can either be written or photographed on to the film before it is developed. The photographic method is efficient and time saving, and is done with a light-proof box in which the electric-light source is enclosed. This box has a flat top (large enough to take the largest size of film) in one corner of which a window about 6 cm by 2·5 cm is provided. A corresponding corner of the x-ray film is protected from the x-rays by means of a piece of lead the same size and 1–2 mm thick fixed permanently on or in the cassette. The patient's name and number are written within a space of 6 cm by 2·5 cm on one corner of a white transparent card, which is placed in front of the window. The x-ray film, exposed but not developed, is placed on the top of the card, and good contact between the film and the card ensured by means of a well-padded hinged flap, which can also be used when pressed down to actuate the electric-light switch. To ensure that the same exposure is given to each film the light must be kept on for the same time, which is best done by some timing device such as a condenser discharge circuit. The film is then developed in the usual manner.

The card used for the purpose of photographing the name of the patient on the film should be of even texture to avoid a granular background. Cards made from cloth pulp are most likely to be suitable in this respect. The name can be written on the card with almost any ink, or with a typewriter—red ink or pencil often giving suitable results. Insufficient opacity of the ink is not usually a cause of illegibility, which is more likely caused by excessive granularity of the card, inadequate light exposure or poor contact between the card and the film during the light exposure.

MARKING ORDER OF FILMS FOR LEGIBILITY WITHOUT TRANSMITTED LIGHT

Unfortunately neither the name photographed nor the date radiographed on the films can easily be read except by transmitted light. To facilitate placing the radiographs rapidly in the correct order according to the dates on which they were taken, a serial numeral 1, 2, 3, 4 and so on should be written clearly in white ink or in yellow, red, or green grease pencil on to each film after development, or better still small numbered adhesive labels should be stuck on (one is shown in Fig. 313). The order in which they were taken can thus be found without the necessity of holding them up in front of a viewing box to read their individual dates.

SELECTION AND MARKING OF KEY RADIOGRAPHS

In some chest diseases a large number of films may be taken over a period of years, and many of these may become of little value to the patient or his physician in the course of time. In this category are films taken over a long interval during which there was no change, or the immediate post-operative radiographs in an uncomplicated case, which may only be of interest for research purposes.

It is sometimes convenient to select a sample from these many radiographs illustrating the important features, particularly when the appearances have changed. These can either be marked in some way to indicate that they are key radiographs (for instance with a small coloured adhesive label) or kept in a separate envelope inserted in the main envelope, or in one side of a partitioned envelope, the remainder being placed in the other side. Tomograms are usually taken on a smaller sized film, and are thus easily placed in smaller envelopes inserted in the main one.

DARK-ROOM TECHNIQUE

A number of chest radiographs of poor quality are still seen each year and in the majority of cases this is due to faults in the dark room causing fogging of the film, most of which could easily be avoided or corrected.

FAULTY STORAGE

Faulty storage may result in a general grey fogging of the films. Before use, films should be kept in a reasonably cool place, and not kept for too long. Boxes should be numbered or dated as they are received, and used in the same order to avoid the risk of an odd box lying around for too long a period. All risk of fogging of the films from stray radiation from diagnostic or therapeutic x-rays or the emanations of radioactive substances in nearby rooms should be eliminated.

EXCESS OF LIGHT

Light fogging may occur if blinds, doors, or light traps are faulty, or the filters of the dark-room lights are defective. A test to eliminate such sources of unwanted light should be made from time to time.

CHEMICAL FOGGING

Chemical fogging can be avoided by keeping the developing solution at the correct strength and temperature, and seeing that the time of development is adjusted to this. Topping up with special replenisher solutions is a help in keeping the developing process reasonably constant, while there are very few departments that are not busy enough to justify thermostatically controlled units.

Washing of films between the developer and the fixer must be carried out with care so that no excess of developer or water is carried from one tank to another.

Fixing solutions must be discarded before they become exhausted or cause staining of the films. Modern electrolytic methods of collecting the unused waste silver from the fixer are efficient and an economic proposition, and will keep the solution in a satisfactory state for months, the level being kept up by the addition of fresh solution, and the pH kept between 4 and 5 (optimum 4·2). This can be checked daily with an indicator paper or a solution of bromocresol purple. A small quantity of 5 per cent acetic acid should be added to the fixing solution until the right colour is registered by the indicator.

UNDERDEVELOPMENT

The film will be underdeveloped if the developing solutions are of incorrect strength, the temperature of the solutions is too low or the time in the developer is too short. Using old style wet developing techniques, these faults are easily corrected. With automatic developing units it is all too readily assumed that development is correct. If there is any doubt about this, two films should be exposed at the same time and each developed in a different unit. The degree of blackening in each radiograph is then compared, and if one is less than the other, the unit concerned should be readjusted.

TOMOGRAPHY

TYPES OF APPARATUS

Many types of apparatus are available for tomography, and the type already installed in the department will be the one to use. Provided that the x-ray tube column and the Potter–Bucky diaphragm run independently, there is no excuse for anyone not employing this valuable method of investigation, since a very simple home-made coupling (such as the one originally introduced by Twining, 1937) can produce very satisfactory tomograms.

Various refinements on this simple principle include vertical coupling, a V-shaped contactor to keep the current on over a given arc of swing, devices for propelling the tube column at a given constant rate of movement, full mechanization with the layer selection and the preparation of the column for its final run controlled electrically with push-button switches, and complications of the x-ray tube or film movements, such as a figure-of-eight swing of the tube and dipping of the Potter–Bucky diaphragm, with or without image magnification.

All these refinements may facilitate the ease with which the investigation is carried out, or contribute to the consistency of the tomograms, but they will not greatly improve their quality, at any rate in tomograms of the chest. The most important factors controlling the quality are smooth running of the tube column and Potter–Bucky diaphragm tray, so that there is no blurring from unwanted movements, and a satisfactory Potter–Bucky grid which produces good contrast, sharp detail, and no visible grid lines.

CHECKING CALIBRATION

The calibration of the apparatus should be checked once to see that the figures marked on the scale do in fact correspond to layers the same distance from the table top. If lead numerals are placed parallel to the film on wooden steps at intervals of, for instance, 3, 4, 5, 6 and 7 cm from the table top, and the layer selector is set for 5 cm and an exposure made, it will be possible to judge from the tomograms whether the 5 cm numeral has come out most clearly and the calibration is therefore correct, or whether some other numeral is the clearest, in which case the appropriate correction of the scale could be made.

MARKING OF LAYER DEPTHS ON FILMS

The layer depths are best marked on the films by placing bold lead numerals, approximately 1·5 cm in size, on the cassette, and radiographing them along with the patient.

THE ARC OF SWING

The arc of swing should be about 25 degrees from the vertical when working at a tube-film distance of 85–100 cm. Increasing it to 50 degrees decreases the contrast slightly without showing cavities or small foci any more clearly. If the swing is much less than 25 degrees the visible layer becomes too wide and the individual shadows too indistinct, so that small cavities or foci may pass undetected.

CENTRING OF THE X-RAY BEAM

Centring of the x-ray beam will of course depend on the information being sought. The level of an abnormal shadow in relation to the clavicle can be measured on the plain radiograph, and the beam centred on to this point. The main bronchial and hilar shadows lie roughly at the level of the sternal angle or second costal cartilage.

Except for comparative tomograms of known localized opacities, quite a large area should be included (18 cm by 24 cm or 24 cm by 30 cm) since features invisible in a plain radiograph are often seen on tomograms. Very accurate centring by means of fluoroscopy has therefore no great advantage over centring in relation to some easily palpable landmark. By omitting fluoroscopy, no time is wasted waiting for the eyes to become adapted to the dark. In any case few radiographers are skilled at fluoroscopy, and few radiologists have the time to do more than inspect the resulting films and see they are adequate.

SELECTION OF LAYERS

The selection of layers depends particularly on the information being sought. If the radiologist cannot be present, the radiographer must be carefully briefed about the purpose of the examination and the layers and region required.

When possible the tomographs should be inspected as soon as they are fixed and before the patient is moved, so that any additional layers found to be necessary can be taken under identical conditions. Once the patient has been moved it is difficult to place him in exactly the same position again, and a cavity seen at a level of 5 cm on one occasion may only be seen at a level of 6 cm on another. Additional layers taken on a second occasion must therefore cover a wider range than would have been necessary had they been taken there and then.

Errors of exposure, faulty centring, or a suspected deficiency in the range of layers can all be best corrected at a single session. In fact the most reliable results can only be obtained if each case is handled separately and given individual attention, the technique being adapted to it with the same skill and care as is used, for instance, in a gastro-intestinal examination personally undertaken by the radiologist.

SIMULTANEOUS MULTISECTION TOMOGRAPHY

Simultaneous multisection tomography is a method whereby five or even seven different layers may be tomographed simultaneously with a single exposure and a single swing of the x-ray tube. The method was considered mathematically by Ziedes de Plantes (1933) and applied practically by Watson (1951, 1953). The author examined a series of patients both by this method and by conventional tomography, and the findings were compared with the specimens after resection. Although the radiographs by the multisection method had rather less contrast and were rather greyer than by the other method, small foci and small cavities were shown equally well by both (Figs. 355 and 356). The saving in time and energy is considerable, and for this reason alone the method is valuable in many cases.

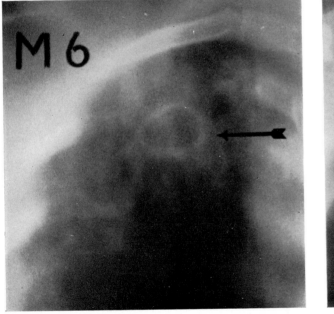

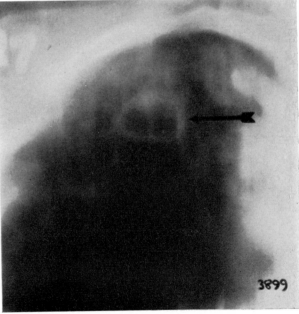

Fig. 355.—Simultaneous multisection tomogram (one of five layers taken simultaneously with a single exposure and a single tube-film movement). Arrow points to the ring shadow of a tuberculous cavity in the right upper zone.

Fig. 356.—Same case. Conventional single-layer tomogram. Same mA and time, but 10 kVp less. The film is rather blacker and has more contrast, but the ring shadow (opposite arrow) is no clearer.

SAVING IN RADIATION DOSAGE

The saving in the amount of radiation received by the patient is also considerable although, in view of the relatively small dose received even in conventional tomography, this is not an important factor generally. In special circumstances, however, when children are being tomographed, or when simultaneous bronchography or aortography and tomography is being done, or when a patient has recently received a lot of radiation, simultaneous multisection tomography has obvious advantages.

Table 13 shows the total skin dosage of radiation received by patients during lateral-view tomograms of the chest taken by both methods under routine working conditions. Obtaining the identical five layers by simultaneous multisection tomography entailed a dose one-quarter of that received during the five separate swings of the conventional tomography.

TABLE 13

TOTAL SKIN DOSAGE OF RADIATION RECEIVED DURING LATERAL-VIEW TOMOGRAPHY
(200 MA SECS)

	Type	*kVp*	*Dose per swing: roentgen units*	*Total dose for five layers: roentgen units*
St. Bartholomew's Hospital (Mr. G. S. Innes)	Conventional	75	4	20
	Multisection (five layers)	85	5·1	5·1
Cancer Hospital (Dr. G. Spiegler)	Conventional	80	8	40
	Multisection (five layers)	90	10	10

THE TECHNIQUE

Simultaneous multisection tomography can be used with most types of x-ray couch provided there is easy access to the clear space beneath the tray of the Potter–Bucky diaphragm.

The five films are placed in a light-proof box with a radio-translucent front. They are spaced 1·1 cm apart by balsa wood or plastic sheets. The tray of the Potter–Bucky diaphragm is withdrawn and the box put in its place so that the uppermost film lies in the same position as the single film would occupy in conventional tomography. The layer reproduced on this top film will then correspond to that to which the layer selector is set, and the other four films will reproduce lower layers, 1, 2, 3, and 4 cm respectively nearer to the table-top level.

Since intensifying screens tend to absorb a lot of x-rays, a special combination of them is indicated to avoid under-exposure of the lower films. The following combination of intensifying screens is satisfactory for a range of 50–90 kVp.

> (1) Single high-definition screen.
> (2) Single ordinary standard screen.
> (3) One pair of high-definition screens.
> (4) One pair of ordinary standard screens.
> (5) One pair of high-voltage screens.

All intensifying screens except the last must be " front screens ". The first screen beneath the front of the box should be facing the floor.

Ilford or Kodak screens, and Kodak " Blue Brand " or Ilford " Red Seal " films, have been found to result in an even density throughout the five-film series.

The exposure will be the same mA seconds as for conventional tomograms, but an increase of 10 kVp will be needed. The side of the first two balsa-wood spacers which lies directly against the first two films should be covered with a thin sheet of paper which will absorb some of the scatter radiation from the spacers. Both paper and screens should be stuck to the spacers to ensure rapid loading and unloading of films in the dark room.

MARKING OF SIMULTANEOUS MULTISECTION TOMOGRAMS

If the upper screen of each layer has a serial number written on it in black marking ink, this number will appear faintly on each of the exposed films, since there will be no fluorescence through the ink. Later, after development, the films are assembled in numerical order, and the depths written on them in white ink or grease pencil starting at number 1 with the depth indicated on the layer selector. Lead markers would tend to show on all five films, and are best avoided. A strip of lead placed in a suitable position on the front of the box will enable the usual photographic name and date identification to be carried out, if this is in routine use.

POSITIONING OF PATIENT WITH SEVERE SCOLIOSIS FOR CHEST RADIOGRAPH

In a patient with severe scoliosis in the thoracic region, the lungs are often obscured by the shadow of the spine and heart (Fig. 357), especially if the patient is positioned with both shoulders against the casette and the clavicles are parallel to the film.

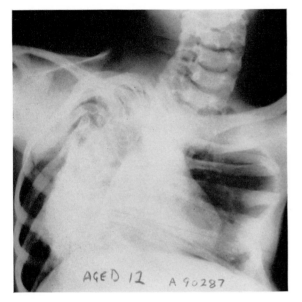

Fig. 357.—Radiograph of the chest. Child aged 12 years, with severe scoliosis. Right lung much obscured by the shadow of the spine, that on the left by the heart.

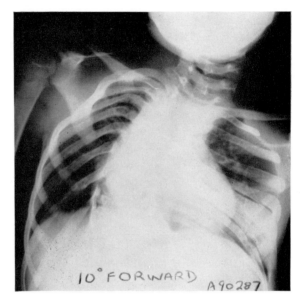

Fig. 358.—Same child, but rotated 10 degrees to bring the spine centrally. Lung fields now well seen.

A satisfactory radiograph of the lungs can often be obtained (Fig. 358) if the patient is positioned somewhat differently. A finger should be placed on the most lateral or prominent part of the spinal curve, and the patient rotated until one's finger (and the spine) arrive more or less opposite the centre of the casette. This is achieved with very little rotation of the patient—often only 10–15 degrees. The radiograph is then taken with the patient in this position.

BIBLIOGRAPHY AND REFERENCES

Annotation. (1950). " The Nomenclature of Broncho-Pulmonary Anatomy ". *Thorax*, **5**, 222.
— (1954). " Observer Error ". *Lancet*, **1**, 87.
— (1955). " Diagnosis of Pericardial Effusion ". *Lancet*, **1**, 91.
Bourne, G. (1949). *An Introduction to Cardiology*, p. 17. London; Arnold.
Boyden, E. A. (1955). *Segmental Anatomy of the Lungs. A Study of the Patterns of the Segmental Bronchi and Related Pulmonary Vessels*. New York; McGraw-Hill.
Brock, R. C. (1954). *The Anatomy of the Bronchial Tree*, 2nd ed. London; Oxford University Press.
Carstairs, L. S. (1961). " The Interpretation of Shadows in a Restricted Area of a Lung Field on the Chest Radiograph ". *Proc. R. Soc. Med.*, **54**, 978.
Cochrane, A. L., and Garland, L. H. (1952). " Observer Error in the Interpretation of Chest Films ". *Lancet*, **2**, 505.
Cunningham, G. J., and Parkinson, T. (1950). " Diffuse Cystic Lungs of Granulomatous Origin ". *Thorax*, **5**, 43.
Dolton, E. G., and Jones, H. E. (1952). " Congenital Anomalies of the Aortic Arch ". *Lancet*, **1**, 537.
Dornhorst, A. C., and Pierce, J. W. (1954). " Pulmonary Collapse and Consolidation ". *J. Fac. Radiol.*, **5**, 276.
Fisher, R. E. W., and Makin, R. (1952). " Pulmonary Haemosiderosis ". *Lancet*, **1**, 540.
Fleischner, F. G. (1941). " Linear Shadows in the Lung ". *Amer. J. Roentgen.*, **46**, 610.
Fletcher, C. M. (1948). " Pneumoconiosis of Coal-Miners ". *Brit. med. J.*, **1**, 1065.
— (1949). " The Classification of Radiographic Appearances in Coalminers' Pneumoconiosis ". *J. Fac. Radiol.*, **1**, 40.
Fraser, R. G., Macklen, P. T. and Thurlbeck, W. M. (1970). *New Engl. J. Med.* (In press).
Garland, L. H. (1950). " On the Reliability of Roentgen Survey Procedures ". *Amer. J. Roentgen.*, **64**, 32.
Glendinning, A. C. (1954). " Occasional Bronchography ". *Lancet*, **2**, 1253.
Greenfield, I. (1943). " ' Spring Water ' Cyst of the Mediastinum ". *J. thorac. Surg.*, **12**, 495.
Hamilton, W. J., Hamilton, S. G. I., and Simon, G. (1971) *Surface and Radiological Anatomy*. Cambridge; Heffer.
Hamman, L., and Rich, A. R. (1944). " Acute Diffuse Interstitial Fibrosis of Lungs ". *Johns Hopk. Hosp. Bull.*, **74**, 177.
Harley, H. R. S., and Drew, C. E. (1950). " Cystic Hygroma of the Mediastinum ". *Thorax*, **5**, 105.
Hodges, F. J., and Eyster, J. A. E. (1926). " Estimation of Transverse Cardiac Diameter in Man ". *Arch. intern. Med.*, **37**, 707. A reproduction of the chart is also given by Bourne (1949).
Hodgman, J. E., Mikity, V. G., Talter, D. and Cleland, R. S. (1969). *Pediatrics*, **44**, 179.
International Labour Office (1959). " Classification of Radiographs of the Pneumoconioses ", *see* Van Mechelen, V., and McLaughlun, A. I. G. (1962). *Ann. Occup. Hyg.*, **4**, 237.
Kerley, P. J. (1951). *See* Shanks, S. C., and Kerley, P. J. (1951).
Liebow, A. A., Steer, A. and Billingsley, J. G. (1965). " Desquamative Interstitial Pneumonia ". *Amer. J. Med.*, **39**, 369.
Livingstone, J. L., Lewis, J. G., Reid, Lynne, and Jefferson, K. E. (1964). " Diffuse Interstitial Pulmonary Fibrosis ". *Quart. J. Med.*, **33**, 71.
Macleod, W. M. (1954). " Abnormal Transradiancy of One Lung ". *Thorax*, **9**, 147.
Morgan, A. D., Lloyd, W. E., and Price-Thomas, C. (1952). " Tertiary Syphilis of the Lung and its Diagnosis ". *Thorax*, **7**, 125.
Newell, R. R., Chamberlain, W. E., and Rigler, L. (1954). " Descriptive Classification of Pulmonary Shadows ". *Amer. rev. Tuberc.*, **69**, 566.
Oswald, N. C., and Parkinson, T. (1949). " Honeycomb Lungs ". *Quart. J. Med.*, **18**, 1.
Philip, W. Paton, Harrison, K., and Cruickshank, D. B. (1954). " A Posterior Mediastinal Dermoid Tumour with Marked Anatomical Differentiation ". *Thorax*, **9**, 245.
Pierce, J. W. (1953). " Pulmonary Manifestations of Fungous Diseases ". In *Modern Trends in Diagnostic Radiology* (Second Series). London; Butterworths.
Pryce, D. M., Sellors, T. H., and Blair, L. G. (1947). " Intralobar Sequestration of Lung Associated with an Abnormal Pulmonary Artery ". *Brit. J. Surg.*, **35**, 18.
Reid, L. M. (1955). " Correlation of certain bronchographic abnormalities seen in chronic bronchitis with the pathological changes ". *Thorax*, **10**, 199; and *Brit. J. Radiol.*, **32**, 291.
Reid, Lynne (1967). *The Pathology of Emphysema*. London; Lloyd-Luke.
Rosen, S. H., Castleman, B., and Liebow, A. A. (1958). " Pulmonary Alveolar Proteinosis." *New Engl. J. Med.*, **258**, 1123.
Scadding, J. G. (1952). " Chronic Lung Disease with Diffuse Nodular or Reticular Radiographic Shadows ". *Tubercle., Lond.*, **33**, 352.
— (1960). " Chronic Diffuse Interstitial Fibrosis of the Lungs ". *Brit. med. J.*, **1**, 443.
— (1964). " Fibrosing Alveolitis ". *Brit. med. J.*, **2**, 686 and 941.
Shanks, S. C., and Kerley, P. J. (1951). *A Text Book of X-Ray Diagnosis*, 2nd ed., **2**, 318. London; Lewis.
Sharp, M. E., and Danino, E. A. (1953). " An Unusual Form of Pulmonary Calcification: Microlithiasis Alveolaris Pulmonum ". *J. Path. Bact.*, **65**, 389.
Simon, G. (1949). *X-Ray Diagnosis*, p. 174. Cambridge; W. Heffer.
— (1952). " The Lateral Position in Chest Tomography ". *J. Fac. Radiol.*, **4**, 77.
— (1968). " The Limitations of the Radiograph for Detecting Early Heart Enlargement ". *Brit. J. Radiol.*, **41**, 863.
— Bonnell, J., Kazantzis, G. and colleagues (1969). " Some Radiological Observations on the Range of Movement of the Diaphragm ". *Clin. Radiol.*, **20**, 231.
Smart, J., and Thompson, V. C. (1947). " Intra-Thoracic Lipomata ". *Thorax*, **2**, 163.

BIBLIOGRAPHY AND REFERENCES

Springett, V. H. (1956). *Minimal Pulmonary Tuberculosis found by Mass Radiography (Fluorography)*. London; Lewis.

Store, S. D. (1954). " A Case of Pulmonary Hamartoma ". *Brit. med. J.*, **1**, 25.

Thomas, C. P., and Drew, C. E. (1953). " Fibroma of the Visceral Pleura ". *Thorax*, **8**, 180.

Thompson, B. C. (1947). " Prognosis of Primary Pleurisy with Effusion ". *Brit. med. J.*, **1**, 487.

Trapnell, D. H. (1963). " The Peripheral Lymphatics of the Lung ". *Brit. J. Radiol.*, **36**, 660.

Turkington, S. I., Scott, G. A., and Smiley, T. B. (1950). " Leiomyoma of the Bronchus ". *Thorax*, **5**, 138.

Twining, E. W. (1937). " Tomography by means of a simple attachment to the Potter-Bucky Couch ". *Brit. J. Radiol.*, **10**, 332.

Van Allen, C. M., Lindskog, G. E., and Richter, H. G. (1931). " Collateral Respiration. Transfer of Air Collaterally between Pulmonary Lobules ". *J. clin. Invest.*, **10**, 559.

Waring, J. J. (1955). " The Pathogenesis and Prognosis of Tuberculous Pleurisy with Effusion ". *Tubercle., Lond.*, **36**, 59.

Watson, W. (1951). " Simultaneous Multisection Tomography ". *Radiography*, **17**, 221.

—— (1953). " Simultaneous Multisection Tomography ". In *Modern Trends in Diagnostic Radiology* (Second Series). London; Butterworths.

Whitaker, W. (1954). " Total Pulmonary Venous Drainage through a Persistent left Superior Vena Cava ". *Brit. Heart J.*, **16**, 177.

White, P. D. (1951). *Heart Disease*, 4th ed., p. 144. New York; Macmillan.

Willis, R. A. (1967). *Pathology of Tumours*, 4th ed., p. 378. London; Butterworths.

Wilson, M. G., and Mikity, V. G. (1960). " A New Form of Respiratory Disease in Premature Infants ". *Amer. J. Dis. Child.*, **99**, 489.

Wood, P. (1960). *Diseases of the Heart and Circulation*, 2nd ed., p. 157. London; Eyre and Spottiswoode.

Ziedses des Plantes, B. G. (1933). " Planigraphie ". *Fortschr. Röntgenstr.*, **47**, 407.

INDEX